AF744213

Brain and Spinal Cord Atrophy in Multiple Sclerosis

Brain and Spinal Cord Atrophy in Multiple Sclerosis

Robert Zivadinov
Rohit Bakshi
(Editors)

Nova Biomedical Books
New York

Editorial Production Manager: Donna Dennis
Senior Production Editor: Susan Boriotti
Production Editors: Marius Andronie, Rusudan Razmadze and Keti Datunashvili
Office Manager: Annette Hellinger
Graphics: Magdalena Nuñez
Editorial Production: Maya Columbus, Vladimir Klestov, Lorna Loperfido and Joanne Overton
Circulation: Ave Maria Gonzalez, Vera Popovic, Luis Aviles, Alexandra Columbus, Raymond Davis, Cathy DeGregory, Melissa Diaz, Marlene Nuñez and Jeannie Pappas

*

Library of Congress Cataloging-in-Publication Data
Available Upon Request

p. cm.
Includes bibliographical references and index.
ISBN: 1-59454-160-4.

An Imprint of Nova Science Publishers, Inc.
400 Oser Ave, Suite 1600
Hauppauge, New York 11788-3619
Tel. 631-231-7269 Fax 631-231-8175
e-mail: Novascience@earthlink.net
Web Site: http://www.novapublishers.com

Printed in the United States of America

Dedication

To my parents, who stayed behind
and Tina, who came with me across the ocean.

Robert Zivadinov

To my family for their unqualified love and support.

Rohit Bakshi

Contents

Acknowledgments ix

List of Contributors xi

Abbreviations xv

Foreword xix
Nancy Richert

Chapter I **Central Nervous System Atrophy in Multiple Sclerosis: Introduction** 1
Robert Zivadinov, Marino Zorzon and Rohit Bakshi

Chapter II **Central Nervous System Atrophy in Multiple Sclerosis: Mechanisms** 5
Alireza Minagar, Eduardo Gonzalez Toledo and J. Steven Alexander

Chapter III **Linear and Regional Measures of Brain Atrophy in Multiple Sclerosis** 15
Jack H. Simon

Chapter IV **Whole Brain Atrophy Measurement and Short-Term Brain Volume Changes** 29
Claudio Gasperini

Chapter V **The Measurement of Brain Atrophy in Multiple Sclerosis: Technical Aspects** 39
Kathleen Garrison, Roland G. Henry and Daniel Pelletier

Chapter VI **Technical Aspects of Spinal Cord Atrophy Measurement** 63
Christopher R. Tench and Cris S. Constantinescu

Chapter VII **MRI Measures of Pathology and their Relationship to Central Nervous System Atrophy in Multiple Sclerosis** **73**
Dominik S. Meier, Howard L. Weiner, Samia J. Khoury and Charles R.G. Guttmann

Chapter VIII **Neurologic Disability and Central Nervous System Atrophy in Multiple Sclerosis** **113**
Robert Zivadinov and Rohit Bakshi

Chapter IX **Brain Atrophy, Cognitive Dysfunction and Emotional Disturbances in Multiple Sclerosis** **137**
Ralph H. B. Benedict and Dominic A. Carone

Chapter X **Relationship Between Central Nervous System Atrophy and Genetic-Immunological Markers in Multiple Sclerosis** **167**
Marino Zorzon and Robert Zivadinov

Chapter XI **Treatment Effects on MRI Measures of Central Nervous System Atrophy in Multiple Sclerosis** **175**
Marco Rovaris and Massimo Filippi

Index **191**

Acknowledgments

I would like to express my gratitude to The Jacobs Neurological Institute, under whose auspices I continue my quest for knowledge about Multiple Sclerosis.

Additional thanks go to Dr. Frederick E. Munschauer III, Chairman of The Jacobs Neurological Institute, for his continuing support and encouragement.

To my research staff at the Buffalo Neuroimaging Analysis Center, I extend heartfelt appreciation for dedication and a job well done.

And particular thanks to my Assistant, Eve Salczynski, for expert technical editing and being the perfect right hand.

Robert Zivadinov

To my colleagues and support staff in Buffalo, Boston and beyond who continue to enrich me with their wisdom, dedication, and friendship.

Rohit Bakshi

List of Contributors

J. Steven Alexander
Department of Cellular and Molecular Physiology
Louisiana State University Health Sciences Center
Shreveport, LA, USA
Email: *jalexa@lsuhsc.edu*

Rohit Bakshi
Center for Neurological Imaging
Partners Multiple Sclerosis Center
Brigham & Women's Hospital
Harvard Medical School
Boston, MA, USA
Email: *rbakshi@bwh.harvard.edu*

Ralph H.B. Benedict
Department of Neurology
The Jacobs Neurological Institute
School of Medicine and Biomedical Sciences
SUNY–University at Buffalo
Buffalo, NY, USA
Email: *benedict@buffalo.edu*

Dominic A. Carone
Department of Neurology
The Jacobs Neurological Institute
School of Medicine and Biomedical Sciences
SUNY–University at Buffalo
Buffalo, NY, USA
Email: *DCaroneJr@aol.com*

Cris S. Constantinescu
Division of Clinical Neurology
Faculty of Medicine
University of Nottingham
Nottingham, UK
Email: *cris.constantinescu@nottingham.ac.uk*

Massimo Filippi
Neuroimaging Research Unit
Department of Neurology
Scientific Institute and University Ospedale San Raffaele
Milan, Italy
Email: *filippi.massimo@hsr.it*

Kathleen Garrison
UCSF Magnetic Resonance Science Center
University of California at San Francisco
San Francisco, CA, USA
Email: *kathleen@mrsc.ucsf.edu*

Claudio Gasperini
Department of Neuroscience
S. Camillo-Forlanini Hospital
Rome, Italy
Email: *c.gasperini@libero.it*

Eduardo Gonzalez Toledo
Department of Radiology
Louisiana State University Health Sciences Center
Shreveport, LA, USA
Email: *Egonz1@lsuhsc.edu*

Charles R.G. Guttmann
Center for Neurological Imaging
Partners Multiple Sclerosis Center
Brigham & Women's Hospital
Harvard Medical School
Boston, MA, USA
Email: *guttmann@bwh.harvard.edu*

Roland G. Henry
Department of Radiology
University of California at San Francisco
San Francisco, CA, USA
Email: *henry@mrsc.ucsf.edu*

Samia J. Khoury
Partners Multiple Sclerosis Center
Brigham & Women's Hospital
Harvard Medical School
Boston, MA, USA
Email: *skhoury@rics.bwh.harvard.edu*

Dominik S. Meier
Center for Neurological Imaging
Partners Multiple Sclerosis Center
Brigham & Women's Hospital
Harvard Medical School
Boston, MA, USA
Email: *meier@bwh.harvard.edu*

Alireza Minagar
Department of Neurology
Louisiana State University Health Sciences Center
Shreveport, LA, USA
Email: *aminag@lsuhsc.edu*

Daniel Pelletier
University of California at San Francisco
San Francisco, CA, USA
Email: *danp@itsa.ucsf.edu*

Marco Rovaris
Neuroimaging Research Unit
Department of Neurology
Scientific Institute and University Ospedale San Raffaele
Milan, Italy
Email: *rovaris.marco@hsr.it*

Jack H. Simon
University of Colorado
Department of Radiology (Neuroradiology)
University of Colorado Health Sciences Center
Denver, CO, USA
Email: *jack.simon@uchsc.edu*

Christopher R. Tench
Division of Clinical Neurology
Faculty of Medicine
University of Nottingham
Nottingham, UK
Email: *msxct@nottingham.ac.uk*

Howard L. Weiner
Partners Multiple Sclerosis Center
Brigham & Women's Hospital
Harvard Medical School
Boston, MA, USA
Email: *hweiner@rics.bwh.harvard.edu*

Robert Zivadinov
Department of Neurology
The Jacobs Neurological Institute
Buffalo Neuroimaging Analysis Center
School of Medicine and Biomedical Sciences
SUNY–University at Buffalo
Buffalo, NY, USA
Email: *rzivadinov@TheJNI.org*

Marino Zorzon
Department of Clinical Medicine and Neurology
University of Trieste
Trieste, Italy
Email: *m.zorzon@fmc.units.it*

Abbreviations

ADC	apparent diffusion coefficient
APP	amyloid precursor protein
BBB	blood-brain barrier
BBSI	brain boundary shift integral
BCR	bicaudate ratio
BICCR	brain to intracranial capacity ratio
BPF	brain parenchymal fraction
BVMT-R	Brief Visuospatial Memory Test – Revised
CA	Cytosine-Adenosine
CHAMPS	Controlled High-Risk Subjects Avonex Multiple Sclerosis Prevention Study
CIS	clinically isolated syndrome
CNS	central nervous system
COV	coefficient of variation
COWAT	Controlled Oral Word Association Test
CSF	cerebrospinal fluid
CT	computerized tomography
CTL	cytotoxic T lymphocyte
CVLT II	California Verbal Learning Test
DI	diffusion imaging
D-KEFS	Delis-Kaplan Executive Function System
DTI	diffusion tensor imaging
ECAM	endothelial cell adhesion molecule
EDSS	Expanded Disability Status Scale
FDG PET	F-labeled fluorodeoxyglucose positron emission tomography
FLAIR	fluid attenuated inversion recovery
FLV	FLAIR lesion volume
FOV	field of view
GM	gray matter
IBA	index of brain atrophy
ICAM-1	intercellular adhesion molecule 1
IFN	interferon
IL	interleukin

iNOS	inducible nitric oxide synthase
IR	inversion recovery
IVIG	intravenous immunoglobulin
IVMP	intravenous methylprednisolone
JLO	Judgment of Line Orientation
LFA-1	lymphocyte function associated antigen
LL	lesion load
MACAM-1	mucosal addressin cell adhesion molecule 1
MACFIMS	Minimal Assessment of Cognitive Function in Multiple Sclerosis
MBP	myelin basic protein
MHC	major histocompatibility complex
MIDAS	Medical Image Display Analysis Software
MOG	myelin oligodendrocyte glycoprotein
MR	magnetic resonance
MRF	Markov random field
MRI	magnetic resonance imaging
mRNA	messenger RNA
MRS	magnetic resonance spectroscopy
MS	multiple sclerosis
MSFC	Multiple Sclerosis Functional Composite
MT	magnetization transfer
MTR	magnetization transfer ratio
NAA	N-acetyl-aspartate
NABT	normal appearing brain tissue
NAWM	normal appearing white matter
NBV	normalized brain parenchymal volume or normalized brain volume
NEO-PI	NEO Personality Inventory
NfH	Neurofilament heavy
NfL	Neurofilament light
NMR	nuclear magnetic resonance
NP	neuropsychology
NPI	Neuropsychiatric Inventory
OLD	semi-automated, non-normalized technique with partial brain coverage
PASAT	Paced Auditory Serial Addition Test
PBVC	percentage brain volume change
PD	proton density
PECAM-1	platelet endothelial cell adhesion molecule-1
PLO	pathological laughter-crying
PLP	proteolipid protein
PP	primary progressive
Rag-1	recombination activating gene 1
RF	radio frequency
RR	relapsing remitting
SDMT	Symbol Digit Modalities Test
SIENA	Structural Image Evaluation, using Normalization, of Atrophy

SIENAX	extension of SIENA
SNR	signal to noise ratio
SP	secondary progressive
SPM	statistical parametric mapping
T1LV	T1 lesion volume
TDS	template-driven segmentation
TLA	total lesion area
TND	targeted neurological deficit
TVW	third ventricle width
VBM	voxel-based morphometry
VCAM	vascular cell adhesion molecule
VCAM-1	vascular cell adhesion molecule 1
VF	ventricular fraction
VLA-4	very late activation antigen 4
WBR	whole brain ratio
WCST	Wisconsin Card Sorting Test
WMSA	white matter signal abnormalities

Foreword

Nancy Richert
Uniformed Services University of Health Sciences, Bethesda, USA

Numerous MRI sequences have been used to quantitate disease activity in patients with multiple sclerosis. Conventional MRI sequences, which measure enhancing lesion number/volume and T2 hyperintense lesion number/volume, primarily reflect the inflammatory component of the disease, and this analysis is often restricted to lesional activity in the cerebral white matter. What is not addressed by these measures is the more insidious neurodegenerative component of the disease, which has been identified in normal appearing white matter, cortical grey matter, deep grey matter and within the spinal cord by histopathology and newer MRI techniques.

Axonal and neuronal loss begin at the earliest stage of the disease e.g. in patients with clinically isolated syndromes, and the loss is progressive throughout the disease course. Because axons and myelin comprise roughly 65% of brain tissue, it follows that an MRI measure of cerebral or spinal cord atrophy would reflect the neurodegenerative process. Validation that atrophy reflects axonal loss has been provided by studies correlating atrophy with MR spectroscopy measures of the neuronal-specific marker N-acetyl aspartate (NAA). During the past 5 years, MRI measures of atrophy have evolved from simple manual tracing of regional structures on hard copy films to sophisticated semiautomated or fully automated computerized programs for brain segmentation and analysis. Because of the robust correlation between axonal loss and clinical disability, atrophy measures have been incorporated into clinical trials of new therapeutic agents and will be essential for future clinical trials investigating neuroprotective agents. Atrophy measures, which initially appeared to be the simplest, most straightforward method for measuring axonal loss, have now become a labyrinth and conflicting results have been reported from some clinical trials, as a result of using different atrophy measures.

I congratulate the authors and editors of this book for assembling this wealth of information into well-organized chapters on the technical aspects of atrophy measures, clinical correlations of atrophy, and therapeutic treatment effects on atrophy. I anticipate that this book will become a reference text for imaging researchers as well as a source of reliable information for the casual observer.

Nancy Richert
Laboratory of Diagnostic Radiology Research, NINDS, NIH
Uniformed Services University of Health Sciences

In: Brain and Spinal Cord Atrophy in Multiple Sclerosis
Editors: R. Zivadinov and R. Bakshi, pp. 1-4
ISBN 1-59454-160-4

Chapter I

Central Nervous System Atrophy in Multiple Sclerosis: Introduction

Robert Zivadinov[1-3*], Marino Zorzon[4] and Rohit Bakshi[5]

[1]Department of Neurology, SUNY–University at Buffalo School of Medicine and Biomedical Sciences, Buffalo, NY, USA; [2]Buffalo Neuroimaging Analysis Center, Buffalo, NY, USA; [3]The Jacobs Neurological Institute, Buffalo, NY, USA; [4]Dept of Neurology, University of Trieste, Trieste, Italy; [5] Center for Neurological Imaging, Partners Multiple Sclerosis Center, Brigham & Women's Hospital, Harvard Medical School, Boston, MA, USA

The purpose of this book is to synthesize current concepts about the pathogenesis, MRI measurement and clinical relevance of central nervous system (CNS) atrophy in multiple sclerosis (MS).

Progressive CNS atrophy in MS has been recognized for many years. Early computed tomography (CT) studies showed that atrophy can develop within one year of the diagnosis in MS patients, and progresses in association with an aggressive clinical course (Gross et al., 1993). Other CT studies correlated brain atrophy in MS patients with dementia (Huber et al., 1987). Magnetic resonance imaging (MRI) emerged as a better tool than CT in the diagnosis and longitudinal monitoring of CNS atrophy. One of the first MRI studies, in vivo, showing a link between atrophy and axonal dysfunction in MS, was published nearly a decade ago by Davie and colleagues (1995). Reduced N-acetyl aspartate (NAA) levels detected by magnetic resonance spectroscopy (MRS) were associated with both cerebellar dysfunction and cerebellar atrophy (Davie et al., 1995).

Early histologic studies established that demyelination alone results in a reduction of axonal diameter, suggesting that atrophy can occur by at least two mechanisms: loss of myelin per se and associated axonal shrinkage (Prineas and Connell, 1978). However, only a few years ago MRI and pathologic studies confirmed that atrophy may occur by at least two mechanisms, one potentially reversible (demyelination) and the other not likely to reverse

* Corresponding Author: Robert Zivadinov, MD, PhD, Department of Neurology, University at Buffalo, SUNY, The Jacobs Neurological Institute, 100 High Street, Buffalo, NY 14203, USA. Tel. 716 859 7031; Fax. 716 859 7874; E-mail: *rzivadinov@thejni.org*

(axonal loss) (Ferguson et al., 1997; Miller et al., 2002; Trapp et al., 1998; Zivadinov and Bakshi, 2004). When severe tissue destruction occurs, the CNS responds by shrinkage and reorganization, leading to reduced volume of brain and spinal parenchyma and enlargement of adjacent cerebrospinal fluid (CSF) spaces. The measurement of progressive atrophy of both the brain and spinal cord is complex and likely reflects the effects of many factors such as inflammatory tissue injury, demyelination, axonal transection, neuronal loss and Wallerian degeneration. Although MS has traditionally been regarded as a chronic inflammatory demyelinating disorder of the CNS that predominantly involves the brain's white matter (WM), a growing body of evidence indicates that irreversible tissue destruction, including widespread axonal and neuronal degeneration in lesional and non-lesion tissue in both WM and gray matter (GM), is a key component of the MS disease process. Using MRI analysis methods, the brain can be segmented into GM, WM, and CSF compartments, providing more detailed information on the topography of atrophy.

Patients exhibit significant brain and spinal cord atrophy from the earliest stages of MS. Whether the rate of brain atrophy varies within the same individual or among subjects in different stages of the disease is still an open question. We do not yet know with certainty when this process begins, whether brain atrophy develops to the same degree in all disease subtypes, or whether the rate of brain atrophy is fairly constant in an individual over time.

The last five years have seen the development and implementation of a variety of computer-assisted analysis approaches to detect progressive atrophy of the brain and spinal cord. Numerous methodologies have been applied to the measurement of CNS atrophy, including assessment of whole-brain and spinal cord atrophy, and regional volume loss. The measurement of brain atrophy seems to be of growing clinical relevance as a biomarker of the disease process. CNS atrophy is a powerful longitudinal predictor of neurologic disability and correlates better with disability than do conventional MRI lesion measures in patients with MS. The clinical relevance of CNS atrophy is reinforced by studies showing that atrophy accounts for more variance than conventional lesion measures in predicting physical disability and neuropsychological dyfunction. Therefore, measurement of atrophy shows promise in providing a clinically relevant surrogate marker of disease and in being able to partially resolve the "clinical–MRI paradox" that has existed for conventional white matter lesion measurements. However, currently available anti-inflammatory immunomodulatory agents and immunosuppressive treatments, while effective at preventing clinical deterioration, have shown, at best, only a partial effect on preventing CNS atrophy.

One of the primary goals of this book is to discuss CNS atrophy in a comprehensive manner in order to educate general neurologists as well as specialists in MS and imaging. The authors and topics of the chapters have been chosen by the Editors to provide a state-of-the-art review of this important field. The chapters focus on several key issues pertaining to CNS atrophy in MS such as pathogenesis and mechanisms, technical aspects of the MRI measurement of brain and spinal cord atrophy, the relationship between CNS atrophy and other MRI metrics, clinical relevance, the association with neurobehavioral and genetic-immunologic components of the disease, and the effects of disease-modifying therapies on tissue atrophy. Pros and cons of different technical approaches are discussed critically. Special attention is devoted to CNS atrophy as a clinically relevant biologic marker of the MS disease process.

In Chapter 2, the group from Louisiana State University reviews the pathophysiology of CNS atrophy in MS, providing a comprehensive review of immunologic and pathologic data and weaving this information into hypotheses on the pathogenesis of atrophy. They focus the reader's attention on newly emerging concepts such as axonal injury and axonal transection in acute and chronic inflammatory lesions, reduced axonal diameter and tissue contraction related to astrogliosis, chronic demyelination and inefficient remyelination, loss of trophic support of axons and sublethal axonal injury, apoptosis, altered electrical conduction, iron deposition in grey matter and direct microscopic injury against myelin and axons mediated by autoreactive T lymphocytes and other immune cells.

The following four chapters review the current approaches to the measurement of brain atrophy in MS. There is no accepted gold standard for measuring CNS atrophy and, there is a need to gain a perspective on the relative pros and cons of the various techniques. A variety of automated and semiautomated methods have been developed using commercially available and proprietary software packages. In Chapter 3, Dr. Simon describes linear and regional measures of brain atrophy, emphasizing the advantages and disadvantages of these approaches. He also discusses regional injury in specific areas of the CNS-such as neuronal fibers crossing the corpus callosum. In Chapters 4 and 5, groups from the University of Rome and the University of California at San Francisco review the technical aspects of measurement of brain atrophy, emphasizing the methodological challenges and limits of different approaches. Particular attention is given to the number of confounding technical factors that may alter image acquisition or the segmentation algorithm, thus potentially introducing error. Moreover, the short-term confounding factors that may influence cerebral volume such as inflammation and edema, steroid therapy, nutritional status, intracranial hypertension, alcohol, anorexia, and dehydration are described. The group from the University of Nottingham describes technical aspects of the measurement of spinal cord atrophy. They focus on emerging technical improvements and the importance of atrophy in the spinal cord in relation to physical disability. This is followed by a discussion in Chapter 7 from the Harvard group on MRI measures of lesions and diffuse pathology and their relationship to CNS atrophy. The authors focus attention on the sensitivity of MRI metrics toward individual pathological processes that participate in the neurodegenerative process leading to tissue loss.

The next two chapters review the literature on the important topic of clinical relevance of CNS atrophy. Written by the editors of this book, Chapter 8 focuses on clinical aspects of CNS atrophy, including the relationship between atrophy and disability, disease course, disease duration, quality of life and fatigue. In Chapter 9, the group from the University at Buffalo summarizes the emerging literature on the correlation between brain atrophy and neurobehavioral components of the MS disease process. They review what is known about neuropsychological syndromes and propose cost-effective methods for objective evaluation. In addition, they also critically review the data on the relationship between MRI and neuropsychological functions in MS.

The expression of a variety of genes may influence the heterogeneity and severity of MS pathological processes measured by the accumulation of disease activity on conventional and non-conventional long-term MRI measures. In Chapter 10, the authors from the University of Trieste and the University of Buffalo assess the correlation between putative disease-modifying genes and immunologic markers, and MRI measures that have been shown to reflect axonal degeneration.

Finally, in Chapter 11, the Milan group summarizes results from trials which assessed the efficacy of disease-modifying MS treatments in the prevention of brain and spinal cord atrophy. They propose that CNS atrophy should be included as a secondary outcome measure in trials of disease-modifying agents aimed at limiting disease progression.

The Editors are hopeful that this book will serve as a useful reference for both scientists and practitioners interested in research into MS, the imaging of MS, and the clinical care of patients with MS.

Acknowledgments

We thank Eve Salczynski for technical support. This work was supported in part by a research grant to R. Bakshi from the National Institutes of Health (NIH-NINDS 1 K23 NS42379).

References

Davie CA, Barker GJ, Webb S, Tofts PS, Thompson AJ, Harding AE, et al. Persistent functional deficit in multiple sclerosis and autosomal dominant cerebellar ataxia is associated with axon loss. *Brain* 1995; 118: 1583-92.

Ferguson B, Matyszak MK, Esiri MM, Perry VH. Axonal damage in acute multiple sclerosis lesions. *Brain* 1997; 120: 393-9.

Gross KR, Tomberg TA, Kokk AA, Kaasik AE. [The prognosis of multiple sclerosis: computed tomographic comparisons]. *Zh Nevropatol Psikhiatr Im S S Korsakova* 1993; 93: 32-5.

Huber SJ, Paulson GW, Shuttleworth EC, Chakeres D, Clapp LE, Pakalnis A, et al. Magnetic resonance imaging correlates of dementia in multiple sclerosis. *Arch Neurol* 1987; 44: 732-6.

Miller DH, Barkhof F, Frank JA, Parker GJ, Thompson AJ. Measurement of atrophy in multiple sclerosis: pathological basis, methodological aspects and clinical relevance. *Brain* 2002; 125: 1676-95.

Prineas JW, Connell F. The fine structure of chronically active multiple sclerosis plaques. *Neurology* 1978; 28: 68-75.

Trapp BD, Peterson J, Ransohoff RM, Rudick R, Mork S, Bo L. Axonal transection in the lesions of multiple sclerosis. *N Engl J Med* 1998; 338: 278-85.

Zivadinov R, Bakshi R. Role of MRI in multiple sclerosis II: brain and spinal cord atrophy. *Front Biosci* 2004; 9: 647-64.

In: Brain and Spinal Cord Atrophy in Multiple Sclerosis
Editors: R. Zivadinov and R. Bakshi, pp. 5-13
ISBN 1-59454-160-4

Chapter II

Central Nervous System Atrophy in Multiple Sclerosis: Mechanisms

Alireza Minagar[1*], *Eduardo Gonzalez Toledo*[2] *and J. Steven Alexander*[3]
From: Departments of Neurology[1], Radiology[2], and Cellular and Molecular Physiology[3]
Louisiana State University Health Sciences Center
1501 Kings Highway, Shreveport, LA 71130

Introduction

Multiple sclerosis (MS) is an immune-mediated disease that affects genetically susceptible individuals following exposure to certain, yet unidentified, environmental factors (viral infection, bacterial lipopolysaccharides, superantigens, reactive metabolites, or metabolic stress). Genetic and environmental factors play a significant role in the pathogenesis of MS. MS remains the most common cause of neurological disability among young adults, and affects more than 350,000 individuals in North America, and more than 1.1 million worldwide. In the United States, the incidence of MS is almost 2-5 cases per 100.000 persons annually. More than two thirds of new cases of MS, particularly relapsing-remitting (RR) MS, are diagnosed in women. The extended course of disease, the early manifestation, and the usually slow but persistent central nervous system (CNS) atrophy imposes an enormous economic and social burden on our society.

MS is multiphasic and approximately 85% of patients initially exhibit an RR course characterized by exacerbations of neurological deficits with intervals of clinical stability. Within 6 to 10 years, half of these patients enter the next phase of MS known as secondary progressive (SP) MS, characterized by less inflammation and exacerbations, but more persistent disability and increasing physical and cognitive impairment. Neuropathology of MS, at least in the initial stages of disease, consists of transendothelial migration of activated

* Corresponding Author: Alireza Minagar, MD, Assistant Professor of Neurology, Department of Neurology, Louisiana State University Health Sciences Center, 1501 Kings Highway, Shreveport, LA 71130. Tel: (318) 675-4679; Fax: (318) 675-7805; Email: aminag@lsuhsc.edu

leukocytes through a failing blood-brain barrier and the development of multifocal demyelinating plaques in the gray and white matter of the optic nerves, cerebral hemispheres, brainstem, and spinal cord. Microscopic examination of these MS plaques reveals sharply demarcated areas of myelin loss with relative sparing of axons, inflammatory infiltrates composed of lymphocytes and macrophages, and astrocytic proliferation.

Progression from a disease with a massive inflammatory component towards a disease with reduced inflammation, chronic disability, progressive neurodegeneration and CNS atrophy is also associated with less therapeutic response to available immunomotherapies. The available disease modifying treatments (interferons, glatiramer acetate, and mitoxantrone) are only partially effective in altering the course of RR MS and just marginally effective in the management of SP MS.

Axonal pathology has been associated with MS since the first reports on MS (Ludwin, 1981). This axonal loss may result from the initial demyelinating attack, or could be an epiphenomenon secondary to demyelination. Demyelination in MS also involves oligodendrocyte loss, which is assessed by counting cells that express oligodendrocytes' specific biomarkers (Butzkueven et al., 2002; Chang et al., 2002). Axonal loss in MS has been closely linked with cytotoxic T lymphocytes (CTLs) with a $CD8^+$ phenotype with the potential to recognize and attack major histocompatibility complex (MHC) class I-expressing brain cells (Neumann et al., 2002) and neurotoxic mediators of inflammation such as glutamate (Geurts et al., 2003; Pitt et al., 2000). Recent studies have shown that axonal loss occurs in the early stages of the MS inflammatory cascade and contributes to the ultimate development of SP MS and neurodegeneration.

Pathogenesis of CNS Atrophy in MS

The inflammatory cascade of MS results in a loss of myelin, causing a loss of tissue volume, and likely contributes to the generalized atrophy observed. However, it is not only this myelin loss but loss of other tissue elements such as axons and glial cells that contributes to CNS atrophy in patients with MS. Indeed, the combination of myelin and axonal loss are likely the major causes of brain atrophy. Both early and recent literature support the concept of axonal loss in chronic MS lesions (Charcot, 1868; Lassmann, 1999). Evidence of axonal loss has also been obtained from studies on acute MS lesions applying amyloid precursor protein staining (Ferguson et al., 1997) and from confocal microscopy, which demonstrated axonal spheroids and transactions (Trapp et al., 1998).

Axonal loss through transection and Wallerian degeneration of the nerve fibers that pass through MS lesions contributes to brain atrophy. Based on the fact that axons compose a large portion of brain volume and because of the severity and extent of axonal loss in MS lesions (Trapp et al., 1998), it appears that axonal loss is a major contributor to CNS atrophy in MS patients.

Gray matter involvement is another potential contributor to CNS atrophy and tissue loss in MS. Gray matter lesions are not usually detected with conventional magnetic resonance imaging (MRI) sequences, however, recent advances in neuroimaging technology have improved our capability to detect these lesions (Bakshi et al., 2001) and atrophy of gray matter areas (Bermel et al., 2003). Diffuse hypometabolism has been shown to involve both cortical and subcortical gray matter of MS patients using 18-FDG PET (Bakshi et al., 1998).

Although gray matter lesions are much less frequent than white matter lesions, axonal loss or myelin breakdown within these lesions could potentially contribute to the global CNS atrophy observed in MS patients.

Axonal Loss in MS: Role of Inflammation

Current evidence indicates that myelin-specific CD4+ T lymphocytes and macrophages are the major players in the initial phases of MS. CD4+ T lymphocytes specific for myelin basic protein (MBP), myelin oligodendrocyte glycoprotein (MOG), or proteolipid protein (PLP), three putative CNS antigens in the pathogenesis of MS precipitate an inflammatory cascade within the CNS that eventually leads to loss of myelin and CNS atrophy. Lymphocyte activation is necessary for CNS penetration of lymphocytes and recent data suggest a "molecular mimicry" where cross-reactivity between the Epstein-Barr virus polymerase peptide associated with MS-susceptible HLA-DR2 molecules (DRB*1501, DQB*0602) activates the myelin-specific CD4+ T lymphocytes (Lang et al., 2002). Activated CD4+ T lymphocytes and macrophage cross the BBB and enter the CNS. This penetration occurs through a unique and specialized continuous endothelial barrier at tight junctions. Activated CD4+ Th1 cells secrete pro-inflammatory cytokines such as IFN-γ, TNF-α, and IL-1β that upregulate endothelial cell adhesion molecules (ECAMs) such as vascular cell adhesion molecule (VCAM), platelet endothelial cell adhesion molecule-1 (PECAM-1), mucosal addressin cell adhesion molecule 1 (MACAM-1), E-selectin, and intercellular adhesion molecule1 (ICAM-1) (Losy et al., 1999; Minagar et al., 2001; Minagar et al., 2003). The upregulated expression of ECAMs is associated with activation of endothelial cells and the release of endothelial microparticles (Minagar 2001), secretion of matrix metalloproteinases (MMPs), and loss of occludin and VE-cadherin in tight and adherens junctions (Minagar et al., 2003). Leukocyte-secreted matrix metalloproteinases (MMPs) facilitate transendothelial migration of these cells into the CNS by degrading extracellular matrix macromolecules. MMPs also have TNF-α convertase activity and cleave membrane-bound TNF-α to its soluble form. Once activated, CD4+ T lymphocytes are in the CNS, recognition of myelin antigens by these cells requires expression of MHC class II molecules on antigen presenting cells. Normally, CNS tissue does not express MHC class II molecules; however, under the influence of IFN-γ, a potent stimulator of class II expression on resident CNS antigen presenting cells including microglia and astrocytes, it is thought that Th1 T lymphocytes promote this stage of MS pathogenesis (Slavin et al., 2001). IFN-γ secretion is also driven by osteopontin, a cytokine generated by neurons and glia in inflamed CNS tissue (Chabas et al., 2001). Activated CD4+ T lymphocytes within the CNS are not able to recognize intact myelin. The myelin sheath undergoes proteolytic processing into peptide fragments by antigen presenting cells prior to binding MHC class II molecules and presentation to CD4+ T lymphocytes. MMPs and other proteolytic enzymes, such as cathepsins (secreted by microglia in response to IFN-γ) are major participants in processing of myelin proteins. Proteolytically derived 13-16 amino acid fragments that bind MHC class II molecules on resident CNS antigen presenting cells are recognized by the antigen-specific T lymphocyte receptors expressed on myelin-specific CD4+ T lymphocytes. This results in new CNS T lymphocyte activation and sustained production and secretion of IFN-γ, which in turn enhances and feeds the cycle of myelin antigen recognition and T lymphocyte activation.

Within the inflammatory cascade of MS, activated macrophages/microglia are the other main effector cells of the immune response within the CNS that are potentially involved in axonal damage and CNS atrophy. These cells generate and secrete both cytotoxic and trophic factors with detrimental effects on neurons and serve to remove myelin debris via phagocytosis. Activated macrophages/microglia release inflammatory mediators such as TNF-α, nitric oxide (NO) and glutamate, which promote both neuronal and axonal injury. TNF-α released by activated macrophages may directly affect neurites and suppress their outgrowth and branching (Neumann et al., 2002; Siebert and Bruck, 2003).

Activation of macrophages/microglia during the inflammatory cascade of MS is also accompanied by the generation of NO [by inducible nitric oxide synthase (iNOS)] and NO metabolites are present at high concentrations within MS lesions (Bo et al., 1994; Brosnan et al., 1994). Experimental exposure to NO can reversibly impair axonal conduction within the CNS (Redford et al., 1997) and demyelinated axons are particularly sensitive to NO (Redford et al., 1997). At higher levels (Kapoor 2001) or in axons that have been physiologically active (Smith et al., 2001), NO will induce persistent conduction block and axonal degeneration. Recently, Kapoor et al. (Kapoor et al., 2003) hypothesized that NO axonal injury may occur through an inhibition of mitochondrial respiration.

In MS patients, glutamate production by macrophages and altered glutamate transport and detoxification by oligodendrocytes have been reported to be potentially responsible for axonal damage and oligodendrocyte destruction in MS lesions (Werner et al., 2001).

Another possible mechanism of inflammatory axonal loss in MS is cytotoxic attack of axons by CD8+ T lymphocytes (Bitsch et al., 2000). CD8+ T lymphocytes are clonally expanded in MS lesions (Babbe et al., 2000) and have been observed in close proximity to demyelinated neurites (Neumann et al., 2002).

Axonal Loss in MS: Molecular Pathogenesis

Neurons and their synaptic connections are critical for maintaining impulse conduction and integrity of the CNS. Despite the fact that neuronal bodies are relatively protected against some inflammatory insults, axons are sensitive to toxic inflammatory mediators (Coleman and Perry, 2002). Axons are vulnerable because of their unusual size and shape and their high metabolic activity. Axons are especially prone to mechanical trauma, ischemic episodes, oxidative stress, and inflammatory mediators. One factor proposed to contribute to CNS atrophy in MS is iron deposition, perhaps through oxidative stress (Bakshi et al., 2001b; Bakshi et al., 2002). Focal damage to an axon leads to the development of "Wallerian degeneration" of the distal segment separated from the cell body, while the proximal segment [still attached to the mother cell body] may die due to isolation from other neurons (Coleman and Perry, 2002). This loss of neurons may cause further loss of neurons that have lost their connections through a retrograde or anterograde trans-neuronal degeneration. This may lead to axonal and neuronal degeneration in regions remote from the primary site of inflammatory focus. Loss of axons and neuronal synapses is a liability in the CNS since axons cannot regenerate. The severity of axonal loss in MS patients is a significant factor in the development of permanent neurological deficits and disability (Matthews et al., 1998; Trapp et al., 1998). MR-spectroscopic examination of MS lesions has linked the severity of axonal dysfunction with permanent disability in MS patients (Lassmann, 2001).

Axonal damage is abundant in initial stages of pathogenesis of MS and correlates with inflammatory reactions within demyelinated lesions. Indeed, axonal loss is a consistent feature of MS neuropathology. Based on MR-spectroscopic studies, axons are lost even in otherwise normal appearing white matter (Bjartmar and Trapp, 2003; De Stefano et al., 2003). Study of the extent of axonal damage in acute and chronic lesions of MS shows a decrease of axonal density of up to 60% (Lovas et al., 2000; Mews et al., 1998). Quantitative measurement of MS tissue at autopsy has shown a loss of 45% of these fibers over long periods of time (Evangelou et al., 2000; Evangelou et al., 2001).

MR-spectroscopic examinations of MS patients have revealed decreased *N*-acetyl aspartate (NAA) [a specific index of axonal integrity detected by MR- spectroscopy] levels in both acute MS lesions (Arnold and Matthews, 2002) and in normal appearing white matter at early stages of the disease process (De Stefano et al., 2001). An in vivo assessment of levels of brain NAA revealed a diffuse decrease in NAA in MS patients with early disease, low white matter lesion load, and no significant clinical disability (De Stefano et al., 2002). This diffuse axonal damage as supported by low levels of brain NAA in MS patients may be an epiphenomenon of acute inflammation, since it may be reversible by treatment with interferon-β1b (Narayanan et al., 2001).

Impaired axonal transport is another abnormality observed in MS lesions. Tissue staining with antibodies against amyloid precursor protein (APP) has been used to detect acute axonal damage and axonal swelling in a number of CNS inflammatory disorders, including MS. The local accumulation of APP as well as axonal swelling at the site of axonal damage in MS lesions indicates a local arrest of physiological axonal transport (Tsunoda and Fujinami, 2002). Accumulation of the pore-forming subunit of neuronal-type voltage-gated calcium channels has been reported in axons within actively demyelinated lesions of MS patients and such ectopic distribution of calcium channels in the axonal membrane may result in increased calcium influx, contributing to axonal degeneration, possibly via the activation of neutral proteases (Kornek et al., 2001).

During CNS inflammation in MS, glutamate is released by activated leukocytes. Glutamate excitotoxicity mediated by AMPA/kinate receptors causes injury to neurons, oligodendrocytes, and axons. In addition, altered expression patterns of metabotropic glutamate receptors in axons within MS lesions has been reported (Geurts et al., 2003). The pattern of mGluR1α axonal IR in MS points to axonal changes in the center of MS lesions and in the surrounding normal appearing white matter (Geurts et al., 2003); such altered presence of mGluR1α IR in MS tissue has been attributed to a disturbance in axonal transport.

Repair and CNS Atrophy

Our evolving understanding of the pathogenesis of MS indicates that repair and regeneration mechanisms that prevent or reverse CNS atrophy in MS are major therapeutic targets. In MS patients, spontaneous remyelination is limited and partial. Only 40% of MS lesions show remyelination extending over more than 10% of the lesion during dynamic inflammation (Prineas et al., 1993; Raine and Wu, 1993); fewer chronic lesions demonstrate remyelination (Ozawa et al., 1994). Both humoral and cell-mediated immune responses have been implicated in the pathogenesis of remyelination and repair in MS patients. Ciric et al.

investigated the role of a human monoclonal IgM antibody (sHIgM22) in the remyelination process and found that the antibody binds to oligodendrocytes, induces calcium signals in cultured glial cells, and promotes remyelination independent of Fc function (Ciric et al., 2003). Rodriguez and colleagues (Bieber et al., 2003) also demonstrated a role for cell-mediated immunity in the spontaneous remyelination of the CNS axons after lysolecithin-induced demyelination in the spinal cord. In their lysolecithin-induced demyelination model of Rag-1-deficient mice (which lack both B cells and T cells), the mice showed significantly reduced spontaneous remyelination compared with control mice of matching genetic background.

The ultrastructural neurohistologic features of repair and remyelination include a shortened internode distance and a decreased myelin thickness to axonal diameter ratio (Perier and Gregoire, 1965; Prineas and Connell, 1979). Repair of demyelinated axons may be complete or incomplete. Uncommonly, if complete, it mainly occurs at the lesion edge, creating a transition zone between normal appearing white matter and the center of the demyelinated lesion. The repair and remyelination process in the pathogenesis of MS shows a close correlation with the presence of oligodendrocytes expressing myelin proteins or myelin proteins mRNA in their cytoplasm (Bruck et al., 1994; Ozawa et al., 1994).

Remyelination and repair are typical features of MS lesions and take place early during the development of acute MS lesions. Substantial repair of injured axons and remyelination requires the presence of a significant number of myelinating oligodendrocytes from the progenitor pool. Despite CNS capability for remyelination, this process eventually fails and this results in permanent disability in MS patients.

Conclusions

CNS atrophy remains the most significant and the least known feature of MS pathogenesis. In recent advances in molecular biology and neuroimaging of the human nervous system, a new under-explored aspect of MS has emerged: atrophy of the CNS. An increasing body of evidence demonstrates that tissue destruction, mainly axonal loss and neurodegeneration is a key element in the pathogenesis of MS and is a significant factor in the development of cognitive decline and permanent disability. Indeed, CNS atrophy commences in early stages of MS and advances relentlessly throughout the course of the disease. Two main components of tissue loss and CNS atrophy are loss of myelin and axonal degeneration. It is a logical assumption that loss of the myelin sheath during the inflammatory cascade results in loss of tissue volume and contributes to CNS atrophy. Axonal degeneration, the other main component of tissue loss, correlates with both permanent disability and brain atrophy in advanced MS. Cumulative data indicate that axonal loss is the major determinant of progressive neurological disability. Multiple neuroimaging studies in MS patients with less than 5 years disease duration indicate axonal damage or loss. The neurodegenerative process and axonal loss, at least initially, is accompanied by a local response from oligodendrocyte progenitor cells and some remyelination. However, such repair mechanisms eventually fail and patients develop generalized brain atrophy, cognitive decline, and permanent disability. The exact mechanisms behind such devastating CNS atrophy remain largely unknown; however, it appears that atrophy may represent an epiphenomenon related to the effects of dynamic inflammation within the CNS, including demyelination, axonal injury, neuronal loss,

Wallerian degeneration, and possibly iron deposition. Untangling the molecular pathogenesis of CNS atrophy will likely assist us in finding new therapies for MS.

References

Arnold DL, Matthews PM. MRI in the diagnosis and management of multiple sclerosis. *Neurology* 2002; 58: S23-31.

Babbe H, Roers A, Waisman A, Lassmann H, Goebels N, Hohlfeld R, et al. Clonal expansions of CD8(+) T cells dominate the T cell infiltrate in active multiple sclerosis lesions as shown by micromanipulation and single cell polymerase chain reaction. *J Exp Med* 2000; 192: 393-404.

Bakshi R, Miletich RS, Kinkel PR, Emmet ML, Kinkel WR. High-resolution fluorodeoxyglucose positron emission tomography shows both global and regional cerebral hypometabolism in multiple sclerosis. *J Neuroimaging* 1998; 8: 228-34.

Bakshi R, Ariyaratana S, Benedict RHB, Jacobs L. Fluid-attenuated inversion recovery magnetic resonance imaging detects cortical and juxtacortical multiple sclerosis lesions. *Arch Neurol* 2001a; 58: 742-748

Bakshi R, Dmochowski J, Shaikh ZA, Jacobs L. Gray matter T2 hypointensity is related to plaques and atrophy in the brains of multiple sclerosis patients. *Journal of the Neurological Sciences* 2001b; 185:19-26

Bakshi R, Benedict RHB, Bermel RA, Caruthers SD, Puli SR, Tjoa CW, Fabiano AJ, Jacobs L. T2 hypointensity in the deep gray matter of patients with multiple sclerosis: a quantitative magnetic resonance imaging study. *Archives of Neurology* 2002;59:62-68

Bermel RA, Innus MD, Tjoa CW, Bakshi R. Selective caudate atrophy in multiple sclerosis: a 3D MRI parcellation study. *NeuroReport* 2003; 14:335-339

Bieber AJ, Kerr S, Rodriguez M. Efficient central nervous system remyelination requires T cells. *Ann Neurol* 2003; 53: 680-4.

Bitsch A, Schuchardt J, Bunkowski S, Kuhlmann T, Bruck W. Acute axonal injury in multiple sclerosis. Correlation with demyelination and inflammation. *Brain* 2000; 123: 1174-83.

Bjartmar C, Trapp BD. Axonal degeneration and progressive neurologic disability in multiple sclerosis. *Neurotox Res* 2003; 5: 157-64.

Bo L, Dawson TM, Wesselingh S, Mork S, Choi S, Kong PA, et al. Induction of nitric oxide synthase in demyelinating regions of multiple sclerosis brains. *Ann Neurol* 1994; 36: 778-86.

Brosnan CF, Battistini L, Raine CS, Dickson DW, Casadevall A, Lee SC. Reactive nitrogen intermediates in human neuropathology: an overview. *Dev Neurosci* 1994; 16: 152-61.

Bruck W, Schmied M, Suchanek G, Bruck Y, Breitschopf H, Poser S, et al. Oligodendrocytes in the early course of multiple sclerosis. *Ann Neurol* 1994; 35: 65-73.

Butzkueven H, Zhang JG, Soilu-Hanninen M, Hochrein H, Chionh F, Shipham KA, et al. LIF receptor signaling limits immune-mediated demyelination by enhancing oligodendrocyte survival. *Nat Med* 2002; 8: 613-9.

Chabas D, Baranzini SE, Mitchell D, Bernard CC, Rittling SR, Denhardt DT, et al. The influence of the proinflammatory cytokine, osteopontin, on autoimmune demyelinating disease. *Science* 2001; 294: 1731-5.

Chang A, Tourtellotte WW, Rudick R, Trapp BD. Premyelinating oligodendrocytes in chronic lesions of multiple sclerosis. *N Engl J Med* 2002; 346: 165-73.

Charcot J-M. Histologie de la sclerose en plaques. Vol 41. Paris, France: *Gaz Hop*, 1868: 554-555, 557-558, 566.

Ciric B, Howe CL, Paz Soldan M, Warrington AE, Bieber AJ, Van Keulen V, et al. Human monoclonal IgM antibody promotes CNS myelin repair independent of Fc function. *Brain Pathol* 2003; 13: 608-16.

Coleman MP, Perry VH. Axon pathology in neurological disease: a neglected therapeutic target. *Trends Neurosci* 2002; 25: 532-7.

De Stefano N, Guidi L, Stromillo ML, Bartolozzi ML, Federico A. Imaging neuronal and axonal degeneration in multiple sclerosis. *Neurol Sci* 2003; 24 Suppl 5: S283-6.

De Stefano N, Narayanan S, Francis GS, Arnaoutelis R, Tartaglia MC, Antel JP, et al. Evidence of axonal damage in the early stages of multiple sclerosis and its relevance to disability. *Arch Neurol* 2001; 58: 65-70.

De Stefano N, Narayanan S, Francis SJ, Smith S, Mortilla M, Tartaglia MC, et al. Diffuse axonal and tissue injury in patients with multiple sclerosis with low cerebral lesion load and no disability. *Arch Neurol* 2002; 59: 1565-71.

Evangelou N, Konz D, Esiri MM, Smith S, Palace J, Matthews PM. Regional axonal loss in the corpus callosum correlates with cerebral white matter lesion volume and distribution in multiple sclerosis. *Brain* 2000; 123: 1845-9.

Evangelou N, Konz D, Esiri MM, Smith S, Palace J, Matthews PM. Size-selective neuronal changes in the anterior optic pathways suggest a differential susceptibility to injury in multiple sclerosis. *Brain* 2001; 124: 1813-20.

Ferguson B, Matyszak MK, Esiri MM, Perry VH. Axonal damage in acute multiple sclerosis lesions. *Brain* 1997; 120: 393-9.

Geurts JJ, Wolswijk G, Bo L, van der Valk P, Polman CH, Troost D, et al. Altered expression patterns of group I and II metabotropic glutamate receptors in multiple sclerosis. *Brain* 2003; 126: 1755-66.

Kapoor R, Davies M, Blaker PA, Hall SM, Smith KJ. Blockers of sodium and calcium entry protect axons from nitric oxide-mediated degeneration. *Ann Neurol* 2003; 53: 174-80.

Kornek B, Storch MK, Bauer J, Djamshidian A, Weissert R, Wallstroem E, et al. Distribution of a calcium channel subunit in dystrophic axons in multiple sclerosis and experimental autoimmune encephalomyelitis. *Brain* 2001; 124: 1114-24.

Lang HL, Jacobsen H, Ikemizu S, Andersson C, Harlos K, Madsen L, et al. A functional and structural basis for TCR cross-reactivity in multiple sclerosis. *Nat Immunol* 2002; 3: 940 3.

Lassmann H. Mechanisms of demyelination and tissue damage in multiple sclerosis. *Acta Neurol Belg* 1999; 99: 6-10.

Lassmann H. Classification of demyelinating diseases at the interface between etiology and pathogenesis. *Curr Opin Neurol* 2001; 14: 253-8.

Losy J, Niezgoda A, Wender M. Increased serum levels of soluble PECAM-1 in multiple sclerosis patients with brain gadolinium-enhancing lesions. *J Neuroimmunol* 1999; 99: 169-72.

Lovas G, Szilagyi N, Majtenyi K, Palkovits M, Komoly S. Axonal changes in chronic demyelinated cervical spinal cord plaques. *Brain* 2000; 123: 308-17.

Ludwin SK. Pathology of demyelination and remyelination. *Adv Neurol* 1981; 31: 123-68.

Matthews PM, De Stefano N, Narayanan S, Francis GS, Wolinsky JS, Antel JP, et al. Putting magnetic resonance spectroscopy studies in context: axonal damage and disability in multiple sclerosis. *Semin Neurol* 1998; 18: 327-36.

Mews I, Bergmann M, Bunkowski S, Gullotta F, Bruck W. Oligodendrocyte and axon pathology in clinically silent multiple sclerosis lesions. *Mult Scler* 1998; 4: 55-62.

Minagar A, Jy W, Jimenez JJ, Sheremata WA, Mauro LM, Mao WW, et al. Elevated plasma endothelial microparticles in multiple sclerosis. *Neurology* 2001; 56: 1319-24.

Minagar A, Ostanin D, Long AC, Jennings M, Kelley RE, Sasaki M, et al. Serum from patients with multiple sclerosis downregulates occludin and VE-cadherin expression in cultured endothelial cells. *Mult Scler* 2003; 9: 235-8.

Narayanan S, De Stefano N, Francis GS, Arnaoutelis R, Caramanos Z, Collins DL, et al. Axonal metabolic recovery in multiple sclerosis patients treated with interferon beta-1b. *J Neurol* 2001; 248: 979-86.

Neumann H, Medana IM, Bauer J, Lassmann H. Cytotoxic T lymphocytes in autoimmune and degenerative CNS diseases. *Trends Neurosci* 2002; 25: 313-9.

Ozawa K, Suchanek G, Breitschopf H, Bruck W, Budka H, Jellinger K, et al. Patterns of oligodendroglia pathology in multiple sclerosis. *Brain* 1994; 117: 1311-22.

Perier O, Gregoire A. Electron microscopic features of multiple sclerosis lesions. *Brain* 1965; 88: 937-52.

Pitt D, Werner P, Raine CS. Glutamate excitotoxicity in a model of multiple sclerosis. *Nat Med* 2000; 6: 67-70.

Prineas JW, Barnard RO, Kwon EE, Sharer LR, Cho ES. Multiple sclerosis: remyelination of nascent lesions. *Ann Neurol* 1993; 33: 137-51.

Prineas JW, Connell F. Remyelination in multiple sclerosis. *Ann Neurol* 1979; 5: 22-31.

Raine CS, Wu E. Multiple sclerosis: remyelination in acute lesions. *J Neuropathol Exp Neurol* 1993; 52: 199-204.

Redford EJ, Kapoor R, Smith KJ. Nitric oxide donors reversibly block axonal conduction: demyelinated axons are especially susceptible. *Brain* 1997; 120: 2149-57.

Siebert H, Bruck W. The role of cytokines and adhesion molecules in axon degeneration after peripheral nerve axotomy: a study in different knockout mice. *Brain Res* 2003; 960: 152-6.

Slavin AJ, Soos JM, Stuve O, Patarroyo JC, Weiner HL, Fontana A, et al. Requirement for endocytic antigen processing and influence of invariant chain and H-2M deficiencies in CNS autoimmunity. *J Clin Invest* 2001; 108: 1133-9.

Smith KJ, Kapoor R, Hall SM, Davies M. Electrically active axons degenerate when exposed to nitric oxide. *Ann Neurol* 2001; 49: 470-6.

Trapp BD, Peterson J, Ransohoff RM, Rudick R, Mork S, Bo L. Axonal transection in the lesions of multiple sclerosis. *N Engl J Med* 1998; 338: 278-85.

Tsunoda I, Fujinami RS. Inside-Out versus Outside-In models for virus induced demyelination: axonal damage triggering demyelination. *Springer Semin Immunopathol* 2002; 24: 105-25.

Werner P, Pitt D, Raine CS. Multiple sclerosis: altered glutamate homeostasis in lesions correlates with oligodendrocyte and axonal damage. *Ann Neurol* 2001; 50: 169-80.

In: Brain and Spinal Cord Atrophy in Multiple Sclerosis
Editors: R. Zivadinov and R. Bakshi, pp. 15-27
ISBN 1-59454-160-4

Chapter III

Linear and Regional Measures of Brain Atrophy in Multiple Sclerosis

Jack H. Simon*

Department of Radiology-Neuroradiology, University of Colorado
Health Sciences Center, Denver, Colorado

Introduction

Many of the linear measures of brain (or spinal cord) atrophy are primarily of historical interest, as they were utilized by necessity before sophisticated computer image processing was well developed, but these measures were important factors in generating interest that led the transition to the more comprehensive measures routinely utilized today including in clinical trials (Simon, 2001). The linear measures had an early obvious advantage in that they could be applied to assessing visually obvious atrophy observed in routine imaging, for example, the enlarged third ventricle in MS so apparent by computerized tomography (Gyldensted, 1976). The linear measures provided some of the first evidence that atrophy could be measured in early MS over short one-to-two year intervals by MRI (Simon et al., 1999). The linear measures remain reasonable approaches for evaluation of focal atrophy in some regions of the brain (third ventricle), but have been largely supplanted by more comprehensive approaches. In contrast, regional measures of atrophy (as opposed to global measures of the full brain or spinal cord) remain important approaches to evaluating the pathology of MS and its functional correlates as they allow us to focus on the anatomical areas where MS pathology is most active (e.g., around the ventricles), without diluting the measure of change with lower magnitude areas of volume loss. The regional measures also allow us to ask specific clinical, functional and pathophysiologic questions about regional injury—such as that occurring in thalamus relating to the numerous passing neuronal tracts (Cifelli et al., 2002). The regional ventricle and multi-slice brain measures are discussed

* Corresponding Author: Jack H. Simon MD, Ph.D., Professor Radiology, Neurology, Neurosurgery, Psychiatry, University of Colorado, Health Sciences Center Denver, Colorado. Phone: 303-372-6222 ; e-mail: *jack.simon@uchsc.edu*

elsewhere in this volume, as are the regional measures applied to the spinal cord and optic nerve.

The pathophysiology underlying regional atrophy and in many cases, global atrophy in MS, is likely a combination of both focal (usually macroscopic) and diffuse microscopic pathology of uncertain etiology, as detected by quantitative MRI techniques in the normal appearing white matter (NAWM) or normal appearing brain tissue (NABT) by magnetization transfer imaging, diffusion–based measures or MR spectroscopy (Filippi et al., 2003). The focal pathology of MS, indicated by the classic acute inflammatory lesion, frequently results over time in local volume loss. This is most evident, for example, by observing the local volume loss along the ventricular surfaces. Volume loss is also observed as a result of other mechanisms, including what appears to be neuronal tract degeneration, which is likely a generalized phenomenon resulting in global volume loss, but is also apparent at times in some regions of the central nervous system (CNS), such as of typical lesions (transcallosal bands) affecting the corpus callosum (Simon et al., 2001) (Fig. 1). In general, local linear measures may be sensitive compared to global measures, where local effects due to focal MS lesions dominate. The more subtle but important global volume loss, which has been described even in the early stages of MS based on increases in ventricle volume (Dalton et al., 2002), or brain parenchymal fraction measures (Rudick et al., 1999) may be best detected by computer-assisted technology, and in groups of patients rather than in individuals. As disease progresses, the global measures may become more important as they reflect numerous smaller contributions of the multi-focal and / or diffuse pathology of MS.

In general, linear or regional measures are accomplished using a computer workstation, with variable degrees of sophistication, with manual interaction by an experienced trained operator. Depending on the task, these measures may be simple and quick (third ventricle width), or laborious (for example manually outlining the brainstem and cerebellum). The regional measures can be augmented by semi-automated or automated computerized methods, for example, based on finding surfaces, common characteristics and connectivity, on single acquisition or based on multispectral (multi-series) acquisitions (Miller et al., 2002). Standard stereological methods (e.g., Cavalieri) can be utilized to define regions within borders. Disadvantages of the manual operator driven methods include errors due to operator bias when the method is not automated, with low precision compared to many automated techniques. However, it should be borne in mind that in many circumstances even a computer algorithm driven segmentation or border determination, though precise, may be inaccurate, and the errors (from inaccuracy) may be uncorrelated from scan-to-scan. Compared to global methods, regional or linear methods may be unduly influenced by focal pathology. However, the argument can be applied that global measures may lose sensitivity as they by necessity include regions of the brain or spinal cord less prone to volume loss.

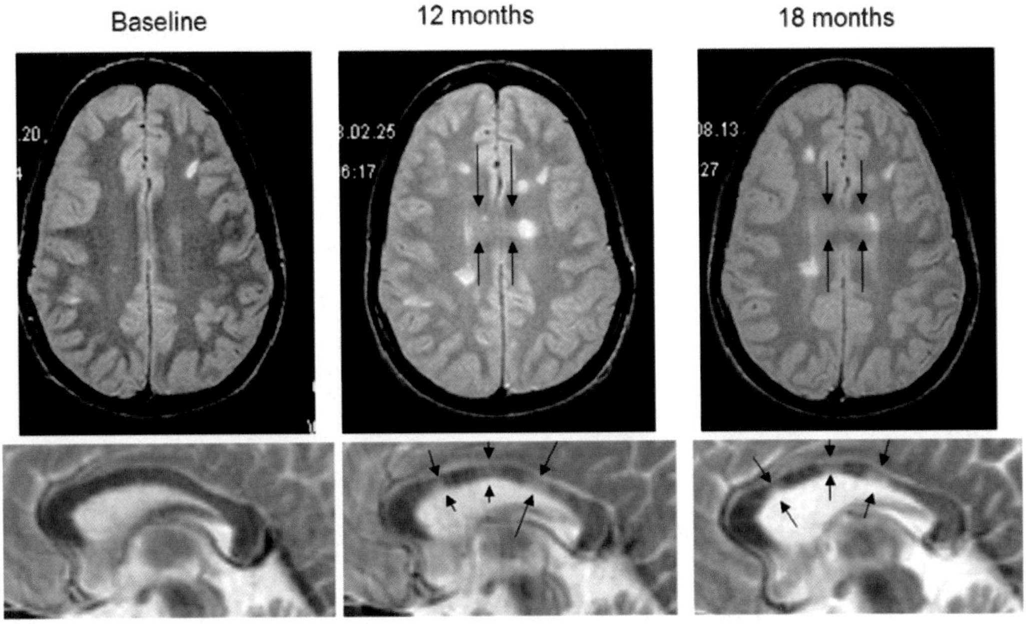

Fig. 1. Atrophy of the corpus callosum associated with transcallosal bands. Top row, axial images show development (at 12 months) and persistence (18) months of transcallosal bands (arrows). On the corresponding sagittal series, the bands account for several of the T2-hyperintense areas in the corpus callosum (arrows). Note that on the sagittal images the corpus callosum can be seen to lose height and area focally in the regions characterized by T2-hyperintensity. Series from a patient presenting with a clinically isolated syndrome and a positive MRI from the CHAMPS Trial.

Linear Measures of Third Ventricle, Lateral Ventricle, Brain Width

Linear measures of the width of the brain, third and lateral ventricle were prospectively acquired as a natural history measure of atrophy in the placebo cohort of the original phase III Trial of interferon beta-1a, a trial designed in the late 1980's (Fig 2) (Simon et al., 1999). The third ventricle measure in particular had an historical basis in observations of regional atrophy in MS, reflected in third ventricle enlargement in MS based on visual criteria in the clinic, as well as informative quantitative studies from the CT literature (Gyldensted, 1976). While it is now argued appropriately that these simple approaches are relatively crude and influenced by slice thickness, slice angle and position (Miller et al., 2002), in fact these studies established for the first time, along with other contemporary reports (Losseff et al., 1996) that atrophy could be measured over relatively short one to two year intervals, including atrophy in patients in the relatively early stages of disease. Changes in third ventricle width (+4.5%/year), exceeded those seen in the brain width (-0.64% /year). Interestingly, the changes in brain width parallel in magnitude those seen by whole brain (global) atrophy measures by modern techniques (summarized in Simon et al. (2001).. Based on these initial observations, atrophy observed based on enlargement of the third ventricle (Fig 3) was hypothesized to be related to fiber loss in the adjacent thalamus from Wallerian or other degeneration, as focal MS lesions were known to be rare in the thalamus (Simon, 1999; Simon et al., 1999). More recent studies confirm thalamic atrophy attributed to neuronal loss in secondary progressive MS (Cifelli et al., 2002). From the same phase III trial discussed above, placebo patients with gadolinium enhancing lesions at baseline exhibited greater atrophy over the next two years (Simon, 1999; Simon et al., 1999) than those without enhancing lesions. That finding, suggesting a link between inflammation and atrophy via myelin or axonal loss, in parallel to the link between inflammation and axonal loss (Trapp et al., 1998) has received only mixed and generally weak confirmation at best from analyses based on global measurers of atrophy. To date, it is not known whether the limited relationship when observed between enhancing lesions and atrophy reflects "better" technique (global measures) or loss of sensitivity by these global measures to important regional atrophy as the global measures potentially dilute out main cause (local volume loss) by summing all tissue, including those unaffected by the inciting, primary pathophysiology (eg inflammation).

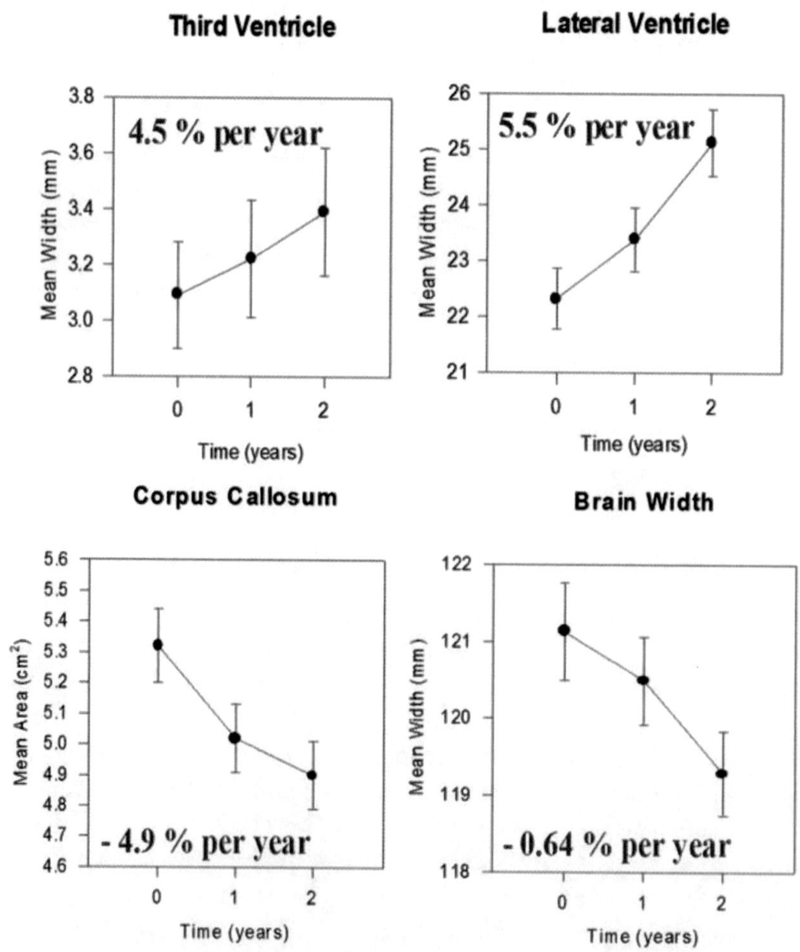

Fig. 2. Longitudinal results for linear (third and lateral ventricle and brain width) and regional (corpus callosum) atrophy measures in placebo patients from the Phase III MS Trial of interferon beta-1a over a two year interval. From Simon et al. (Simon et al., 1999).

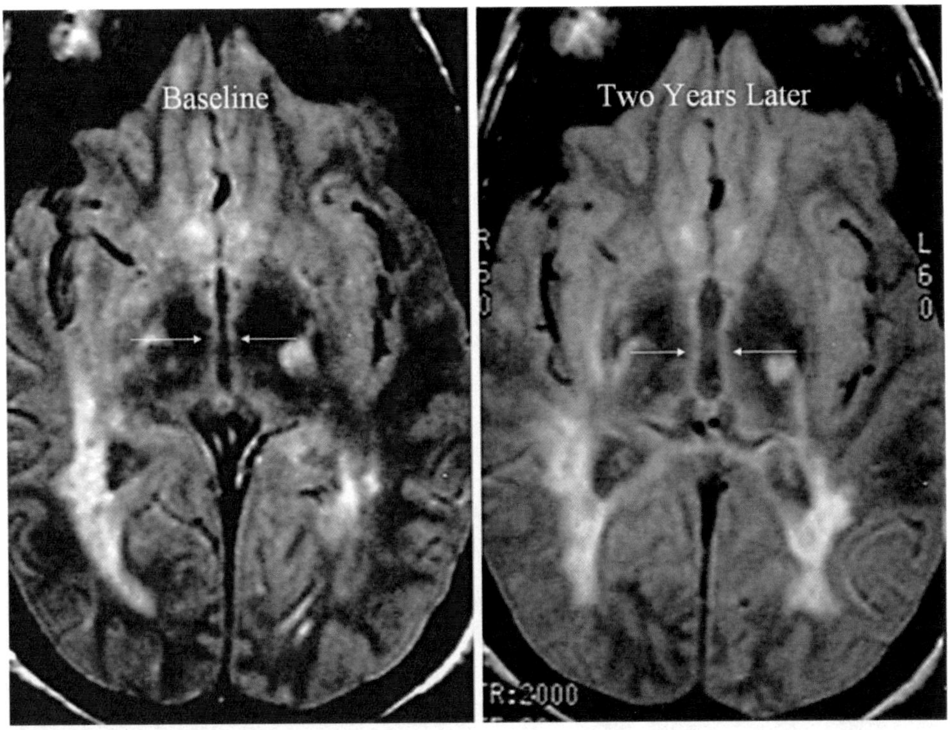

Fig. 3. Increase in third ventricle width (arrows) over two years on proton density weighted images. The increased width is thought to be related to volume loss in the adjacent thalamus, and/or more lateral tissues, possibly the result of neuronal degeneration. From Simon et al. (Simon, 1999).

In contrast to population studies, in an individual patient, linear measures are practical measures of structure size (brain width, third ventricle width, or bicaudate width [see below] and may be useful in supporting more qualitative (visual) impressions. Unfortunately, in structures such as lateral ventricle with rapidly varying contour, the linear measures may fail. When feasible another projection (e.g., coronal) may benefit determination of the maximal width of a ventricle.

Regional Measure of Corpus Callosum

Measures of the corpus callosum area have been applied in a large number of studies in MS, with some of the more interesting relationships suggested between corpus callosum area and cognitive function. Measures of corpus callosum area rather than volume are obtained as the lateral margins of callosum cannot be defined (Fig 4). The sharp borders between the callosum and adjacent tissues on T1 or T2 weighted images make area measurements relatively straightforward, accurate and reproducible. Area or volume loss in the corpus callosum may reflect typical focal lesions, which are common (Simon et al., 1986; Simon et al., 1987), the effects of fiber tract injury, including those visible as transcallosal bands (Simon et al., 2001), and likely the result of more generalized injury in the NAWM of the corpus callosum. Several studies have shown that the NAWM fraction of the corpus callosum has markedly reduced axonal density and total axonal content (Evangelou et al., 2000a;

Evangelou et al., 2000b) accompanying its volume loss. Intrinsic injury to the corpus callosum can be detected based on MR spectroscopy (Inglese et al., 2003; Ranjeva et al., 2003). The precise details of axonal versus myelin loss contributions to corpus callosum atrophy have not been determined. In one study of early MS (Ranjeva et al., 2003), changes in the corpus callosum were speculated to be more so the result of myelin pathology (increased diffusivity, decreased MTR, increased choline) rather than the result of axonal loss (NAA not reduced), at a time when the corpus callosum did not show a statistically significant decrease in area. In later stages of disease, axonal loss is a main contributor to corpus callosum atrophy (Evangelou et al., 2000a; Evangelou et al., 2000b). While we consider the corpus callosum as a measure of regional atrophy, it is in fact a potentially powerful measure of global injury in MS, as at least in theory, any injury affecting interhemispheric fibers that pass through the callosum may cause callosum volume loss, which is readily measured in vivo. (Coombs et al., 2004). The relative rate of corpus callosum versus brain atrophy has not been comprehensively evaluated using modern global measures and at multiple stages of disease. In one earlier study corpus callosum atrophy appeared to precede brain atrophy (Dietemann et al., 1988). However, future studies with current best technology will be required to determine how the global information potentially within the corpus callosum (interhemisheric fibers) compares to the global information provided by whole brain measures.

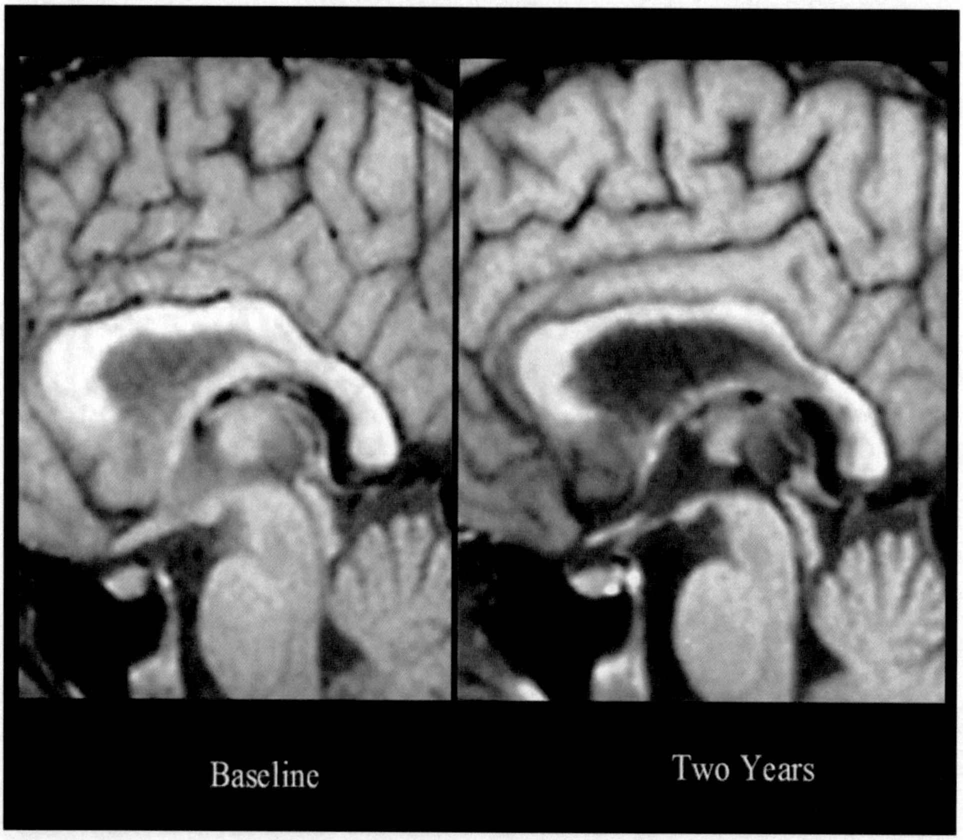

Fig. 4. Diffuse atrophy of the corpus callosum over a two year interval. From Simon et al. (Simon, 1999).

Several studies have addressed the functional consequences of generalized corpus callosum injury as indicated by atrophy, as it relates to interhemispheric transfer of information (Pelletier et al., 1993; Pelletier et al., 2001; Pozzilli et al., 1991; Rao et al., 1989). Regionalized atrophy within the corpus callosum has also been found associated with specific functional consequences. In one study (Pelletier et al., 1993), corpus callosum volume loss in the posterior callosum was found to be associated with left ear dichotic suppression abnormality, alternate finger tapping with the anterior region, and cross-lateralization abnormality with the mid-anterior and posterior regions.

A relationship has also been observed between corpus callosum atrophy and neuropsychological performance (Comi et al., 1993; Edwards et al., 2001; Huber et al., 1992) and dementia (Huber et al., 1987). As corpus callosum atrophy may reflect global injury, it provides a morphological marker of cognitive impairment (Huber et al., 1992).

Regional Measures of Thalamus/Basal Ganglia

Interest in measuring the volume of the thalamus in MS is based on the extensive reciprocal connections between the thalamus and cortex and subcortical structures, and studies showing accumulation of iron-containing material resulting in T2 shortening (Black-T2) in the thalamus and other deep gray matter in MS hypothesized to be related to neuronal degeneration (Bakshi et al., 2002). The thalamus is potentially sensitive to effects from pathology in widespread areas of the CNS (Cifelli et al., 2002). The finding of expansion of the third ventricle in relatively early MS was originally hypothesized to be the result of neuronal tract injury in the thalamus with secondary (ex vacuo) expansion of third ventricle, as focal MS lesions are rare in the thalamus (Simon, 1999; Simon et al., 1999). In a study of regional injury to the medial dorsal nucleus of the thalamus using NAA as a measure of axonal density and atrophy based on tracing the borders, both in vivo and in autopsy specimens, Cifelli et al. (Cifelli et al., 2002) found a significant (17%) decrease in (normalized) thalamic volume and a twofold increase in mean third ventricle width, with these measures modestly correlated.

Another linear and regional measure likely affected by deep gray matter atrophy is the bicaudate ratio (Aylward et al., 1991; Doraiswamy et al., 1994). This class of atrophy ratios is based on the minimum intercaudate distance divided by brain width along the same line, and has also been described as an inter-caudate distance (Caon et al., 2003) measured as the distance based on the width from the medial border of the caudate nucleus divided by the width to the inner table of the skull (Fig 5). These methods are simple, do not require sophisticated processing, and are relatively unaffected by acquisition technique. As for third ventricle width, some variation in this measure may occur due to variation in slice selection. For example, the ratios are sometimes based on selecting a mostly caudal slice containing caudate nucleus and lateral ventricle, and the inner table is not always distinct by MRI. Nevertheless, this relatively simple approach has shown some of the stronger published results relating atrophy to EDSS, as well as neuropsychological correlations.

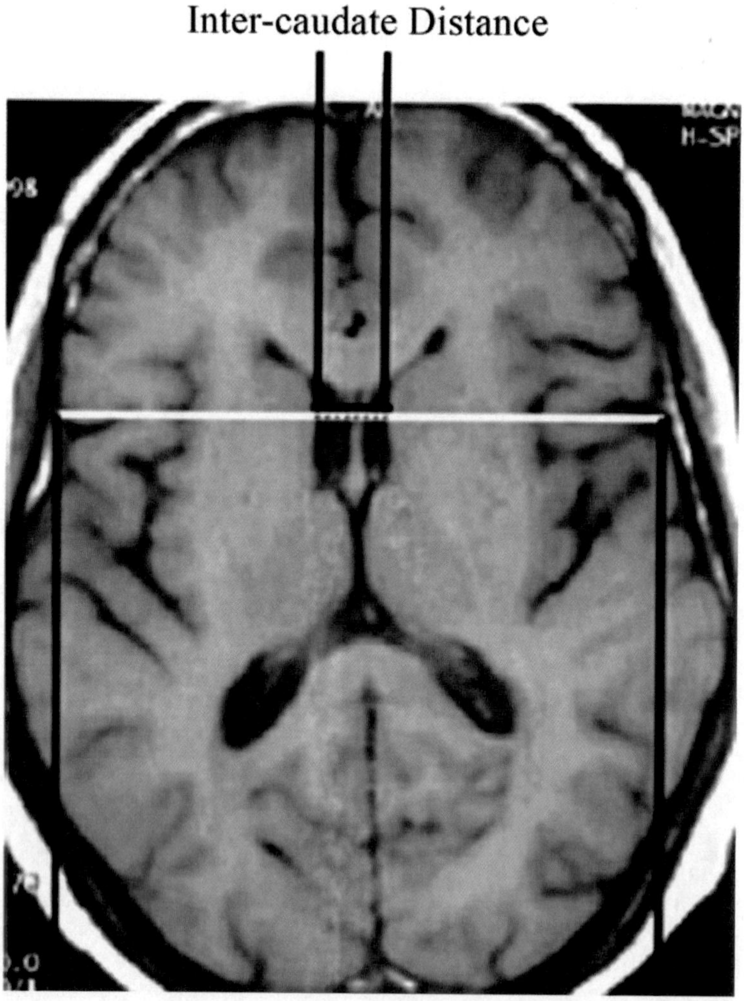

Fig. 5. Methodology for intercaudate ratio based on intercaudate distance divided by the transverse width of the inner table of the skull. An alternative approach is based on the width of the brain at the same level. Figure from Caon et al. (Caon et al., 2003).

Several pathologic factors may contribute to the abnormal bicaudate ratio in MS such as localized subcortical volume loss, decreased caudate nucleus volume, or loss of brain width based on all intervening structures (Bermel et al., 2002). In Huntington disease the bicaudate ratio increases primarily from caudate volume loss, but in one study of 60 MS patients and 50 controls caudate volume loss did not explain the decreased ratio (Bermel et al., 2002).

In an eloquent study of caudate volume based on 3D acquisitions and manual tracing, Bermel et al. (Bermel et al., 2003) detected a substantial decrease in volume in MS patients compared to controls, the caudate atrophy appearing selective and not associated with disease duration, physical disability, or other MR measures (T1 or T2 lesion load) theorized as indicating that selective caudate atrophy in MS may occur through direct mechanisms.

Regional Cortical Atrophy

Gray matter has been the focus of numerous recent investigations in MS as it has been recognized that the pathology can be extensive, both focal and diffuse (Bo et al., 2003), yet conventional MRI techniques have virtually no sensitivity to gray matter pathology. The focal pathology, characterized by a relatively low level of inflammation compared to white matter, nevertheless is characterized by demyelination, neuronal transection and apoptosis . Cortical gray matter volume loss can be detected in the early course of the disease by automated volumetric measures (De Stefano et al., 2003). Technical issues, however, remain as borders between gray matter and white matter, and gray matter and CSF are not necessarily accurately separated by computerized methods in part due to quality of the input data, including voxel size, tissue contrast, and signal inhomogeneity. These factors also affect linear approaches, which are time consuming and difficult to standardize among observers. Nevertheless, Bakshi et al. (Bakshi et al., 2001) were able to demonstrate regional brain atrophy based on ordinal scales of volume loss, the atrophy correlated with measures of disability and clinical course. Regional variation in cortical atrophy has recently been shown in a cross-sectional study using a computerized segmentation, where frontal and temporal loss was found earlier in MS, and motor strip tissue loss detected later in the course of disease (Sailer et al., 2003).

Cerebellum/Brain Stem

Cerebellar and infratentorial atrophy is common in relapsing-remitting (RR) and secondary progressive (SP) MS (Bakshi et al., 2001; Filippi et al., 1998; Lin et al., 2003). Generally, the approach to measuring volume in these areas is based on expert operators either manually outlining the structures or using semi-automated methods. Liu et al. (Liu et al., 1999) and Edwards et al. (Edwards et al., 1999) have applied semi-automated stereological techniques (Cavalieri) to assess atrophy in the cerebellum and brainstem of MS patients. Based on these approaches, correlations between cerebellar and brain stem atrophy and functional disturbances have been described. In one study, both greater atrophy of cerebellum and greater axonal loss (based on N-acetylaspartate) were observed in the MS group with severe cerebellar (functional) deficit compared to a matched (cerebellum) unimpaired MS group (Davie et al., 1995). Edwards et al. (Edwards et al., 1999) measured brainstem and cerebellum volume using the Cavalieri method and found that the volume of cerebellum and brainstem correlated with the Scripp's Neurological Disability Scale scores. In one study (Liu et al., 1999), no relationship was found between volume loss in the supratentorial compared to the infratentorial compartments.

Normalizing Brain Atrophy Measures in Linear and Regional Measures

As for global brain measures, normalized linear and regional brain atrophy measures have been described. Normalization may be based on a denominator containing the width of the intracranial cavity (inner surface of skull) or the outer surface of the brain (bicaudate ratio). The effectiveness of this normalization approach in cross-sectional studies relates to known influences of gender and body size on brain volume (Zivadinov et al., 2003), but these approaches have also been utilized successfully in longitudinal series (Zivadinov et al., 2003). A normalization approach has been described for the corpus callosum (Schreiber et al., 2001) and thalamus in MS (Cifelli et al., 2002).

Conclusion

While primarily of historical interest, the linear measures of atrophy (e.g., third ventricle) may have some theoretical advantage in measuring change in regions of great focal volume loss. There is strong and increasing evidence for diffuse injury in MS that is best measured by global methods (brain volume or brain parenchymal fraction), but the regional measures, like the linear measures, at least have the theoretical advantage of evaluating disease undiluted by unaffected regions. The regional measures also add to our understanding by providing insight into specific brain function (cerebellum) or injury, or injury to specific components of the CNS-such as neuronal fibers crossing the corpus callosum.

References

Aylward EH, Schwartz J, Machlin S, Pearlson G. Bicaudate ratio as a measure of caudate volume on MR images. *AJNR Am J Neuroradiol* 1991; 12: 1217-22.

Bakshi R, Benedict RH, Bermel RA, Caruthers SD, Puli SR, Tjoa CW, et al. T2 hypointensity in the deep gray matter of patients with multiple sclerosis: a quantitative magnetic resonance imaging study. *Arch Neurol* 2002; 59: 62-8.

Bakshi R, Benedict RH, Bermel RA, Jacobs L. Regional brain atrophy is associated with physical disability in multiple sclerosis: semiquantitative magnetic resonance imaging and relationship to clinical findings. *J Neuroimaging* 2001; 11: 129-36.

Bermel RA, Bakshi R, Tjoa C, Puli SR, Jacobs L. Bicaudate ratio as a magnetic resonance imaging marker of brain atrophy in multiple sclerosis. *Arch Neurol* 2002; 59: 275-80.

Bermel RA, Innus MD, Tjoa CW, Bakshi R. Selective caudate atrophy in multiple sclerosis: a 3D MRI parcellation study. *Neuroreport* 2003; 14: 335-9.

Bo L, Vedeler CA, Nyland HI, Trapp BD, Mork SJ. Subpial demyelination in the cerebral cortex of multiple sclerosis patients. *J Neuropathol Exp Neurol* 2003; 62: 723-32.

Caon C, Zvartau-Hind M, Ching W, Lisak RP, Tselis AC, Khan OA. Intercaudate nucleus ratio as a linear measure of brain atrophy in multiple sclerosis. *Neurology* 2003; 60: 323 5.

Cifelli A, Arridge M, Jezzard P, Esiri MM, Palace J, Matthews PM. Thalamic neurodegeneration in multiple sclerosis. *Ann Neurol* 2002; 52: 650-3.

Comi G, Filippi M, Martinelli V, Sirabian G, Visciani A, Campi A, et al. Brain magnetic resonance imaging correlates of cognitive impairment in multiple sclerosis. *J Neurol Sci* 1993; 115 Suppl: S66-73.

Coombs BD, Best A, Brown, MS, Miller DE, Corboy J, Baier M, and Simon JH Multiple sclerosis pathology in the normal and abnormal appearing white matter of the corpus callosum by diffusion tensor imaging. *Mult Scler* 2004 ; 10 : 392-7.

Dalton CM, Brex PA, Jenkins R, Fox NC, Miszkiel KA, Crum WR, et al. Progressive ventricular enlargement in patients with clinically isolated syndromes is associated with the early development of multiple sclerosis. *J Neurol Neurosurg Psychiatry* 2002; 73: 141-7.

Davie CA, Barker GJ, Webb S, Tofts PS, Thompson AJ, Harding AE, et al. Persistent functional deficit in multiple sclerosis and autosomal dominant cerebellar ataxia is associated with axon loss. *Brain* 1995; 118: 1583-92.

De Stefano N, Matthews PM, Filippi M, Agosta F, De Luca M, Bartolozzi ML, et al. Evidence of early cortical atrophy in MS: relevance to white matter changes and disability. *Neurology* 2003; 60: 1157-62.

Dietemann JL, Beigelman C, Rumbach L, Vouge M, Tajahmady T, Faubert C, et al. Multiple sclerosis and corpus callosum atrophy: relationship of MRI findings to clinical data. *Neuroradiology* 1988; 30: 478-80.

Doraiswamy PM, Patterson L, Na C, Husain MM, Boyko O, McDonald WM, et al. Bicaudate index on magnetic resonance imaging: effects of normal aging. *J Geriatr Psychiatry* Neurol 1994; 7: 13-7.

Edwards SG, Gong QY, Liu C, Zvartau ME, Jaspan T, Roberts N, et al. Infratentorial atrophy on magnetic resonance imaging and disability in multiple sclerosis. *Brain* 1999; 122: 291-301.

Edwards SG, Liu C, Blumhardt LD. Cognitive correlates of supratentorial atrophy on MRI in multiple sclerosis. *Acta Neurol Scand* 2001; 104: 214-23.

Evangelou N, Esiri MM, Smith S, Palace J, Matthews PM. Quantitative pathological evidence for axonal loss in normal appearing white matter in multiple sclerosis. *Ann Neurol* 2000a; 47: 391-5.

Evangelou N, Konz D, Esiri MM, Smith S, Palace J, Matthews PM. Regional axonal loss in the corpus callosum correlates with cerebral white matter lesion volume and distribution in multiple sclerosis. *Brain* 2000b; 123: 1845-9.

Filippi M, Mastronardo G, Rocca MA, Pereira C, Comi G. Quantitative volumetric analysis of brain magnetic resonance imaging from patients with multiple sclerosis. *J Neurol Sci* 1998; 158: 148-53.

Filippi M, Rocca MA, Comi G. The use of quantitative magnetic-resonance-based techniques to monitor the evolution of multiple sclerosis. *Lancet Neurol* 2003; 2: 337-46.

Gyldensted C. Computer tomography of the cerebrum in multiple sclerosis. *Neuroradiology* 1976; 12: 33-42.

Huber SJ, Bornstein RA, Rammohan KW, Christy JA, Chakeres DW, McGhee RB. Magnetic resonance imaging correlates of neuropsychological impairment in multiple sclerosis. *J Neuropsychiatry Clin Neurosci* 1992; 4: 152-8.

Huber SJ, Paulson GW, Shuttleworth EC, Chakeres D, Clapp LE, Pakalnis A, et al. Magnetic resonance imaging correlates of dementia in multiple sclerosis. *Arch Neurol* 1987; 44: 732-6.

Inglese M, Li BS, Rusinek H, Babb JS, Grossman RI, Gonen O. Diffusely elevated cerebral choline and creatine in relapsing-remitting multiple sclerosis. *Magn Reson Med* 2003; 50: 190-5.

Lin X, Blumhardt LD, Constantinescu CS. The relationship of brain and cervical cord volume to disability in clinical subtypes of multiple sclerosis: a three-dimensional MRI study. *Acta Neurol Scand* 2003; 108: 401-6.

Liu C, Edwards S, Gong Q, Roberts N, Blumhardt LD. Three dimensional MRI estimates of brain and spinal cord atrophy in multiple sclerosis. *J Neurol Neurosurg Psychiatry* 1999; 66: 323-30.

Losseff NA, Wang L, Lai HM, Yoo DS, Gawne-Cain ML, McDonald WI, et al. Progressive cerebral atrophy in multiple sclerosis. A serial MRI study. *Brain* 1996; 119: 2009-19.

Miller DH, Barkhof F, Frank JA, Parker GJ, Thompson AJ. Measurement of atrophy in multiple sclerosis: pathological basis, methodological aspects and clinical relevance. *Brain* 2002; 125: 1676-95.

Pelletier J, Habib M, Lyon-Caen O, Salamon G, Poncet M, Khalil R. Functional and magnetic resonance imaging correlates of callosal involvement in multiple sclerosis. *Arch Neurol* 1993; 50: 1077-82.

Pelletier J, Suchet L, Witjas T, Habib M, Guttmann CR, Salamon G, et al. A longitudinal study of callosal atrophy and interhemispheric dysfunction in relapsing-remitting multiple sclerosis. *Arch Neurol* 2001; 58: 105-11.

Pozzilli C, Bastianello S, Padovani A, Passafiume D, Millefiorini E, Bozzao L, et al. Anterior corpus callosum atrophy and verbal fluency in multiple sclerosis. *Cortex* 1991; 27: 441-5.

Ranjeva JP, Pelletier J, Confort-Gouny S, Ibarrola D, Audoin B, Le Fur Y, et al. MRI/MRS of corpus callosum in patients with clinically isolated syndrome suggestive of multiple sclerosis. *Mult Scler* 2003; 9: 554-65.

Rao SM, Bernardin L, Leo GJ, Ellington L, Ryan SB, Burg LS. Cerebral disconnection in multiple sclerosis. Relationship to atrophy of the corpus callosum. *Arch Neurol* 1989; 46: 918-20.

Rudick RA, Fisher E, Lee JC, Simon J, Jacobs L. Use of the brain parenchymal fraction to measure whole brain atrophy in relapsing-remitting MS. Multiple Sclerosis Collaborative Research Group. *Neurology* 1999; 53: 1698-704.

Sailer M, Fischl B, Salat D, Tempelmann C, Schonfeld MA, Busa E, et al. Focal thinning of the cerebral cortex in multiple sclerosis. *Brain* 2003; 126: 1734-44.

Schreiber K, Sorensen PS, Koch-Henriksen N, Wagner A, Blinkenberg M, Svarer C, et al. Correlations of brain MRI parameters to disability in multiple sclerosis. *Acta Neurol Scand* 2001; 104: 24-30.

Simon JH. From enhancing lesions to brain atrophy in relapsing MS. *J Neuroimmunol* 1999; 98: 7-15.

Simon JH. Brain and spinal cord atrophy in multiple sclerosis: role as a surrogate measure of disease progression. *CNS Drugs* 2001; 15: 427-36.

Simon JH, Holtas SL, Schiffer RB, Rudick RA, Herndon RM, Kido DK, et al. Corpus callosum and subcallosal-periventricular lesions in multiple sclerosis: detection with MR. *Radiology* 1986; 160: 363-7.

Simon JH, Jacobs L, Kinkel RP. Transcallosal bands: a sign of neuronal tract degeneration in early MS? *Neurology* 2001; 57: 1888-90.

Simon JH, Jacobs LD, Campion MK, Rudick RA, Cookfair DL, Herndon RM, et al. A longitudinal study of brain atrophy in relapsing multiple sclerosis. The Multiple Sclerosis Collaborative Research Group (MSCRG). *Neurology* 1999; 53: 139-48.

Simon JH, Schiffer RB, Rudick RA, Herndon RM. Quantitative determination of MS-induced corpus callosum atrophy in vivo using MR imaging. *AJNR Am J Neuroradiol* 1987; 8: 599-604.

Trapp BD, Peterson J, Ransohoff RM, Rudick R, Mork S, Bo L. Axonal transection in the lesions of multiple sclerosis. *N Engl J Med* 1998; 338: 278-85.

Zivadinov R, Locatelli L, Stival B, Bratina A, Grop A, Nasuelli D, et al. Normalized regional brain atrophy measurements in multiple sclerosis. *Neuroradiology* 2003; 45: 793-8.

In: Brain and Spinal Cord Atrophy in Multiple Sclerosis
Editors: R. Zivadinov and R. Bakshi, pp. 29-38
ISBN 1-59454-160-4

Chapter IV

Whole Brain Atrophy Measurement and Short-Term Brain Volume Changes

*Claudio Gasperini**
Department of Neuroscience, S. Camillo-Forlanini Hospital, Rome, Italy

Introduction

The nature of the process responsible for the atrophy in multiple sclerosis (MS) is uncertain, but it is thought to be a combination of demyelination and perhaps, more importantly, axonal loss. Axonal loss may be caused by Wallerian degeneration, diffuse low-grade inflammation, or neurodegeneration. Moreover, abnormalities are reported in normal appearing white matter (NAWM) and the cortex using quantitative magnetic resonance imaging (MRI) methods, and pathological studies confirm the presence of disease in these regions.

With this background, brain volume measurements on MRI in MS have been proposed as a surrogate marker for axonal loss, the presumed underlying pathological process leading to irreversible disability in MS. Interest in this technique has been stimulated by the development of a range of methods that are sensitive and reproducible in measuring even small changes in tissue volume and by observations of more robust correlations that use measures of atrophy to assess a patient's level of disability than had been previously obtained by examining correlations with lesion volume or activity measures.

Several problems have been underlined in the use of this surrogate marker. First, the major problem with cross-sectional studies of cerebral atrophy is the natural variation in brain volume in normal subjects. Serial assessment is essential to enable the measurement of progressive atrophy but since the changes expected to occur are extremely small, the measurement technique needs to be both sensitive and highly reproducible. Second, other factors such the segmentation process, MR pulse sequence, and MRI scanner upgrades may influence the quantitative measurement of brain volume. Finally, other confounding factors

* Corresponding Author: Claudio Gasperini, M.D., Department of Neuroscience, S. Camillo-Forlanini Hospital, Circonvallazione Giannicolense 87, Rome, Italy. 00390658704272; e-mail: c.gasperini@libero.it

that are known to influence cerebral volume must also be considered: alcohol, and corticosteroids.

In light of these problems, this chapter will focus on the role of automated analysis, use of different segmentation methods, absolute vs. normalized brain atrophy measures, gray/white matter segmentation, and confounding factors that are known to influence cerebral volume. More details about the technical aspects of brain atrophy measurement are provided in the chapter presented by the group from the University of California at San Francisco (Garrison et al., 2004).

Role of Automation and Gray/Matter Segmentation

Manual and Semiautomated Methods

Manual outlining or linear measurements of tissues easily permit measurement of changes in volume or dimensions over time. However, in order to get good reproducibility, this method needs an experienced observer familiar with normal central nervous system (CNS) neuroanatomy.

Manual segmentation of the whole brain from multislice or 3D image sets is laborious and rarely used; it is more practical for outlining or defining small structures or selected regions, for example, outlining the cross section of the spinal cord or measuring third ventricle dimensions.

Techniques requiring a high degree of manual input typically have the following advantages: they are methodologically simple; little specialized software is required; and the segmentation results relate well to the operator's perceptions of the limits of particular structures. Typical disadvantages include: they are prone to operator bias; the precision is low when compared with many automated techniques, and analysis times can be long.

Semiautomated methods can supplement or replace manual outlining methods, resulting in improved speed and reproducibility. Brain volume may be analysed using semiautomated seed-growing software based on local thresholding (Bermel et al., 2003). Parenchymal and ventricular volumes are usually measured on T1-weighted images and intracranial volume is measured on the corresponding T2-weighted images. Parenchymal volume consists of combined supra and infratentorial parenchyma (whole-brain parenchyma). Images below the cerebellum are not taken into account. Ventricular measurements include all four ventricles. In this case, two ratios for brain volumes are calculated: (I) parenchymal fraction defined as whole-brain parenchyma divided by intracranial volume and (II) ventricular fraction defined as ventricular volume divided by whole-brain parenchyma.

The use of regional segmentation algorithms, such as seed growing (Rovaris et al., 2000), local edge detection algorithms and contouring (Plummer, 1992) has assisted in outlining lesions and also small structures such as the spinal cord, optic nerve and ventricles (Losseff et al., 1996; Nijeholt et al., 1998). Measurement reproducibility improves from 3-5% for manual outlining to 1-3% for semiautomated approaches for measuring the spinal cord and ventricles.

Automated Methods and Gray/White Matter Segmentation

Unfortunately, detection of small volume changes from serial MRI is difficult with conventional method of atrophy measurement that rely on manual outlining of regions of interest or on semiautomated thresholding. This is true because results are critically dependent on the reproducibility of the outlining of the structure being measured. Such measurements are time consuming, observer dependent and susceptible to segmentation error. Registration of serial MRI may offer a useful alternative in that cerebral losses may be measured directly from automated subtraction of brain volumes. All analyses are performed after acquisition and so do not increase scanning time. The main advantage of the technique is that accurate positional matching allows digital subtraction of serial imaging that is not critically dependent on the accuracy of segmentation. Individuals serve as their own control and change in brain volume is calculated directly from the registered MRI. This method provides a measure of net volume loss over the whole brain, so that small positional shifts or shape changes do not affect the total calculated atrophy. Automated methods provide good reproducibility and reduced reliance on time-consuming operator input (Fox et al., 2000).

Many automated methods allow the segmentation of the brain parenchyma into brain white and gray matter and CSF compartments (Sanfilipo et al, 2004). Few proven approaches exist for automated segmentation of individual brain structures or for the spinal cord or optic nerve.

Both single contrast acquisitions (Chard et al., 2002) and multi-spectral data (Ge et al., 2000; Udupa et al., 1997) have been utilized for whole brain segmentation and volumetry. Usually the difference in signal intensity between brain parenchyma and CSF on a single contrast acquisition is enough to drive the segmentation process. Methods for removing any residual signal from the scalp in the resulting segmentation include automated detection of the intracranial contour (Zijdenbos and Dawant, 1994) and segmentation based on probabilistic spatial tissue distributions (Ashburner and Friston, 2000).

The segmentation of gray and white matter volumes may again be accomplished utilizing either single-contrast or multi-spectral data, although additional sophistication is required to separate the two tissue types. Methods include statistical parametric mapping (SPM)-based segmentation (Ashburner and Friston, 2000; Sharma et al., 2004) and the fuzzy C-means algorithm, as described by (Pham and Prince, 1999b).

A method for determining the regions of tissue occupied by MS lesions is necessary if misclassification of these regions is to be avoided and accurate tissue volumes are to be determined. Automated segmentation of multiple sclerosis lesions has been investigated by a number of researchers (Guttmann et al., 1999; Kikinis et al., 1999; Udupa et al., 1997; Zijdenbos and Dawant, 1994); if total lesion load is small, manual segmentation may be a reasonable alternative. In the case of negligible lesion volume, lesion segmentation may be unnecessary (Miller et al., 2002; Zivadinov and Bakshi, 2004; Sharma et al., 2004).

Unfortunately, brain tissue segmentation in any disease process may be complicated by both changes in tissue signal intensity characteristics and, in the case of MS, the presence of lesions. There are a number of strategies that may improve the analysis, although each method could be associated with differing susceptibilities to disease-related segmentation bias. In addition, there is no accepted standard technique for measuring brain tissue volumes, so it is not possible to validate and calibrate any segmentation method fully. Given this, it is important that multiple segmentation methods are implemented independently and applied to different scan acquisition methods, as each will have its own advantages and disadvantages.

Comparison of Segmentation Algorithms for Volume Analysis and Pulse Sequences

The principal aspects of data acquisition that influence the efficacy of volume measurements are image resolution in three dimensions and image contrast. The desirability of high resolution scans to reduce partial volume errors means that 3D (volumetric) acquisitions are attractive, although both 2D (Molyneux et al., 2000; Bermel et al., 2003; Horsfield et al., 2003) and 3D (Liu et al., 1999; Horsfield et al., 2003) sequences have been used successfully to derive volume measures in the CNS. 3D sequences also allow more accurate re-slicing of datasets when registering volumes between serial acquisitions.

The choice of image contrast is also important in reliable volume measurements. The choice of contrast weighting methods depends on the study's aims and, to an extent, on the choice of analysis technique. For whole-brain atrophy measurements, segmentation of the brain is necessary, meaning that suppression of CSF, for example using fluid-attenuated inversion recovery (FLAIR) sequences, is desirable to generate a sharp distinction in signal between cerebral and extra-axial tissue. For this reason, the most widely used 3D sequence is a T1-weighted gradient echo, with or without added CSF suppression, the latter provided by an inversion recovery pre-pulse (Sanfilipo et al., 2004).

Studies focusing on the measurement of atrophy of individual structures within the CNS may require alternative imaging strategies. For instance, a study of white matter atrophy requires good contrast between white matter, gray matter, CSF and possibly lesions. Segmentation may be aided by multiple contrast (multi-spectral) acquisitions, typically T1-weighted, T2-weighted and proton-density-weighted data acquisitions.

It is clear that many promising techniques have been developed with which to measure global and regional brain tissue volumes; these offer high reproducibility and sensitivity to small changes over time. Few studies have focused on comparing different segmentation analysis techniques for determining brain volumes (Leigh et al., 2002; Horsfield et al., 2003; Sharma et al., in press).

In a recent study (Leigh et al., 2002), three different pulse sequences and three different segmentation methods were used to measure change in brain volume over 2 years in 10 patients with relapsing-remitting multiple sclerosis and five healthy controls. T1-weighted, FLAIR and PD/T2-weighted sequences were analyzed. Image segmentation to determine brain volume was performed using the following: a histogram segmentation algorithm, an adaptive fuzzy c-means algorithm and an adaptive Bayesan segmentation with a K means clustering. In MS patients, significant atrophy was seen after 1 and 2 years compared with baseline; however, for various combinations of acquisition sequence and segmentation algorithm the percentage change in brain volume varied markedly. The reduction ranged from 0.34 to 1.67% comparing month 12 with baseline and from 0.79 to 3.11% comparing month 24 with baseline. This study underlines the important differences that one can observe when using various imaging and image segmentation techniques to quantify the change in brain volume over time, thereby making it difficult to compare results from different populations.

A considerable number of specific methods for measuring tissue volume in the brain have been developed and applied in multiple sclerosis. A summary of the benefits and limitations of current methods for brain volume measurements is provided in Table 1 (Miller et al., 2002) and has been reviewed recently (Zivadinov and Bakshi, 2004).

Table 1. Methods used for measuring cerebral atrophy.

Location/generic methodology	Method	Advantages	Disadvantages
Brain/linear and regional measures	Third ventricle width Third ventricle volume Brain width Corpus callosum width Volume on central brain slices Stereology CSF volumes Bicaudate ratio	Easy to implement; rapid analysis;standard acquisition methods; enables targeting of eloquent regions	Limited anatomical scope; may miss subtle effects; may exhibit user bias; high user input
Brain/whole-brain segmentation	BPF WBR BICCR Fuzzy connectedness Probabilistic segmentation TDS SIENAX MIDAS	Increased automation reduces user bias and user input; Generally higher measurements precision	Complex analysis methods,possibly more complex acquisition schemes
Brain/registration-based methods	Voxel-based morphometry SIENA	Regional atrophy may become apparent	Complex analysis methods; limited application to multiple sclerosis to date

Adapted from Miller DH Brain 2002

Absolute vs. Normalized Brain Atrophy Measures

The Use of Relative Volumes

Comparison between groups of patients is confounded by the presence of substantial inter-subject variations in head size that can mask differences attributable to atrophy. Normalizing the volumes of brain, specific tissues and structures to head sizes may be successful in reducing these confounding effects (Mathalon et al., 1993; Whitwell et al., 2001). Relative volumes also remove variability in volume data due to scanner instability, as all structures in the image will experience the same amount of scaling due to such effects.

A number of normalization methods have emerged: the scalp (Freeborough and Fox, 1997), total intracranial capacity determined by the sum of the volumes of gray matter, white matter and CSF (Guttmann et al., 2000) and the sum of the brain, and ventricular and sulcal CSF (Rudick et al., 1999; Bermel et al., 2003), have all been used to create volumes against which normalization can be performed.

There is still a controversy regarding the best regional brain atrophy measure in MS studies. In a recently published study, Zivadinov et al. (2003) investigated in a cross-sectional study whether normalized measures of regional brain atrophy correlated with MRI defined regional brain lesions better than did absolute measures of regional brain atrophy. Generally, they found that normalized measures of regional brain atrophy correlated with regional brain volumes and disability better than did absolute measures. The magnitude of correlation between disability (EDSS score) and normalized regional brain atrophy measures was more than two-fold higher than the correlation between EDSS and absolute measures of the same regions. These data suggest that normalized regional brain atrophy measures are preferable to absolute regional measures in cross-sectional studies.

Confounding Factors that Are Known to Influence Cerebral Volume

Little is known about the mechanisms underlying cerebral atrophy, but loss of neurons, axons, and oligodendrocytes, the formation of glial scars, and the effect of medications may contribute to the reduction of brain volume. Because of the unknown underlying mechanisms, any research using brain volume as an outcome parameter must consider other factors that could produce temporary or permanent atrophy, including systemic illnesses, alcohol use, changes in hydration and nutrition, and use of corticosteroids.

Corticosteroids

The mechanism by which steroids affect cerebral volume is not clearly understood. There appear to be different reasonable explanations: (a) it has been implied that steroid-induced protein catabolism may lead to a loss in cerebral tissue, since atrophic changes are seen in several tissues; (b) a more likely explanation is that loss of brain volume is secondary to loss of water, since steroids have an effect on water and electrolyte balance, inducing reduction of abnormal vascular permeability and/or promoting water and sodium diuresis with measurable decreases of each in the brain; (c) finally, the proposed mechanism of action of intravenous methylprednisolone (IVMP) in MS includes the downregulation of adhesion molecule expression on endothelial cells, decreased cytokine and matrix metalloproteinases secretion, decreased autoreactive T-cell mediated inflammation, the closing of the blood-brain barrier, inhibition of demyelination and the promotion of remyelination. Some of these mechanisms directly contribute to alterations in proton density and MR relaxation properties of the brain, resulting in a partial volume effects within a given voxel, which may ultimately affect the brain volume. This does not represent an artefact because the potential alteration in relaxation times of tissues would represent the physiologic effect of steroids on the brain and therefore may result in a different classification of the voxel by the segmentation algorithm, especially at tissue interfaces.

The net effect of IVMP on brain volume fluctuations in MS patients is not completely clear. The short-term effect of IVMP on brain volume has been studied in two recently published studies (Hoogervorst et al., 2002; Rao et al., 2002). In 26 RR MS patients who were followed by monthly MRI, a total of 56 courses of IVMP were given during the follow-up, 40 while taking interferon-beta and 16 with no other disease-modifying treatment (Rao et al., 2002). In the 3 months prior to IVMP, brain fractional volume was stable, but when all 56 events were combined, there was a significant reduction at months 1 and 2 following IVMP. A significant reduction in brain fractional volume was also observed when patients were classified according to prior treatment status. This study suggests that MRI should be delayed by 2 months following IVMP to avoid a reversible steroid effect on brain volume. Another study demonstrated that short courses of IVMP (restricted to three or five days) have no major impact on brain volume (Hoogervorst et al., 2002). However, steroids may have a protective effect on brain volume (limiting atrophy) over the long term due to immunomodulatory and anti-inflammatory effects that impact on disease progression (Zivadinov et al., 2001). In a recently published study, we evaluated the long-term effect of treatment with pulses of IVMP in RR MS patients and demonstrated that IVMP limits the development of global brain atrophy over a five-year period (Zivadinov et al., 2001).

Anorexia

Several studies reported widened cerebral sulci and enlarged lateral and third ventricles in patients with anorexia nervosa. Moreover, white matter volume and gray matter volume are reported to be reduced in patients with anorexia nervosa.

A number of hypotheses have been presented to explain the reduction in brain volume that occurs in the underweight anorexic state. These have included such factors as decreased serum proteins resulting in decreased colloidal osmotic pressure and a shift of fluid from the intravascular space into the subarachnoid spaces, partial regeneration of damaged neurons and their axons with possible regeneration of myelin, loss of lean body tissue mass, increased urine and serum cortisol levels, decreased protein synthesis resulting in loss of dendritic spines, a reduction in the number of synaptic junctions, and delayed synaptogenesis. More recently, Swayze et al. (2003) hypothesized that insulin-like growth factor –1 (IGF) may be related to changes in brain tissue. The authors suggest that IGF may be involved not only in the regulation of growth during fetal and childhood development but also serves a vital function in the maintenance of mature cells. It is involved in the proliferation, differentiation, and survival of oligodendrocyte progenitors in cell culture and therefore is crucial in the development and myelination of the central nervous system

Intercurrent Illness and Alochol Use

Atrophy is the loss of mass per unit volume and its progression is the rate of change of tissue loss with time. Axonal loss, demyelination, apoptosis, Wallerian degeneration, gliosis, changes in the size of extracellular space and orientation of axons may all contribute to cerebral atrophy in MS patients. Remyelination should in principle stabilize or possibly increase brain mass, thus slow the progression of cerebral atrophy, whereas inflammation and oedema may actually increase brain volume yet at the same time potentially decrease the cellular components per unit volume of tissue. Rudick et al. (1999) reported that 9.8% of RRMS patients in the placebo arm had a small increase in their brain parenchymal fraction over two years. Although no specific details were provided about these patients, it is possible that they had active acute inflammatory MS disease on MRI that resulted in an increase in water content of the brain and thus an increase in brain volume (Leigh et al., 2002).

Alcohol ingestion (Pfefferbaum et al., 1994) and hemodialysis (Walters et al., 2001) can cause shifts in brain volume resulting in brain shrinkage and thus appearing as atrophy on MRI.

References

Ashburner J, Friston KJ. Voxel-based morphometry--the methods. *Neuroimage* 2000; 11: 805-21.

Bermel RA, Sharma J, Tjoa CW, Puli SR, Bakshi R. A semiautomated measure of whole-brain atrophy in multiple sclerosis. *J Neurol Sci* 2003; 208: 57-65

Chard DT, Griffin CM, Parker GJ, Kapoor R, Thompson AJ, Miller DH. Brain atrophy in clinically early relapsing-remitting multiple sclerosis. *Brain* 2002; 125: 327-37.

Fox NC, Jenkins R, Leary SM, Stevenson VL, Losseff NA, Crum WR, et al. Progressive cerebral atrophy in MS: a serial study using registered, volumetric MRI. *Neurology* 2000; 54: 807-12.

Freeborough PA, Fox NC. The boundary shift integral: an accurate and robust measure of cerebral volume changes from registered repeat MRI. *IEEE Trans Med Imaging* 1997; 16: 623-9.

Garrison K, Henry R, Pelletier D. In: Zivadinov R, Bakshi R, eds. *Brain and Spinal Cord Atrophy in Multiple Sclerosis. Technical Aspects of Brain Atrophy Measurement.* New York: Nova Science Publisher 2004; (p39-61).

Ge Y, Grossman RI, Udupa JK, Fulton J, Constantinescu CS, Gonzales-Scarano F, et al. Glatiramer acetate (Copaxone) treatment in relapsing-remitting MS: quantitative MR assessment. *Neurology* 2000; 54: 813-7.

Guttmann CR, Benson R, Warfield SK, Wei X, Anderson MC, Hall CB, et al. White matter abnormalities in mobility-impaired older persons. *Neurology* 2000; 54: 1277-83.

Guttmann CR, Kikinis R, Anderson MC, Jakab M, Warfield SK, Killiany RJ, et al. Quantitative follow-up of patients with multiple sclerosis using MRI: reproducibility. *J Magn Reson Imaging* 1999; 9: 509-18.

Hoogervorst EL, Polman CH, Barkhof F. Cerebral volume changes in multiple sclerosis patients treated with high-dose intravenous methylprednisolone. *Mult Scler* 2002; 8: 415-9.

Horsfield MA, Rovaris M, Rocca MA, Rossi P, Benedict RHB, Filippi M, Bakshi R. Whole brain atrophy in multiple sclerosis measured by two segmentation processes from various MRI sequences. *J Neurol Sci* 2003; 216:169-177

Kikinis R, Guttmann CR, Metcalf D, Wells WM, 3rd, Ettinger GJ, Weiner HL, et al. Quantitative follow-up of patients with multiple sclerosis using MRI: technical aspects. *J Magn Reson Imaging* 1999; 9: 519-30.

Leigh R, Ostuni J, Pham D, Goldszal A, Lewis BK, Howard T, et al. Estimating cerebral atrophy in multiple sclerosis patients from various MR pulse sequences. *Mult Scler* 2002; 8: 420-9.

Liu C, Edwards S, Gong Q, Roberts N, Blumhardt LD. Three dimensional MRI estimates of brain and spinal cord atrophy in multiple sclerosis. *J Neurol Neurosurg Psychiatry* 1999; 66: 323-30.

Losseff NA, Wang L, Lai HM, Yoo DS, Gawne-Cain ML, McDonald WI, et al. Progressive cerebral atrophy in multiple sclerosis. A serial MRI study. *Brain* 1996; 119: 2009-19.

Mathalon DH, Sullivan EV, Rawles JM, Pfefferbaum A. Correction for head size in brain-imaging measurements. *Psychiatry Res* 1993; 50: 121-39.

Miller DH, Barkhof F, Frank JA, Parker GJ, Thompson AJ. Measurement of atrophy in multiple sclerosis: pathological basis, methodological aspects and clinical relevance. *Brain* 2002; 125: 1676-95.

Molyneux PD, Kappos L, Polman C, Pozzilli C, Barkhof F, Filippi M, et al. The effect of interferon beta-1b treatment on MRI measures of cerebral atrophy in secondary progressive multiple sclerosis. European Study Group on Interferon beta-1b in secondary progressive multiple sclerosis. *Brain* 2000; 123: 2256-63.

Nijeholt GJ, van Walderveen MA, Castelijns JA, van Waesberghe JH, Polman C, Scheltens P, et al. Brain and spinal cord abnormalities in multiple sclerosis. Correlation between MRI parameters, clinical subtypes and symptoms. *Brain* 1998; 121: 687-97.

Pfefferbaum A, Mathalon DH, Sullivan EV, Rawles JM, Zipursky RB, Lim KO. A quantitative magnetic resonance imaging study of changes in brain morphology from infancy to late adulthood. *Arch Neurol* 1994; 51: 874-87.

Pham DL, Prince JL. An adaptive fuzzy C-means algorithm for image segmentation in the presence of intensity inhomogeneities. *Patt Recog Leti* 1999; 20: 57-68.

Plummer DL. Displmage: a display and analysis tool for medical images. *Revist Neuroradiol* 1992; 5: 489-95.

Rao AB, Richert N, Howard T, Lewis BK, Bash CN, McFarland HF, et al. Methylprednisolone effect on brain volume and enhancing lesions in MS before and during IFNbeta-1b. *Neurology* 2002; 59: 688-94.

Rovaris M, Inglese M, van Schijndel RA, Sormani MP, Rodegher M, Comi G, et al. Sensitivity and reproducibility of volume change measurements of different brain portions on magnetic resonance imaging in patients with multiple sclerosis. *J Neurol* 2000; 247: 960-5.

Rudick RA, Fisher E, Lee JC, Simon J, Jacobs L. Use of the brain parenchymal fraction to measure whole brain atrophy in relapsing-remitting MS. Multiple Sclerosis Collaborative Research Group. *Neurology* 1999; 53: 1698-704.

Sanfilipo MP, Benedict RHB, Zivadinov R, Bakshi R. Correction for intracranial volume in analysis of whole brain volume in multiple sclerosis: the proportion vs. residual method. *Neuroimage* 2004; 1732-1743.

Sharma J, Sanfilipo MP, Benedict RHB, Weinstock-Guttman B, Munschauer FE, Bakshi R. Whole brain atrophy in multiple sclerosis measured by automated versus. semiautomated MR imaging segmentation. *AJNR: American Journal of Neuroradiology 2004; 25: 985-996.*

Swayze VW, 2nd, Andersen AE, Andreasen NC, Arndt S, Sato Y, Ziebell S. Brain tissue volume segmentation in patients with anorexia nervosa before and after weight normalization. *Int J Eat Disord* 2003; 33: 33-44.

Udupa JK, Wei L, Samarasekera S, Miki Y, van Buchem MA, Grossman RI. Multiple sclerosis lesion quantification using fuzzy-connectedness principles. *IEEE Trans Med Imaging* 1997; 16: 598-609.

Walters RJ, Fox NC, Crum WR, Taube D, Thomas DJ. Haemodialysis and cerebral oedema. *Nephron* 2001; 87: 143-7.

Whitwell JL, Crum WR, Watt HC, Fox NC. Normalization of cerebral volumes by use of intracranial volume: implications for longitudinal quantitative MR imaging. *AJNR Am J Neuroradiol* 2001; 22: 1483-9.

Zijdenbos AP, Dawant BM. Brain segmentation and white matter lesion detection in MR images. *Crit Rev Biomed Eng* 1994; 22: 401-65.

Zivadinov R, Bakshi R. Role of MRI in multiple sclerosis II: brain and spinal cord atrophy. *Front Biosci* 2004; 9: 647-64.

Zivadinov R, Locatelli L, Stival B, Bratina A, Grop A, Nasuelli D, et al. Normalized regional brain atrophy measurements in multiple sclerosis. *Neuroradiology* 2003; 45: 793-8.

Zivadinov R, Rudick RA, De Masi R, Nasuelli D, Ukmar M, Pozzi-Mucelli RS, et al. Effects of IV methylprednisolone on brain atrophy in relapsing-remitting MS. *Neurology* 2001; 57: 1239-47.

In: Brain and Spinal Cord Atrophy in Multiple Sclerosis
Editors: R. Zivadinov and R. Bakshi, pp. 39-61
ISBN 1-59454-160-4

Chapter V

The Measurement of Brain Atrophy in Multiple Sclerosis: Technical Aspects

Kathleen Garrison, Roland G. Henry and Daniel Pelletier*
University of California San Francisco, CA

Introduction

Brain atrophy reflects the net result of irreversible and destructive pathological processes in multiple sclerosis (MS). Axonal damage and loss, chronic demyelination and gliosis cause a reduction in brain parenchymal tissue volume and a corresponding expansion of cerebrospinal fluid (CSF) spaces. These gross morphological changes can be accurately quantified using standard magnetic resonance imaging (MRI) acquisitions and various image-analysis tools. Measurement of whole brain atrophy from MRI has emerged as an objective and reliable marker of disease progression in MS, and a potential outcome measure in clinical treatment-related trials. Conventional MRI sequences can be used to estimate volumes of intracranial compartments, which are then used to quantify whole brain atrophy in cross-sectional or longitudinal comparisons. Because brain volume changes over time are small, accurate calculation of whole brain atrophy requires a highly reproducible measurement, and MRI can detect subtle changes in brain structure. While the optimal method for quantifying whole brain atrophy in MS has not been established, current approaches and considerations in the measurement are reviewed here. A summary of the specific methods to be discussed is provided in Table 1. In the following, the methodological concepts used in the determination of atrophy from MRI are addressed, followed by examples of current methods and a discussion of technical and other considerations affecting utility and efficacy of these methods. Lastly, the contribution of gray and white matter loss to whole brain atrophy is only briefly discussed as it is still under active investigation.

* Corresponding Author: Daniel Pelletier, M.D., UCSF Multiple Sclerosis Center, 350 Parnassus Avenue, Suite 908, San Francisco, CA 94117. Telephone: (415) 514-1684; Fax: (415) 514-2443; Email: danp@itsa.ucsf.edu

Methodologic Concepts

The basic concept underlying all methods for the measurement of brain atrophy from MRI is the quantification of some or all of the volume of brain tissue. While there are many methods employed (see 'Current Methods' section below), there are a few fundamental concepts and techniques that serve as the defining characteristics of those atrophy assessment methods. These concepts are described below and include normalization, automation and registration.

Normalization

An important distinction between volumetric measurements of whole brain atrophy is whether brain size is reported as the actual volume or as a normalized volume. In general, absolute volume measurements are of limited value for cross-sectional studies due to confounding effects of substantial variation in intracranial volume that exists between subjects. This normal biological variability can mask volume changes attributable to atrophy and obscure subtle disease-related volume differences. Absolute measurements of cerebral volume have poorer scan-rescan reproducibility, thus limiting their usefulness in longitudinal studies. Normalized measurements, calculated as the brain parenchymal volume divided by an estimate of total intracranial volume, have been developed to overcome these pitfalls. Normalization corrects for intracranial volume and may also minimize the effects of patient positioning in the scanner, as all structures in an image will experience the same amount of artefactual scaling due to such effects.

There are several normalized methods available for the measurement of whole brain atrophy, including those for which normalization is based on volume measures of the scalp (Freeborough and Fox, 1997), total intracranial capacity determined by the sum of tissue-specific volumes of gray matter, white matter, and CSF (Chard et al., 2002a; Guttmann et al., 2000b), and the sum of the brain parenchyma and CSF (Rudick et al., 1999; Bermel et al., 2003a). Recently, in a cross-sectional study, Zivadinov et al. (2003) evaluated whether normalized measures of regional brain atrophy correlated with MRI-defined regional brain lesions better than the absolute measures of regional brain atrophy. Their cross-sectional data suggested that normalized regional brain atrophy measures are preferable to absolute regional measures. In a cross-sectional study of Alzheimer's disease (Whitwell et al., 2001), it was shown that normalization using intracranial volume increased sensitivity in distinguishing disease from control groups. To date, there are no longitudinal studies that compared absolute and normalized measurements of whole brain atrophy.

Automation

In order to evaluate whole brain or white and gray matter atrophy, pixels from MRI scans must be classified into specific tissue components such as non-brain tissue, white and gray matter or CSF. Many techniques have been described to segment brain scans into these three components and subsequently assess volume change (Miller et al., 2002; Zivadinov and Bakshi, 2004). These segmentation algorithms and analysis methods differ in the degree of operator input required to perform the measurements, ranging from completely subjective rating scales to fully automated volumetric calculations.

Manual segmentation techniques are typically methodologically simple, require little specialist software, and generate measurements that relate well to the observer's perceptions of structural limits. Methods include the use of an ordinal rating scale, graded calipers to measure distance between anatomic landmarks on films, image analysis software requiring manual selection of anatomic landmarks, stereology, and manual tracing tools in image analysis packages. Manual segmentation of the whole brain is rarely used, however, due to low precision, high measurement variability, heavy time demands and potential for operator bias. Subjective rating of whole brain atrophy is also limited in terms of sensitivity and is thus not very useful in detecting changes over time. However, manual outlining using a stereotactic atlas has been used to detect cerebral atrophy in MS (Filippi et al., 1998) and to correlate atrophy with clinical deterioration (Inglese et al., 1999).

Semiautomated segmentation and atrophy analysis methods offer a more rapid assessment of areas and volumes and potentially increase accuracy due to the operator interaction, ensuring precision throughout the algorithm and subsequent calculation of volume change. Commercially available edge-finding and thresholding software has been adapted to a semiautomated method of atrophy assessment and used to detect whole brain atrophy in MS patients versus age-matched controls (Bermel et al., 2003b) with a magnitude of decreased brain parenchymal fraction (BPF) similar to that found using automated techniques (Rudick et al., 1999; Smith et al., 2002). Using a semi-automated measure, decreases in BPF were also seen in even the youngest of MS patients compared to age-matched controls (Kassubek et al., 2003).

To increase objectivity, reproducibility and efficiency, both the segmentation algorithm and the atrophy analysis method should be as automated as possible, although one study demonstrated that a semiautomated measure of brain parenchymal fraction (see section 'BPF' below) was more accurate than a fully automated BPF method in MS (Zivadinov et al., in press). Many automated methods exist for segmentation and thus volume measurement; most are intensity-based, with segmentation driven by the difference in signal intensity between brain parenchyma and CSF alone. Automated measurements reduce analysis time and reliance on an operator familiar with neuroanatomy and the appearance of tissue pathology in MS. However automated measurements may be critically dependent on the pulse sequence employed (Horsfield et al., 2003; Sharma et al., 2004).

Registration

Automated measurement of whole brain atrophy using image subtraction is an attractive alternative method (to manual methods) of identifying small changes between equivalent pairs of images. For subtraction to yield meaningful results, however, baseline and follow-up scans need to be positionally matched, or registered. Even with careful patient positioning in the scanner upon repeat acquisitions, signal changes due to whole brain atrophy can be small compared to systematic differences or differences due to patient movement and orientation. Recent developments in registration methods have improved the accuracy of post-acquisition positional matching of serial 3-dimensional volumetric MRI scans, allowing whole brain volumes to be registered to within a fraction of a voxel of each other, thereby revealing relevant volume changes (Freeborough et al., 1996; Hajnal et al., 1995). Non-linear registration is the set of techniques resulting in deformation fields that provide information about global atrophy (Freeborough and Fox, 1998), from which statistical analysis of group differences may help characterize whole brain atrophy in MS (Ashburner and Friston, 2000). Rigid-body registration, on the other hand, involves the estimation of a voxel-based map between pairs of images in which one image is assumed stationary and the other image is spatially transformed to match it, thus tracking displacement of the brain during atrophy, for example using the inner table of the skull as a reference (Freeborough and Fox, 1997).

Current Methods

The current methods used to assess whole brain atrophy in MS can be classified into two groups based on their reliance on segmentation and registration, though most methods use a combination of both steps. As described in previous sections, segmentation-based methods rely on an algorithm that classifies voxels into white and gray matter and CSF, while registration-based methods focus on the measurement of volume differences between serial scans. Linear indexes, for example the measurement of ventricular width, have also been applied in several MS studies to establish the relationship between cerebral atrophy and cognitive impairment (Benedict et al., 2004), but these measures are limited to regional brain atrophy and thus will not be discussed here.

Segmentation-Based Methods

Segmentation-based methods employed to measure whole brain atrophy in MS are described below and include brain parenchymal fraction (BPF), index of brain atrophy (IBA), whole brain ratio (WBR), brain to intracranial capacity ratio (BICCR), Fuzzy connectedness/Udupa's method, the Alfano method, and SIENAX.

Brain Parenchymal Fraction

While the term BPF has been applied to many normalization methods, (Rudick et al., 1999) originally introduced the measure as the ratio of brain parenchymal tissue to the sum of brain and ventricular CSF volumes in a study describing progressive cerebral atrophy in relapsing-remitting (RR) MS (Rudick et al., 1999). Both brain parenchymal and total brain volume were obtained automatically by software designed to segment the brain on MRI scans with no special acquisition or repositioning required. The BPF algorithm consisted of a sequence of 3D image processing operations that detected the outer surface of the brain (Fig 1, area in red) and the brain parenchymal tissue within that outer surface (Fig 1, area in green), with volume calculation accounting for partial volume effects.

There are a number of inherent advantages to using this approach for the quantification of whole brain atrophy in MS. First, the normalization procedure takes into account inter-individual variation in head size, thus requiring a single measurement in cross-sectional studies. Secondly, this automated BPF has a high test-retest reproducibility, with a coefficient of variation (COV-standard deviation/mean*100%), of 0.2% for BPF and 0.6% for both outer contour and brain parenchymal volumes. This is due in part to the performance of a single segmentation (for example, a baseline segmentation), thus errors introduced during repeat image acquisitions are present in both the numerator (baseline scan) and denominator (follow-up scan), and cancel out. Finally, BPF may be applied to several MRI scans commonly acquired during clinical examination or clinical trial studies, such as T_2/PD or FLAIR images. Disadvantages of BPF include the potential for outer volume change over time, as this method does not include CSF external to the outer surface of the brain, where CSF volume can increase with progressive brain atrophy and/or gray matter volume loss (De Stefano et al., 2003).

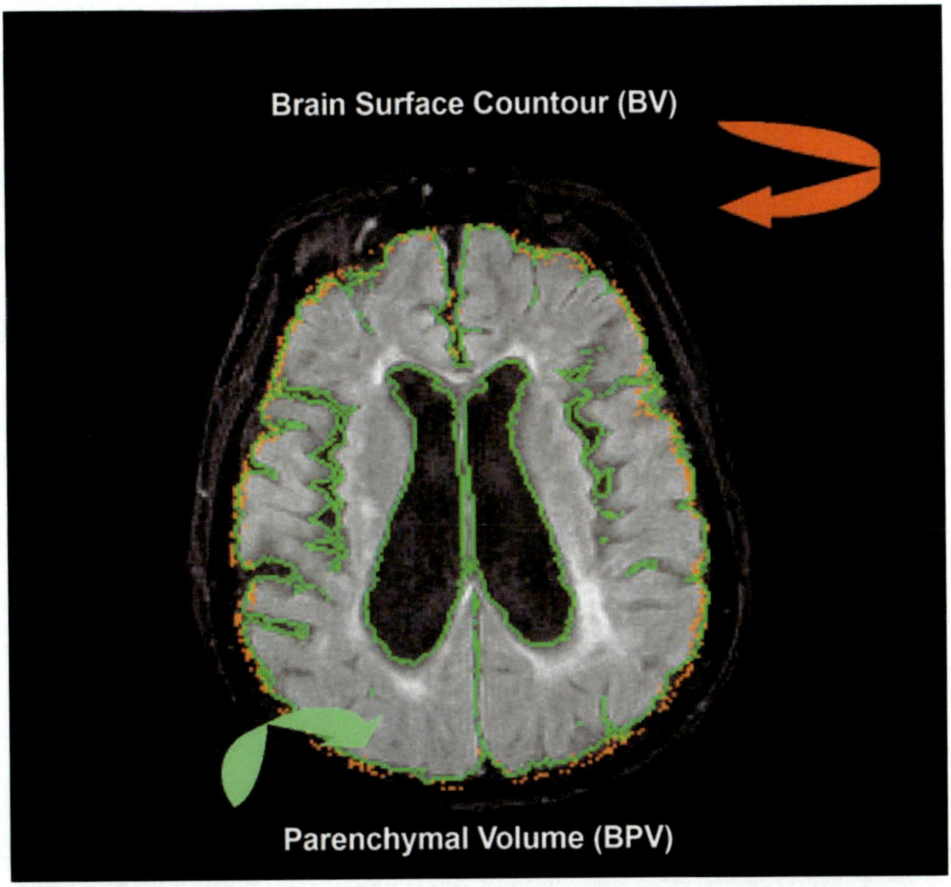

Figure 1. The BPF algorithm detects the outer surface of the brain (area in red) and the brain parenchymal tissue within that outer surface (area in green) (reproduced with permission of Elizabeth Fisher, Ph.D. (Rudick et al., 1999).

The relationship between whole brain atrophy and clinical measures is described in detail in a chapter presented by Zivadinov & Bakshi (2004), but it is interesting to note here that a significant correlation between disability and BPF at baseline was reported in the original study by Rudick et al. (1999), where a treatment effect of INF-1ba on atrophy progression in year two of follow-up was also demonstrated. Decreased BPF and worsening EDSS scores continued to correlate in the same patient cohort over eight years (Fisher et al., 2000; Fisher et al., 2002). BPF thus serves as a useful surrogate marker of the global pathological processes occurring in MS by revealing atrophy compared to normal controls, and detecting disease-related longitudinal changes (Figure 2). Variations on the method include a semiautomated measurement of BPF that includes the outer CSF contour (Bermel et al., 2003), IBA, WBR, and BICCR (see sections below).

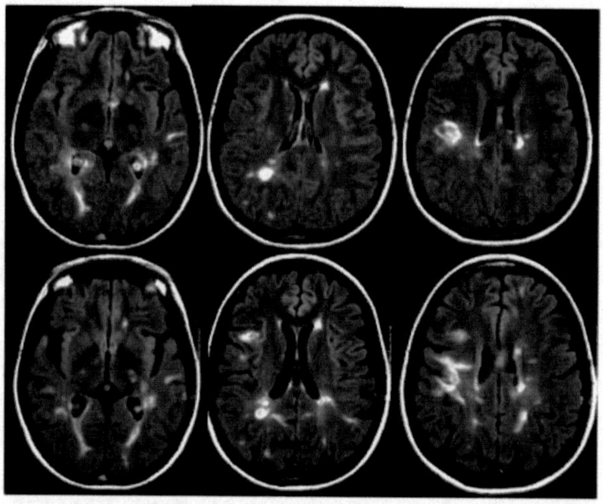

Figure 2. Progressive brain atrophy in RR MS over 18 months is shown on representative MRI scans. BPF was performed at the Buffalo Neuroimaging Analysis Center. For the initial MRI, BPF was calculated at 0.88, which is normal relative to the patient's age. Mild physical disability was demonstrated on the Expanded Disability Status Scale (EDSS) of 1.0. Between MRI scans, the patient experienced frequent relapses and disease progression. At 18 months, EDSS measure of physical disability had increased to 4.0, and BPF decreased by 4.5% to 0.84 (~5 standard deviations below normal). Enlargement of CSF spaces is also evident, including the cortical sulci, sylvian fissures, and third and lateral ventricles (reproduced with permission of Rohit Bakshi, MD) (Zivadinov et al., 2004).

Index of Brain Atrophy

An IBA is defined as supratentorial brain parenchyma)/(supratentorial parenchyma + ventricles) x 100%.

Supratentorial brain and CSF ventricle masks are created from high-resolution T_1-weighted 3D gradient echo and conventional PD/T_2-weighted images. The mask is multiplied by the T_1-weighted image and thresholding is then applied to separate CSF and brain regions.

Scan-rescan COV is 0.9%, representing about 99% reproducibility. However, IBA estimates atrophy from the top of the brain to the top of the midbrain only (defined by an operator), unlike BPF (Rudick et al., 1999), which covers the whole brain. Another difference is that IBA does not remove sulcal CSF regions for normalization. IBA was used to detect significant brain atrophy in primary progressive (PP) patients versus healthy controls (Pelletier et al., 2003), whereas no significant correlation was found between T2 lesion load and atrophy measurement or metabolite ratios (NAA/Cr). A two-year placebo-controlled clinical trial in PP MS is underway using this method as the primary outcome measure.

Whole Brain Ratio

Calculation of the WBR uses anisotropic noise filtering, after which the inverse tangent of the ratio of the filtered T_2-weighted long echo image divided by the filtered T_2-weighted short echo volume is used to create an "angle image", and a histogram of the angle images for all slices is computed. Gaussian distributions of the main peak (representing the brain) are fitted and thresholding determines masks of both the intradural space (width of the histogram main peak) and CSF space (values greater than the main peak). The brain is extracted by the application of an additional threshold of about 60% maximum signal intensity value. WBR is calculated as: (intradural volume – CSF volume)/(intradural volume).

Manual editing is often needed to remove extraneous areas from the intradural mask and also to reclassify lesions into brain if the software misclassifies them as CSF. In a two-year multi-center study of RR MS (Jones et al., 2001), a decrease in WBR was seen after the first year, with an even more significant decrease measured after two years. WBR demonstrated high reproducibility, with a COV of <1%.

Brain to Intracranial Capacity Ratio

BICCR is a fully automated, head-size-normalized measure of whole brain volume from the Montreal Neurological Institute. This method is applied to PD/T_2-weighted images, and involves correction of image intensity non-uniformities; stereotactic registration and resampling of MRI data; intensity normalization to a standard average PD or T_2 volume; cropping inferior and superior slices to leave an anatomically equivalent 80-mm-thick slice in all objects; digital morphometry to identify the intracranial cavity, and Bayesian tissue classification for volume from the resultant mask. The BICCR metric is defined as the ratio of brain tissue volume to total intracranial volume, or (gray matter + white matter + lesions)/(gray matter + white matter + lesions + CSF) x 100%.

This measure varies from BPF (Rudick et al., 1999) by including all external CSF (between the cortex and dura) in addition to CSF within the sulci. Coefficient of variation for this method is 0.21% and is related to scan time, being lower for shorter scan times (and thus thicker slices). Precise repositioning is unnecessary with BICCR, and the measure also accounts for problems from partial head coverage during scanning. Using BICCR to quantify whole brain atrophy in MS, it was demonstrated that more brain atrophy was seen in secondary-progressive (SP) than RR MS or healthy controls, and BICCR was inversely correlated to EDSS and disease duration in patients with SP MS (Collins et al., 2001). BICCR was only slightly lower in RR MS patients than controls despite a significantly lower NAA/Cr ratio in patients versus controls, suggesting that early in the course of MS, axonal injury and atrophy may proceed independently.

3DVIEWNIX/Fuzzy Connectedness

The theory and algorithms of fuzzy connectedness are based on the premise that object information, such as that regarding lesions on PD and T_2-weighted images, is inherently "fuzzy," and local image properties within an object exhibit spatial contiguity that is also fuzzy, hence "fuzzy connectedness" (Udupa and Samarasekera, 1996a). Gray matter, white matter and CSF fluid regions are segmented by treating each as a fuzzy-connected three-dimensional object. An intracranial content mask including gray matter, white matter, ventricular CSF and sulcal CSF is also created. Any residual extracranial components are excluded, if needed, by an operator. The value for total brain parenchymal volume is then calculated by subtracting the CSF fluid volume from the volume of intracranial contents. To normalize for baseline differences in brain parenchymal volume among subjects, the percentage of brain parenchymal volume (PBV) = (brain parenchymal volume) / (volume of intracranial contents) x 100%.

Fuzzy connectedness segmentation theory is based on the notion that computers outperform humans in delineating objects and humans outperform computers in recognition tasks (Miki et al., 1997; Miki et al., 1999; Samarasekera et al., 1997; Udupa et al., 1996b; Udupa et al., 1997). This method has the advantage of normalizing intensity for individual scans and subsequent increased segmentation accuracy, while disadvantages include reliance on time-consuming operator input and required familiarity with neuroanatomy and the appearance of CNS tissue pathology in MS. This method has been described in detail (Udupa and Samarasekera, 1996a; Udupa et al., 1996b) and validated in several studies (Miki et al., 1999; Phillips et al., 1998; Udupa et al., 1997; van Buchem et al., 1997) and in more than 500 data sets. The fuzzy connectedness algorithm has been used to successfully measure whole brain atrophy in both natural history and treatment trials (Ge et al., 2000; Saindane et al., 2000).

3DVIEWNIX (Medical Image Processing Group, Department of Radiology, University of Pennsylvania) is a semiautomated whole brain segmentation software program based on thin-section fast spin echo imaging with two echo times to determine the rate of volumetric change in the brain parenchyma. The "CSF-only" image is obtained by creating an "angle image" of CSF using the equation: $I_{angle} = \tan^{-1}(I_{T2}/I_{INT})$, where I_{angle}, I_{T2}, and I_{INT} are the signal intensities of the voxels on the angle, T_2- and intermediate-weighted images, respectively. This step effectively eliminates CSF signal intensity variation common on PD and T_2-weighted images due to magnetic field inhomogeneity, resulting in an angle image with a relatively homogenous signal intensity value that can be segmented by thresholding into the CSF-only image. The brain parenchyma image is then generated and volume is calculated by image subtraction after segmentation.

Alfano Method

Whole brain atrophy measurement using the fully automated Alfano segmentation method requires utilization of both quantitative relaxometry values and geometric features of MS lesions. The Alfano method provides quantitative assessment of global brain atrophy using calculated R_1 (=T1), R_2 (=T2) and proton density [N(H)] maps from conventional spin-echo studies, combined with spatial contiguity analysis. The technique was originally applied to Alzheimer's disease (Brunetti et al., 2000), where it was found that the unsupervised method improved separation of patients from normal controls. When applied to MS, the Alfano method was a sensitive and reliable measure of compartmentalized intracranial volume (Alfano et al., 2000), though the coefficient of variability for this method was addressed only in regard to the reliability of lesion load measurement. Previous assessment of the inter-study variability of the Alfano method determined a standard deviation of 1.1% in repeat tissue fractional volume measurements in normal control studies (Alfano et al., 1998). Subsequently, the method was refined for whole brain volume measurement to include normalization for intracranial volume content (Quarantelli et al., 2003).

SIENAX

SIENAX is an extension of the longitudinal atrophy measure SIENA (see section 'SIENA' below), adapted for cross-sectional measurements. Images from the segmentation of brain and non-brain tissue and estimates of the external surface of the skull are registered to a standard space brain and skull image pair, thus normalizing for head size and eliminating the need to measure CSF. MRF (MRI random field model)-based tissue type segmentation (Zhang et al., 2001) is then carried out to produce a brain volume estimate. Brain volume is measured with accuracy between 0.50 and 1.00% (Smith et al., 2002) and a test-retest reproducibility of $<1\%$. SIENAX has been used to document significant atrophy in cross-sectional studies of MS patients (Miller et al., 2002), and a correlation has been suggested between SIENAX measures of normal brain volume and other MRI measures, including diffusion (mean diffusivity, $r=-0.58$, $p=0.007$) and spectroscopic imaging (NAA/Cr, $r=0.67$, $p<0.001$) in patients with MS (De Stefano et al., 2002). SIENAX also performs brain tissue segmentation based on the Markov random field (MRF). It was used to detect neocortical gray matter atrophy in RR and PP patients (De Stefano et al., 2003). In that study, both groups showed decreased neocortical gray matter volumes compared to controls, but this decrease was not associated with white matter lesions in the PP group.

Registration-Based Methods

Current registration-based methods used to measure whole brain atrophy in MS are described below and include the brain boundary shift integral (BBSI), Medical Image Display Analysis Software (MIDAS), SIENA, statistical parametric mapping (SPM), template-driven segmentation (TDS), and voxel-based morphometry (VBM).

Brain Boundary Shift Integral

BBSI uses serial MR image co-registration to derive cerebral volume directly (Fox and Freeborough, 1997; Fox et al., 1996). Accurate positional matching is followed by digital subtraction of serial images, and brain volume changes are measured by integrating the lateral shifts of the edges of the brain and ventricles that result from cerebral atrophy. The calculated BBSI represents the total volume traversed by the brain boundaries across serial scans. This method is highly automated, sensitive and reproducible, with reduced image-analysis time, observer dependence, and effect of segmentation error. Because the method gives a measure of net volume loss over the whole brain, small positional shifts or shape changes do not affect the BBSI. The method was applied to measure the rate of cerebral atrophy in MS patients over a one-year period, where it was demonstrated that the rate of atrophy in MS was three times that of age-matched controls, and the rate of ventricular enlargement was five times greater in MS versus controls (Fox et al., 2000). However, no correlation was found between atrophy and disability. BBSI measurement variability compared well with previously described segmentation techniques at 0.16% (root mean square difference) brain volume. An automated version of BBSI, with similar measurement variability, has been developed, and utilizes a full affine registration to correct for pixel size variation by aligning the skull in serial images, then calculates the brain boundary shift using an edge-based rather than intensity-based method.

SIENA

Structural Image Evaluation, using Normalization, of Atrophy (SIENA) is a fully automated method of longitudinal (temporal) brain change analysis. SIENA segments brain from non-brain and estimates the outer skull surface to constrain scaling, using these results to register serial images while normalizing. The registered segmented brain images are used to measure atrophy on the basis of the movement of image edges using the correlation of differentiated normal vectors. Output is converted into percentage brain volume change (PBVC) with precision and sub-voxel accuracy of 0.15% brain volume change error (Smith et al., 2001; Smith et al., 2002). SIENA can be employed for a range of slice thickness, achieving better precision of PBV with thicker slices, probably because of reduced acquisition time and subsequently reduced motion artifacts. A range of MRI sequences can be used, though the external skull surface used for normalization of head size can usually be clearly seen on T_1-weighted images. This method has been used to document significant atrophy in MS patients (Miller et al., 2002), and a close correlation between brain volume and EDSS score has been found with SIENA, particularly when a categorical distribution is used (Smith et al., 2001).

SPM

SPM was developed to quantify brain volume as a fraction of intracranial volume, using a stereotactically normalized atlas to classify voxels as CSF, white matter or gray matter, according to location and signal intensity (Ashburner and Friston, 2000). SPM-based segmentation can be applied to 2D or 3D images and can be used to generate reproducible results suitable for both cross-sectional and longitudinal whole brain volume studies (Chard et al., 2002b, Sharma et al., 2004). Widely available SPM software (SPM99, SPM01; Wellcome Department of Cognitive Neurology, London, UK; (Friston et al., 1995) revealed significant white and gray matter atrophy early in the clinical course of MS (Chard et al., 2002a; Kassubek et al., 2003), accounting for age- and gender-related effects (Chard et al., 2002a). Manual editing or application of a local threshold may be required to avoid misclassification of voxels.

TDS

TDS yields brain volume estimates by projecting anatomically labeled images of a template brain from a reference atlas onto images of the patient's brain (Guttmann et al., 2000a). TDS matches a standard space template onto a patient image, rather than placing the image in stereotactic space like alternate registration algorithms; it is likely that the effect is the same. Matching of images is achieved using a combination of automated linear and nonlinear registration algorithms. Whole brain volumes can be obtained and used in serial studies to evaluate atrophy. TDS was used to measure short-term changes in the BPF from conventional dual-echo scans (Guttmann et al., 2000a), where it was found that such short-term changes were greater than the average change for a one-year period, and greater in RR than SP MS patients. This study suggests exercising caution when using atrophy as a measure of short-term disease progression.

VBM

VBM methods for the measure of brain volume involve the characterization of neuroanatomy based on local composition of brain tissue after macroscopic differences in shape have been discounted. VBM involves a voxel-wise image comparison after deformation fields have been used to spatially normalize the images. Brain volume and tissue "concentration" differences are then measured in structural MR images for the whole brain, outputting a statistical parametric map highlighting regions where gray matter concentration differs significantly between groups. VBM permits unbiased comparison of the whole brain, allowing assessment of differences throughout, and in serial studies a measurement of volumetric change over time can be obtained (Good et al., 2001). However, aspects of the algorithm, including registration to a template (warping) and smoothing, may reduce sensitivity to longitudinal changes. VBM was developed initially for the detection of gray matter changes. How well VBM deals with the white matter changes seen in MS is unknown.

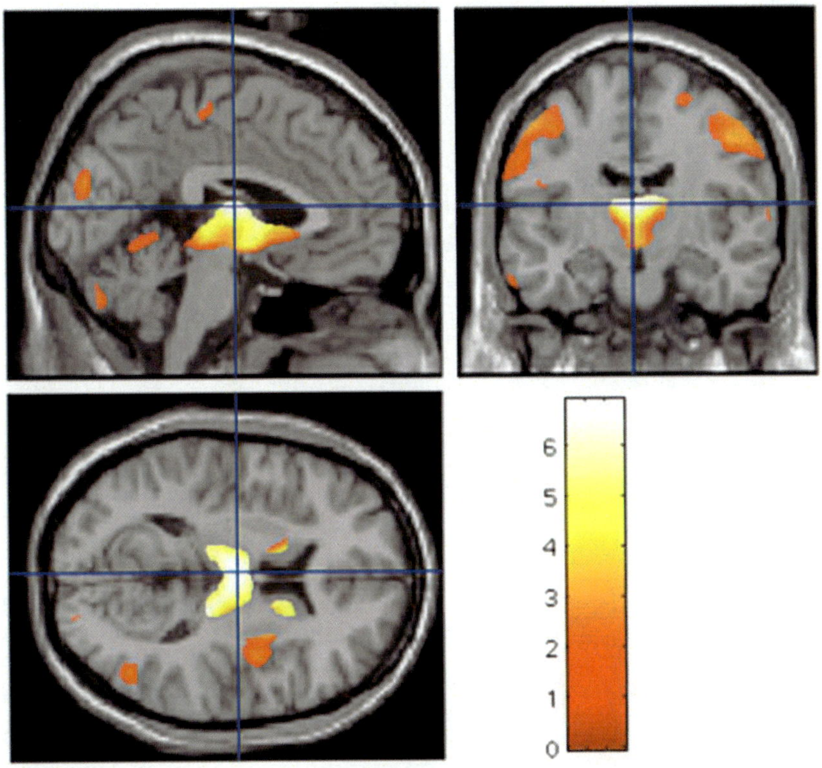

Figure 3: The color indicates the z-score (the higher the z-score the whiter the color) and is overlaid on the single-subject volume of the Montreal Neurological Institute (MNI) template provided with the Statistical Parametric Mapping (SPM) software. The most significant regions include the thalami, basal ganglia, cerebellum, and precentral gyri.

In a study of 25 RR MS patients (mean age=42.2 years, female/male=16/9, mean EDSS=2.3, mean disease duration=4.8 years) and 25 age and gender matched controls (mean age=42.1 years, female/male=16/9) (Henry, unpublished data), VBM analysis of gray matter using the optimized algorithm (Good et al., 2001) indicated significant atrophy of the bilateral thalami (Fig 3 and Table 1). The model included age and sex as confounding variables. Other regions detected (uncorrected $P< 0.001$) included basal ganglia, right cerebellum, and bilateral precentral gyri. The basal ganglia regions were right caudate, putamen, globus pallidus, and left caudate. These preliminary results agree with thalamic abnormalities observed with proton spectroscopic imaging and pathology (Cifelli et al., 2002), T1 relaxation times in SPMS (Parry et al., 2003), diffusion MRI (Fabiano et al., 2003), and T2 hypointensity (Bakshi et al., 2002). The findings of pre-central gyri involvement is also reasonable given the importance of corticospinal tract abnormalities to disability (Pantano et al., 2002; Wilson et al., 2003), and functional deficits observed in fMRI studies (Rocca et al., 2003). While technical issues relating to the effects of lesions on brain segmentation need to be addressed, these results suggest great promise for the contribution of VBM to the analysis of brain atrophy in multiple sclerosis.

Table 1. Methods used for whole brain atrophy measurement.

Method	Segmentation	Registration	Normalization	Automation	Comments
BPF	brain parenchyma, ventricular CSF	No	brain + ventricular CSF	FULL	-used on commonly acquired MR images -includes only ventricular and sulcal CSF
IBA	brain parenchyma, ventricular CSF	No	brain + ventricular and sulcal CSF	SEMI	-only measures above midbrain -high resolution images
WBR	intradural volume, CSF volume	No	Intradural volume	SEMI	-manual editing of lesions
BICCR	gray matter, white matter, lesions, CSF; Bayesan tissue classification	Yes	Intracranial volume	FULL	-limited coverage in reported cases -intensity correction
3DVIEWNIX	gray matter, white matter, lesions, CSF; fuzzy connectedness based thresholding	Yes	Intracranial volume	SEMI	-time-consuming operator input -intensity correction
SPM	gray matter, white matter, CSF; stereotactic space	Yes	intracranial volume	SEMI for MS lesions	-manual editing of misclassified voxels
TDS	template-driven, brain parenchyma, CSF	Yes	intracranial volume	FULL	-limited application in MS
Alfano	gray matter, white matter, lesions, CSF; relaxometric characterization	No	intracranial volume	FULL	-intensity correction
SIENAX/ SIENA	Brain and skull; MRF-based tissue type segmentation	Yes	head size	FULL	-no CSF segmentation needed
BBSI	No	Yes	brain size	SEMI and FULL versions	-strongly depends on accuracy of registration -no segmentation needed
VBM	gray matter, white matter, CSF	Yes	Intracranial volume (possible)	FULL	-lesion mask needed for white matter analysis -complex statistical analysis

Other Considerations

Other important considerations when measuring whole brain atrophy from MR images include choice of pulse sequence used, both biological and technical factors affecting atrophy measurements, and reliability assessment. An additional point of consideration covered here is the contribution of gray and white matter loss to whole brain atrophy in MS. Finally, future directions are discussed.

Pulse Sequences

A number of pulse sequences can be used to generate MR images for the measurement of whole brain atrophy in MS, each with its own features and image contrast. Contrast weighting selection depends on the aims of a particular study, and to a degree on the choice of analysis technique. Measurement of whole brain atrophy requires good contrast between CSF and brain parenchyma, thus atrophy is often measured using a T_1-weighted gradient echo, with or without an inversion recovery pre-pulse for added CSF suppression. Such an acquisition allows voxels with dimensions on the order of 1 x 1 x 1 mm and requires a short scan time. Several alternative MRI pulse sequences have been proposed or used to measure whole brain atrophy, including conventional T_1-weighted spin echo (Losseff et al., 1996; Paolillo et al., 2000; Zivadinov et al., 2001b), fluid-attenuated inversion recovery (FLAIR; (Bermel et al., 2003b; Horsfield et al., 2003; Leigh et al., 2002), 3D gradient echo (Fox et al., 2000; Liu et al., 2001; Pelletier et al., 2003), and a method that uses double-echo PD/T_2-weighted images in a subtraction technique that produces an image with T_1-like contrast (Atkins and Mackiewich, 1998; Horsfield et al., 2003). Using the FLAIR sequence for suppression of CSF is beneficial because it generates a sharp definition of the brain parenchyma. FLAIR sequences are now widely applied to MS patient atrophy measurements for this reason, and also for an increased conspicuity of white matter lesions using this sequence. Because the amount of intracranial CSF is an important indicator of the degree of atrophy, however, it may be useful to retain some signal from CSF.

More importantly, there seem to be statistically significant differences in calculated brain volume that depend on the pulse sequence used to acquire the MR images and the segmentation algorithm used to analyze the data, as compared using the rate of atrophy progression in RR MS patients and healthy controls over two years (Leigh et al., 2002). While whole brain atrophy can be measured using a variety of pulse sequences with marked contrast between brain parenchyma and CSF, unreliable images have occasionally been produced using a dual-echo T_2-weighted sequence on some scanners (Horsfield et al., 2003). This can be explained by the specific algorithm used in this study, for which segmentation is unreliable when fully automated analysis is attempted (Sharma et al., 2004). Resulting poor quality images should be taken as a warning to test reproducibility on several scanners in large multi-centered clinical trials. Because pulse sequence and acquisition parameters seem to have an effect on reproducibility measures, it may be useful to attempt these measures on multiple scanners, thus obtaining a better idea of overall reproducibility in a given context.

MRI sequences are produced based on a unique combination of nuclear magnetic resonance relaxation properties of tissues and proton densities along with contributions of the pulse sequence including echo time, repetition time, echo train length and resulting point-spread function for each voxel, radio frequency pulse flip angle, slice thickness, slice-to-slice cross talk and magnetization transfer effects. Because each set of images depicts the boundaries of the brain parenchyma and CSF differently, these contributing factors may affect whole brain atrophy measurement and can be manipulated by MRI technique. Three dimensional (volumetric) measures, for example, eliminate cross-talk between slices and may reduce the effects of patient repositioning on atrophy measurements. 3D acquisitions also allow more accurate re-slicing of data sets for registration of serial scans, and demonstrate high interscan within-subject reliability (Horsfield et al., 2003). Both 2D (Molyneux et al., 2000) and 3D (Liu et al., 1999) sequences have been used to successfully calculate CNS volumes, though fully automated 3D measures of whole brain atrophy are of limited availability. One- and two-dimensional acquisitions, however, require precise patient repositioning and careful landmark selection and are thus more difficult to use in longitudinal studies. Choice of slice thickness can also affect atrophy measures, as fast scans may reduce motion artifacts.

Biological Factors Affecting Atrophy Measurements

Serial short- and long-term MRI studies that account for the effects of fluid status, nutrition, and body habitus on brain volume fluctuations in MS are still lacking. More detailed information about short-term brain volume changes are presented in the Gasperini chapter (Gasperini, 2004).

Potential non-destructive biological factors contribute to brain-volume loss and influence cerebral volume measurement, including inflammation and edema (Molyneux et al., 2000), steroid therapy (Benston et al., 1978; Hoogervorst et al., 2002; Rao et al., 2002; Zivadinov et al., 2001a), nutritional status (Patel and Finch, 2002), intracranial hypertension (Neville and Wilson, 1970), alcohol (Ron et al., 1982), anorexia (Kohlmeyer et al., 1983), dehydration (Mellanby and Reveley, 1982), cerebral vascular disease and normal aging, to mention some.

The net effect of steroid treatment on fluctuations in brain volume is not completely clear. Steroid-induced protein catabolism may occur with long-term treatment and have systemic effects. Cerebral dehydration due to decreased vascular permeability has also been observed with short-term steroid treatment or rapid dose change, in studies of electrolyte balance and osmolarity (Mellanby and Reveley, 1982; Neville and Wilson, 1970). Steroids may alternatively have a positive effect on brain volume, thus limiting atrophy due to longer-term immunomodulatory and anti-inflammatory impact on disease progression (Miller et al., 2002). The long-term effect of pulse treatment with intravenous methylprednisolone (IVMP) in RR MS has been examined (Zivadinov et al., 2001a), where it has been demonstrated that IVMP limits progressive whole brain atrophy over five years. In the short-term, IVMP caused a significant reduction of brain fractional volume at month one and month two following treatment (Hoogervorst et al., 2002; Rao et al., 2002). Overall, carefully designed serial studies that account for steroid treatment effect and other contributions to brain volume loss in MS are lacking. A period of at least one month following steroid therapy is recommended before measurement of brain atrophy and up to two months if high dose IVMP (500 to 1,000 mg) is being used.

Technical Considerations in Atrophy Measurement

A number of confounding technical factors may alter image acquisition, influence the segmentation algorithm, and ultimately introduce error into the measurement of volume change in the brain. These sources of error include patient positioning in the scanner, minor and major differences in software or hardware, partial volume averaging effects, motion artifacts, dental artifacts, protocol or sequence variation, alterations in magnetic field inhomogeneity, machine-dependent image-to-image variation in MR image intensity scales, and voxel size calibration. Each of these factors can be addressed in study design to eliminate, control or account for their influence on brain volume measurement. For example, image-to-image non-uniformity due to spatially varying electromagnetic fields common to most imaging coils can be corrected using data acquired from phantoms within the head coil in question and using the sequence used for atrophy measurement. As sources of error are eliminated, other technical factors may become more relevant. Voxel size inconsistencies exist and may affect volume measurement, even using modern scanners (Freeborough et al., 1996). Voxel drift can be partially corrected by using phantoms and consistent calibration procedures throughout longitudinal studies, or by normalizing measures of atrophy. Finally, partial volume effects can be minimized with a decrease in voxel size or by accounting for this effect in volume calculations.

Measurement Variation

Reliability of MRI measures of whole brain atrophy in MS is expressed in terms of accuracy and precision. In general, measurement variation arises from both random and systematic error (Sanfilipo et al., 2004) and biological variability. Random error may reduce both accuracy and precision, while systematic error may not affect precision. While precision is easier to verify by way of reproducibility measurements, accuracy is generally difficult to assess for a given method. It is especially important for segmentation to be accurate in studies for which atrophy is a clinical outcome measure, in order to have valid interpretation of results; for example, when investigating white versus gray matter volume loss. Accuracy is also important for comparison between cohorts scanned at multiple institutions with multiple protocols and techniques. At present, such comparisons are not possible due to the lack of gold standards for estimating accuracy. Perhaps in the future, phantoms of known shape and volume, similar to the human brain, can be used to assess accuracy in such trials. Overall, small errors in accuracy are probably insignificant in most atrophy studies, especially if they are consistent between subjects and over time, and as long as they do not impact the sensitivity or precision of the method.

Random measurement errors contribute to the precision of atrophy assessment, and are expressed in terms of reproducibility. The coefficient of variation (COV) between repeated measures is commonly used to report reproducibility, and is usually calculated as: COV = (standard deviation/mean) x 100%.

COV should convey the potential of a method to detect differences at a given level, for example 1% volume loss per year. For whole brain atrophy assessment, a useful method should detect the occurrence of significant change in volume over a given time interval. Measurement variation in the detection of volume change over time includes intra-individual biological variability and time-dependent acquisition and processing variability. For example, a given method may be sensitive to subject head size, angulation of the brain, or subject head placement within the coil. Typically, studies utilize group comparisons of volume changes between controls and patients. In order to detect a significant change in a group, the impact of inter-individual biological variability on precision also needs to be addressed. Therefore, the most useful measure of COV for a given method should depend on the eventual statistical analysis model used. For quantification of whole brain atrophy, this means addressing both intra- and inter-individual variability. In most cases, the COV considers the ratio of the standard deviation of brain volume change to the mean change in brain volume for a group, using a specific method. It may be useful instead to calculate the standard deviation of an individual patient from the mean of that patient's change in brain volume for a particular method, and then assess the COV by dividing the mean of the group into a pool of these individual standard deviations, as calculated in: $COV = squareroot\ (\sum(standard\ deviation_i)^2 /_1) / (\sum(mean_i)/_i)$ X 100, where $_i$ represents the number of controls.

The use of the COV is based partly on the observation that a mean and a standard deviation tend to change together in an experiment. In order to get a good estimate of reproducibility for a given method, repeated measurements should be performed on scan-rescan data rather than reprocessing the same image data, as this simulates conditions in serial studies. For clinical trials, the optimal technique for measuring whole brain atrophy should take into account the small annual percent volume change and the effect size of a given treatment to reduce this percent volume change. Thus, the COV of a given method should be as low as possible within the respective percentage range. Outside of this range, a method that has a COV greater than the annual percent volume change common in MS can still detect a treatment effect, but will require a larger sample size. In addition, most COVs have been calculated and quoted from single center scan-rescan measurements. Ideally, reproducibility of a method should be assessed from multiple centers, accounting for image quality variability, if the measure is to be applied in a multi-center study.

Gray Matter Contribution to Whole Brain Atrophy

Consensus regarding a common pathology in RR, SP and PP MS has been elusive, due in part to the presumption that MS is predominantly a white matter disease. Because the pathology of white matter inflammatory lesions seemed to explain the characteristic RR course of early MS in most patients, focus remained on white matter to offer an explanation for the overall disease process. Yet white matter lesions do not singularly account for the neurological impairment associated with MS, thus the disease process is not limited to the involvement of lesional white matter. Even early studies of MS demonstrated an involvement of gray matter pathology (Greenfield and King, 1936), a topic also more recently revisited (Bo et al., 2003). Advances in neuroimaging have revealed more of the lesional, atrophic or diffuse changes in gray matter (Bakshi et al., 2001; Bakshi et al., 2002; Bermel et al., 2003a; Chard et al., 2002a; Cifelli et al., 2002; De Stefano et al., 2003; Ge et al., 2001; Rovaris et al., 2002; Sharma et al., 2001). Because MR can measure gray matter volumes with some precision, the segmentation algorithms discussed here contribute to a clearer understanding of the topography of atrophy in MS, demonstrating whole brain volume loss due in some part to gray matter pathology. Gray matter damage and atrophy have been shown to occur early in the course of RR MS (Chard et al., 2002a) and may be related to disability (Cifelli et al., 2002; De Stefano et al., 2003; Bakshi et al., 2002), though it remains unclear whether gray matter atrophy occurs subsequent to white matter pathology, or as a consequence of direct pathologic mechanisms. Measurement is dependent on slice thickness and image resolution, and gray matter volume data are currently limited to cross-sectional studies. Relative to the thickness of gray matter cortices and gyri, our current imaging tools offer low image resolution. Even with MR imaging, the study of gray matter would require substantial research and new development to better appreciate the involvement of gray matter in MS.

The relative contribution of white and gray matter volume loss to whole brain atrophy in RR MS has been assessed using T_2 dual-echo fast spin echo images (Ge et al., 2001). Significant decreased white matter (NAWM+lesions volumes) fraction was found compared to age-matched normal controls (-6.4%, $p<0.0001$), suggesting that white matter loss contributes more to the reduction of BPF seen in RR MS. Conversely, using the Alfano method (Quarantelli et al., 2003), a significant decrease (-3.8%, $p < 0.0001$) in fractional gray matter was found in RR MS patients compared to normal controls, suggesting that whole brain atrophy is mainly related to gray matter volume loss. More studies are needed to confirm these findings. In addition, the contribution of gray and white matter volume loss to whole brain atrophy in PP and SP MS patients also requires further investigation.

Table 2: All anatomical regions have a corrected *P* < 0.05 (uncorrected *P* < 0.0001). Stereotactic coordinates are Statistical Parametric Mapping (SPM) based on the Montreal Neurological Institute (MNI) template.

Volume (cc)	Anatomical Location of Maximum Voxel	Coordinates			Z-Score
		X	Y	Z	
R thalamus	R thalamus/Pulvinar	18	-28	10	5.34
R thalamus	R thalamus	12	-15	15	5.06
R thalamus	R thalamus/ LPN	14	-20	14	4.99
L thalamus	L thalamus/Pulvinar	-13	-24	12	4.72
L thalamus	L thalamus/Pulvinar	-16	-29	9	4.64

Future Directions

Research should focus on establishing the time course of atrophy in relation to tissue pathology in the different stages and subgroups of MS; the relationship between inflammation and atrophy, including anti-inflammatory treatment effect on intracranial volume; the pathological mechanisms underlying atrophy; the contribution of axonal loss, myelin loss and gliosis; and whether atrophy in MS results in permanent physical and cognitive disability. Other MR modalities such as MR spectroscopy (NAA and myo-inositol), myelin water measurement using T2 relaxation time, and diffusion tensor imaging can be used in conjunction with brain atrophy measures to elucidate the contribution of major brain components (axons/neurons, glial cells, myelin) to overall tissue loss. Additional MRI/histopathological correlation studies of brain tissue are greatly needed.

Conclusions

It is now possible to accurately and reproducibly measure whole brain atrophy in MS using a variety of MR image analysis methods. While the specific pathology of atrophy in MS has yet to be elucidated, global brain atrophy reflects irreversible tissue loss caused by MS, and is thus a promising surrogate marker of disease progression. Most of the methods presented here are sensitive to subtle changes in brain structures and have been successfully applied to MS as measures of whole brain atrophy. Yet comparative studies of these methods are limited and are complicated by the lack of a gold standard for image acquisition, segmentation algorithm, image analysis method, or reproducibility measure. Overall, the measure of whole brain atrophy from MR images contributes to an appreciation of the dynamics of MS pathology and its relationship to the clinical course of MS. Atrophy appears to correlate more closely with measures of disability evaluation than lesion burden, but the strength of that correlation is dependent upon the method used. Determination of the relative reproducibility, precision, sensitivity, and validity of these methods will promote the use of whole brain atrophy measures as components of comprehensive MRI-based outcome assessment in MS clinical trials. Using MRI analysis to measure whole brain atrophy in MS will aid understanding, monitoring of disease progression, and treatment, and may serve as a useful outcome measure in clinical trials.

References

Alfano B, Brunetti A, Larobina M, Quarantelli M, Tedeschi E, Ciarmiello A, et al. Automated segmentation and measurement of global white matter lesion volume in patients with multiple sclerosis. *J Magn Reson Imaging* 2000; 12: 799-807.

Alfano B, Quarantelli M, Brunetti A, Larobina M, Covelli EM, Tedeschi E, et al. Reproducibility of intracranial volume measurement by unsupervised multispectral brain segmentation. *Magn Reson Med* 1998; 39: 497-9.

Ashburner J, Friston KJ. Voxel-based morphometry--the methods. *Neuroimage* 2000; 11: 805-21.

Atkins MS, Mackiewich BT. Fully automatic segmentation of the brain in MRI. *IEEE Trans Med Imaging* 1998; 17: 98-107.

Bakshi R, Ariyaratana S, Benedict RH, Jacobs L. Fluid-attenuated inversion recovery magnetic resonance imaging detects cortical and juxtacortical multiple sclerosis lesions. *Arch Neurol* 2001; 58: 742-8.

Bakshi R, Benedict RH, Bermel RA, Caruthers SD, Puli SR, Tjoa CW, et al. T2 hypointensity in the deep gray matter of patients with multiple sclerosis: a quantitative magnetic resonance imaging study. *Arch Neurol* 2002; 59: 62-8.

Benedict RHB, Weinstock-Guttman B, Fishman I, Sharma J, Tjoa CW, Bakshi R. Prediction of neuropsychological impairment in multiple sclerosis: comparison of conventional magnetic resonance imaging measures of atrophy and lesion burden. *Arch Neurol* 2004;61:226-230

Benston J, Reza M, Winter J, Wilson G. Steroids and apparent cerebral atrophy on computed tomography scans. *JCAT* 1978; 2: 16-23.

Bermel RA, Sharma J, Tjoa CW, Puli SR, Bakshi R. A semiautomated measure of whole-brain atrophy in multiple sclerosis. *J Neurol Sci* 2003a; 208: 57-65

Bermel RA, Innus MD, Tjoa CW, Bakshi R. Selective caudate atrophy in multiple sclerosis: a 3D MRI parcellation study. *Neuroreport* 2003b; 14: 335-9.

.Bo L, Vedeler CA, Nyland HI, Trapp BD, Mork SJ. Subpial demyelination in the cerebral cortex of multiple sclerosis patients. *J Neuropathol Exp Neurol* 2003; 62: 723-32.

Brunetti A, Postiglione A, Tedeschi E, Ciarmiello A, Quarantelli M, Covelli EM, et al. Measurement of global brain atrophy in Alzheimer's disease with unsupervised segmentation of spin-echo MRI studies. *J Magn Reson Imaging* 2000; 11: 260-6.

Chard DT, Griffin CM, Parker GJ, Kapoor R, Thompson AJ, Miller DH. Brain atrophy in clinically early relapsing-remitting multiple sclerosis. *Brain* 2002a; 125: 327-37.

Chard DT, Parker GJ, Griffin CM, Thompson AJ, Miller DH. The reproducibility and sensitivity of brain tissue volume measurements derived from an SPM-based segmentation methodology. *J Magn Reson Im*aging 2002b; 15: 259-67.

Cifelli A, Arridge M, Jezzard P, Esiri MM, Palace J, Matthews PM. Thalamic neurodegeneration in multiple sclerosis. *Ann Neurol* 2002; 52: 650-3.

Collins DL, Montagnat J, Zijdenbos AP, Evans AC, Arnold DL. Automated estimation of brain volume in multiple sclerosis with BICCR. *Lect Notes Comput Sci* 2001: 141-147.

De Stefano N, Iannucci G, Sormani MP, Guidi L, Bartolozzi ML, Comi G, et al. MR correlates of cerebral atrophy in patients with multiple sclerosis. *J Neurol* 2002; 249: 1072-7.

De Stefano N, Matthews PM, Filippi M, Agosta F, De Luca M, Bartolozzi ML, et al. Evidence of early cortical atrophy in MS: relevance to white matter changes and disability. *Neurology* 2003; 60: 1157-62.

Fabiano AJ, Sharma J, Weinstock-Guttman B, Munschauer FE, 3rd, Benedict RH, Zivadinov R, et al. Thalamic involvement in multiple sclerosis: a diffusion-weighted magnetic resonance imaging study. *J Neuroimaging* 2003; 13: 307-14.

Filippi M, Mastronardo G, Rocca MA, Pereira C, Comi G. Quantitative volumetric analysis of brain magnetic resonance imaging from patients with multiple sclerosis. *J Neurol Sci* 1998; 158: 148-53.

Fisher E, Rudick RA, Cutter G, Baier M, Miller D, Weinstock-Guttman B, et al. Relationship between brain atrophy and disability: an 8-year follow-up study of multiple sclerosis patients. *Mult Scler* 2000; 6: 373-7.

Fisher E, Rudick RA, Simon JH, Cutter G, Baier M, Lee JC, et al. Eight-year follow-up study of brain atrophy in patients with MS. *Neurology* 2002; 59: 1412-20.

Fox NC, Freeborough PA. Brain atrophy progression measured from registered serial MRI: validation and application to Alzheimer's disease. *J Magn Reson Imaging* 1997; 7: 1069-75.

Fox NC, Freeborough PA, Rossor MN. Visualisation and quantification of rates of atrophy in Alzheimer's disease. *Lancet* 1996; 348: 94-7.

Fox NC, Jenkins R, Leary SM, Stevenson VL, Losseff NA, Crum WR, et al. Progressive cerebral atrophy in MS: a serial study using registered, volumetric MRI. *Neurology* 2000; 54: 807-12.

Freeborough PA, Fox NC. The boundary shift integral: an accurate and robust measure of cerebral volume changes from registered repeat MRI. *IEEE Trans Med Imaging* 1997; 16: 623-9.

Freeborough PA, Fox NC. Modeling brain deformations in Alzheimer disease by fluid registration of serial 3D MR images. *J Comput Assist Tomogr* 1998; 22: 838-43.

Freeborough PA, Woods RP, Fox NC. Accurate registration of serial 3D MR brain images and its application to visualizing change in neurodegenerative disorders. *J Comput Assist Tomogr* 1996; 20: 1012-22.

Friston KJ, Ashburner J, Poline JB, Frith CD, Heather JD, Frackowiak RSJ. Spatial registration and normalisation of images. *Hum Brain Mapp* 1995; 2: 165-189.

Gasperini C. In: Zivadinov R, Bakshi R, eds. *Brain and Spinal Cord Atrophy in Multiple Sclerosis. Whole Brain Atrophy Measurement and Short-term Brain Volume Changes.* New York: Nova Science Publisher 2004; (p29-38).

Ge Y, Grossman RI, Udupa JK, Babb JS, Nyul LG, Kolson DL. Brain atrophy in relapsing-remitting multiple sclerosis: fractional volumetric analysis of gray matter and white matter. *Radiology* 2001; 220: 606-10.

Ge Y, Grossman RI, Udupa JK, Wei L, Mannon LJ, Polansky M, et al. Brain atrophy in relapsing-remitting multiple sclerosis and secondary progressive multiple sclerosis: longitudinal quantitative analysis. *Radiology* 2000; 214: 665-70.

Good CD, Johnsrude I, Ashburner J, Henson RN, Friston KJ, Frackowiak RS. Cerebral asymmetry and the effects of sex and handedness on brain structure: a voxel-based morphometric analysis of 465 normal adult human brains. *Neuroimage* 2001; 14: 685-700.

Guttmann CR, Benson R, Warfield SK, Wei X, Anderson MC, Hall CB, et al. White matter abnormalities in mobility-impaired older persons. *Neurology* 2000a; 54: 1277-83.

Guttmann CR, Warfield SK, Guimond A, Kikinis R, Albert MS, Jolesz FA. Variability of brain atrophy estimates in multiple sclerosis (abstract). *Proc Int Soc Magn Reson Med* 2000b; 8: 1188.

Hajnal JV, Saeed N, Oatridge A, Williams EJ, Young IR, Bydder GM. Detection of subtle brain changes using subvoxel registration and subtraction of serial MR images. *J Comput Assist Tomogr* 1995; 19: 677-91.

Hoogervorst EL, Polman CH, Barkhof F. Cerebral volume changes in multiple sclerosis patients treated with high-dose intravenous methylprednisolone. *Mult Scler* 2002; 8: 415-9.

Horsfield MA, Rovaris M, Rocca MA, Rossi P, Benedict RH, Filippi M, et al. Whole-brain atrophy in multiple sclerosis measured by two segmentation processes from various MRI sequences. *J Neurol Sci* 2003; 216: 169-77.

Inglese M, Rovaris M, Giacomotti L, Mastronardo G, Comi G, Filippi M. Quantitative brain volumetric analysis from patients with multiple sclerosis: a follow-up study. *J Neurol Sci* 1999; 171: 8-10.

Jones CK, Riddehough A, Li DKB, Zhao G, Paty DW, Group PSGUMMR. MRI cerebral atrophy in relapsing-remitting MS: results from the PRISMS trial (abstract). *Neurology* 2001; 56: A379.

Kassubek J, Tumani H, Ecker D, Kurt A, Ludolph AC, Juengling FD. Age-related brain parenchymal fraction is significantly decreased in young multiple sclerosis patients: a quantitative MRI study. *Neuroreport* 2003; 14: 427-30.

Kohlmeyer K, Lehmkuhl G, Poutska F. Computed tomography of anorexia nervosa. *AJNR Am J Neuroradiol* 1983; 4: 437-8.

Leigh R, Ostuni J, Pham D, Goldszal A, Lewis BK, Howard T, et al. Estimating cerebral atrophy in multiple sclerosis patients from various MR pulse sequences. *Mult Scler* 2002; 8: 420-9.

Liu C, Edwards S, Gong Q, Roberts N, Blumhardt LD. Three dimensional MRI estimates of brain and spinal cord atrophy in multiple sclerosis. *J Neurol Neurosurg Psychiatry* 1999; 66: 323-30.

Liu XF, Fawcett JR, Thorne RG, DeFor TA, Frey WH, 2nd. Intranasal administration of insulin-like growth factor-I bypasses the blood-brain barrier and protects against focal cerebral ischemic damage. *J Neurol Sci* 2001; 187: 91-7.

Losseff NA, Wang L, Lai HM, Yoo DS, Gawne-Cain ML, McDonald WI, et al. Progressive cerebral atrophy in multiple sclerosis. A serial MRI study. *Brain* 1996; 119: 2009-19.

Mellanby AR, Reveley MA. Effects of acute dehydration on computerized tomographic assessment of cerebral density and ventricular volume. *Lancet* 1982; 2: 874.

Miki Y, Grossman RI, Udupa JK, Samarasekera S, van Buchem MA, Cooney BS, et al. Computer-assisted quantitation of enhancing lesions in multiple sclerosis: correlation with clinical classification. *AJNR Am J Neuroradiol* 1997; 18: 705-10.

Miki Y, Grossman RI, Udupa JK, Wei L, Polansky M, Mannon LJ, et al. Relapsing-remitting multiple sclerosis: longitudinal analysis of MR images--lack of correlation between changes in T2 lesion volume and clinical findings. *Radiology* 1999; 213: 395-9.

Miller DH, Barkhof F, Frank JA, Parker GJ, Thompson AJ. Measurement of atrophy in multiple sclerosis: pathological basis, methodological aspects and clinical relevance. *Brain* 2002; 125: 1676-95.

Molyneux PD, Kappos L, Polman C, Pozzilli C, Barkhof F, Filippi M, et al. The effect of interferon beta-1b treatment on MRI measures of cerebral atrophy in secondary progressive multiple sclerosis. European Study Group on Interferon beta-1b in secondary progressive multiple sclerosis. *Brain* 2000; 123: 2256-63.

Neville BG, Wilson J. Benign intracranial hypertension following corticosteroid withdrawal in childhood. *Br Med J* 1970; 3: 554-6.

Pantano P, Mainero C, Iannetti GD, Caramia F, Di Legge S, Piattella MC, et al. Contribution of corticospinal tract damage to cortical motor reorganization after a single clinical attack of multiple sclerosis. *Neuroimage* 2002; 17: 1837-43.

Paolillo A, Pozzilli C, Gasperini C, Giugni E, Mainero C, Giuliani S, et al. Brain atrophy in relapsing-remitting multiple sclerosis: relationship with 'black holes', disease duration and clinical disability. *J Neurol Sci* 2000; 174: 85-91.

Parry A, Clare S, Jenkinson M, Smith S, Palace J, Matthews PM. MRI brain T1 relaxation time changes in MS patients increase over time in both the white matter and the cortex. *J Neuroimaging* 2003; 13: 234-9.

Patel NV, Finch CE. The glucocorticoid paradox of caloric restriction in slowing brain aging. *Neurobiol Aging* 2002; 23: 707-17.

Pelletier D, Nelson SJ, Oh J, Antel JP, Kita M, Zamvil SS, et al. MRI lesion volume heterogeneity in primary progressive MS in relation with axonal damage and brain atrophy. *J Neurol Neurosurg Psychiatry* 2003; 74: 950-2.

Phillips MD, Grossman RI, Miki Y, Wei L, Kolson DL, van Buchem MA, et al. Comparison of T2 lesion volume and magnetization transfer ratio histogram analysis and of atrophy and measures of lesion burden in patients with multiple sclerosis. *AJNR Am J Neuroradiol* 1998; 19: 1055-60.

Quarantelli M, Ciarmiello A, Morra VB, Orefice G, Larobina M, Lanzillo R, et al. Brain tissue volume changes in relapsing-remitting multiple sclerosis: correlation with lesion load. *Neuroimage* 2003; 18: 360-6.

Rao AB, Richert N, Howard T, Lewis BK, Bash CN, McFarland HF, et al. Methylprednisolone effect on brain volume and enhancing lesions in MS before and during IFNbeta-1b. *Neurology* 2002; 59: 688-94.

Rocca MA, Gavazzi C, Mezzapesa DM, Falini A, Colombo B, Mascalchi M, et al. A functional magnetic resonance imaging study of patients with secondary progressive multiple sclerosis. *Neuroimage* 2003; 19: 1770-7.

Ron MA, Acker W, Shaw GK, Lishman WA. Computerized tomography of the brain in chronic alcoholism: a Survey and follow-up study. *Brain* 1982; 105: 497-514.

Rovaris M, Bozzali M, Iannucci G, Ghezzi A, Caputo D, Montanari E, et al. Assessment of normal-appearing white and gray matter in patients with primary progressive multiple sclerosis: a diffusion-tensor magnetic resonance imaging study. *Arch Neurol* 2002; 59: 1406-12.

Rudick RA, Fisher E, Lee JC, Simon J, Jacobs L. Use of the brain parenchymal fraction to measure whole brain atrophy in relapsing-remitting MS. Multiple Sclerosis Collaborative Research Group. *Neurology* 1999; 53: 1698-704.

Saindane AM, Ge Y, Udupa JK, Babb JS, Mannon LJ, Grossman RI. The effect of gadolinium-enhancing lesions on whole brain atrophy in relapsing-remitting MS. *Neurology* 2000; 55: 61-5.

Samarasekera S, Udupa JK, Miki Y, Wei L, Grossman RI. A new computer-assisted method for the quantification of enhancing lesions in multiple sclerosis. *J Comput Assist Tomogr* 1997; 21: 145-51.

Sanfilipo MP, Benedict RHB, Zivadinov R, Bakshi R. Correction for intracranial volume in analysis of whole brain volume in multiple sclerosis: the proportion vs. residual method. *Neuroimage* 2004;22: 1732-1743.

Sharma J, Sanfilipo MP, Benedict RHB, Weinstock-Guttman B, Munschauer FE, Bakshi R. Whole brain atrophy in multiple sclerosis measured by automated versus. semiautomated MR imaging segmentation. *AJNR: American Journal of Neuroradiology 2004; 25: 985-996.*

Sharma R, Narayana PA, Wolinsky JS. Gray matter abnormalities in multiple sclerosis: proton magnetic resonance spectroscopic imaging. *Mult Scler* 2001; 7: 221-6.

Smith SM, De Stefano N, Jenkinson M, Matthews PM. Normalized accurate measurement of longitudinal brain change. *J Comput Assist Tomogr* 2001; 25: 466-75.

Smith SM, Zhang Y, Jenkinson M, Chen J, Matthews PM, Federico A, et al. Accurate, robust, and automated longitudinal and cross-sectional brain change analysis. *Neuroimage* 2002; 17: 479-89.

Udupa JK, Samarasekera S. Fuzzy connectedness and object definition: theory, algorithms and applications in image segmentation. *Graphical Models and Image processing* 1996a; 58: 246-261.

Udupa JK, Wei L, Samarasekera S, Miki Y, van Buchem MA, Grossman RI. Detection and quantification of MS lesions using fuzzy topolofical principles. *Proc SPIE* 1996b; 2710: 81-91.

Udupa JK, Wei L, Samarasekera S, Miki Y, van Buchem MA, Grossman RI. Multiple sclerosis lesion quantification using fuzzy-connectedness principles. *IEEE Trans Med Imaging* 1997; 16: 598-609.

van Buchem MA, Udupa JK, McGowan JC, Miki Y, Heyning FH, Boncoeur-Martel MP, et al. Global volumetric estimation of disease burden in multiple sclerosis based on magnetization transfer imaging. *AJNR Am J Neuroradiol* 1997; 18: 1287-90.

Whitwell JL, Crum WR, Watt HC, Fox NC. Normalization of cerebral volumes by use of intracranial volume: implications for longitudinal quantitative MR imaging. *AJNR Am J Neuroradiol* 2001; 22: 1483-9.

Wilson M, Tench CR, Morgan PS, Blumhardt LD. Pyramidal tract mapping by diffusion tensor magnetic resonance imaging in multiple sclerosis: improving correlations with disability. *J Neurol Neurosurg Psychiatry* 2003; 74: 203-7.

Zhang Y, Brady M, Smith S. Segmentation of brain MR images through a hidden Markov random field model and the expectation-maximization algorithm. *IEEE Trans Med Imaging* 2001; 20: 45-57.

Zivadinov R, Bakshi R. Role of MRI in multiple sclerosis II: brain and spinal cord atrophy. *Front Biosci* 2004; 9: 647-64.

Zivadinov R, Bakshi R. In: Zivadinov R, Bakshi R, eds. *Brain and Spinal Cord Atrophy in Multiple Sclerosis. Neurological disability and central nervous system atrophy in multiple sclerosis.* New York: Nova Science Publisher 2004;(p113-137).

Zivadinov R, Locatelli L, Stival B, Bratina A, Grop A, Nasuelli D, et al. Normalized regional brain atrophy measurements in multiple sclerosis. *Neuroradiology* 2003; 45: 793-8.

Zivadinov R, Grop A, Sharma J, Bratina A, Tjoa CV, Dwyer M, Zorzon M. Reproducibility and accuracy of quantitative MRI techniques to measure whole brain atrophy in relapsing-remitting multiple sclerosis. *J Neuroimaging* (in press).

Zivadinov R, Rudick RA, De Masi R, Nasuelli D, Ukmar M, Pozzi-Mucelli RS, et al. Effects of IV methylprednisolone on brain atrophy in relapsing-remitting MS. *Neurology* 2001a; 57: 1239-47.

Zivadinov R, Sepcic J, Nasuelli D, De Masi R, Bragadin LM, Tommasi MA, et al. A longitudinal study of brain atrophy and cognitive disturbances in the early phase of relapsing-remitting multiple sclerosis. *J Neurol Neurosurg Psychiatry* 2001b; 70: 773-80.

In: Brain and Spinal Cord Atrophy in Multiple Sclerosis
Editors: R. Zivadinov and R. Bakshi, pp. 63-71
ISBN 1-59454-160-4

Chapter VI

Technical Aspects of Spinal Cord Atrophy Measurement

Christopher R. Tench and Cris S. Constantinescu*
Division of Clinical Neurology, University of Nottingham, United Kingdom

Introduction

It is estimated that magnetic resonance imaging (MRI) detectable spinal cord pathology occurs in up to 90% of patients with multiple sclerosis (MS). Conventional T2 weighted spinal cord MRI is sensitive in detecting focal lesions and their changes over time (Rocca et al., 1999). This can be important in a diagnostic setting, for example, where brain MRI appears normal (Thorpe et al., 1996) (about 5% of clinically definite MS patients). However, measures of T2 lesion load in the cord do not correlate with clinical scores of disability (Kidd et al., 1993), limiting the role of the spinal cord lesion measure in monitoring progression of the disease. This may result from the lack of histopathological specificity of conventional MRI (Matthews and Arnold, 2001), as well as its inability to detect changes in normal appearing white matter (NAWM) and gray matter.

Atrophy of the spinal cord may reflect overall pathological change. Axonal loss in both lesions (Barnes et al., 1991) and NAWM (Evangelou et al., 2000; Ganter et al., 1999) is thought to contribute significantly to white matter (WM) atrophy, and has been observed in pathological studies of the spinal cord in MS (Ganter et al., 1999; Lovas et al., 2000). Axonal loss is also thought to be an important contributing factor to neurologic disability in MS. Indeed, MRI measures of cervical spinal cord cross-sectional area (CSA) or volume, which represent relative atrophy in group comparison studies or rates of atrophy in longitudinal studies, have correlated with disability (Losseff et al., 1996; Vaithianathar et al., 2003), or changes in disability (Lin et al., 2003b), assessed using the Expanded Disability Status Scale

* Corresponding Author: Constantinescu S. Cris, Division of Clinical Neurology, University of Nottingham, Derby Road, Nottingham, United Kingdom. Phone number: +44 115 875 4598; e-mail: cris.constantinescu@nottingham.ac.uk

(EDSS) (Kurtzke, 1983). The fact that pathology in such a small part of the central nervous system (CNS) reflects disability emphasizes the significance of this site in MS.

The importance of the spinal cord in MS, combined with improvements in spinal cord MRI, has led to an increased interest in cord atrophy measurement (Hickman et al., 2003; Lin et al., 2003b; Losseff et al., 1996). This is particularly true of the cervical spinal cord, where 60% of spinal cord pathology is reported to occur (Kidd et al., 1993). Emphasis has been placed on the acquisition of high-resolution images, and on devising highly reproducible methods of measuring the CSA or the volume of a section of cord. The techniques available to measure the cord CSA or volume are the main topic of this chapter. Limitations of the current methods are also described.

Image Analysis Methods Review

Despite the common occurrence of demyelinating lesions in the spinal cord (Oppenheimer, 1978), imaging of the cord is not part of routine assessment as frequently as is imaging of the brain, largely because of technical difficulties (Lycklama et al., 2003). Recent developments in fast imaging and receiver coil design, and the use of cardiac gating, have partially eliminated these issues (Lycklama et al., 2003).

A further hindrance to the accurate and precise measurement of spinal cord area or volume by MRI has been the lack of suitable image analysis techniques. High scan rescan variability has meant that only cross-sectional studies were feasible previously. However, group comparisons in such studies suffered from the variability inherent in the normal population as well as gender differences. Normalization to the total intracranial volume (Liu et al., 1999; Zivadinov et al., 2003) and the largest skull cross sectional area (Vaithianathar et al., 2003) has been used to reduce these errors. Longitudinal studies require much greater sensitivity to detect the small changes seen over periods short on the scale of typical disease duration. With improvements in spinal cord MRI and an increased appreciation of the cord's significance in MS, new and highly reproducible techniques are being developed to measure cord atrophy.

The CSA of a normal adult spinal cord is approximately 90mm^2. Current high resolution MRI achieves voxel dimensions of 1mm, or 10% of the typical cord width. Thus, accurate measurement of the spinal cord CSA or volume is challenging. Furthermore, the low rate of spinal cord atrophy in MS (CSA reduction approximately 2% per year) places demands on the precision of the measurement procedure. To date, MRI-based studies of cord atrophy have demonstrated a considerable variability in reliability of the results and several factors have been found to affect sensitivity: anatomical region measured (Losseff et al., 1996), image analysis procedures, and scanner drift (Leary et al., 1999; Stevenson et al., 1998).

The Cavalieri method of modern design stereology provides an unbiased estimate for the volume of a three-dimensional structure (Roberts et al., 2000) by counting randomly placed points on two-dimensional sections through the structure. The algorithm is implemented in commercially available software (such as ANALYZE, Biomedical Imaging Resource, Mayo Foundation, MN, USA) and has been used to estimate both brain and spinal cord atrophy in MS (Liu et al., 1999). This method produces accurate estimates of volume and a theoretical measurement error, enabling testing for statistical differences between groups. However, the precision required for longitudinal studies means an increase in workload beyond that of other automated or semi-automated methods. Nevertheless, the technique has been used to demonstrate a reduced cervical cord volume in MS patients, compared to age and sex matched controls (Liu et al., 1999).

The simplicity of the cord shape means that the process of monitoring atrophy may be conveniently reduced to performing two-dimensional CSA measurements. This also eliminates variability due to distance between landmarks, which is subject dependent. MRI-based estimates of spinal cord area were initially produced by manual outlining on axially acquired gradient echo images (Kidd et al., 1993). A study of 80 patients [20 relapsing remitting (RR), 20 secondary progressive (SP), 20 primary progressive (PP) and 20 benign] detected significant reduction in cord area at vertebral levels C5, T2, T7 and T11 (Kidd et al., 1993); significant reduction was defined as an area more than two standard deviations below the mean area in normal control subjects. A subsequent two-year longitudinal study of 60 MS patients established a scan-rescan coefficient of variation (COV) of 6%, rendering the method unsuitable for serial monitoring (Losseff and Miller, 1998). Apart from the variance due to manual outlining, inability to precisely locate anatomic landmarks at these vertebral levels contributed to the limited precision.

The reproducibility issues of manual outlining have been addressed utilizing a semi-automated intensity-based contouring algorithm (Losseff et al., 1996). The method is applied to a short length of cord (approximately 15mm long) with the most caudal slice located at the C2/3 intervertebral disc. In this section of the spine, landmarks have minimal anatomic variability and can be reliably identified on the images. Also at this level, cerebrospinal fluid (CSF) space around the cord is particularly large, which enhances the image contrast and improves the reliability of the algorithm. To further improve experimental reproducibility, patients are positioned carefully so that the cord is straight and fully surrounded by CSF. On an axial image, a manually defined region of interest (ROI) locates the cord and provides an estimate of mean cord intensity, while a second ROI delineating the CSF and cord provides an estimate of mean CSF intensity. Voxels affected by partial volume averaging at the cord-CSF interface have intensity midway between the mean cord and CSF intensities on average, and are detected automatically on all slices by the computer, given a single-user-provided seed point placed at the interface. A rapid, high resolution, volume acquisition gradient echo sequence is used, along with post-processing inhomogeneity correction to ensure uniform intensity of both cord and CSF. The scan-rescan COV for an experienced user is 0.79%, making it suitable for longitudinal studies, although a parallel phantom study established that accuracy is limited by a systematic overestimation of the area by 4.5%-10% due to inclusion of edge voxels affected by partial volume averaging. The method has been employed in a serial study and was able to detect significant reduction in cord area over one year (Stevenson et al., 1998); however, no correlation between change in area and change in disability was observed. The sensitivity of intensity based contouring is such that a significant apparent change in the cord area of normal controls has been observed following a scanner hardware upgrade (Stevenson et al., 1998). This has highlighted the need for quality assurance in longitudinal studies, using sequential scanning of a standard phantom (Leary et al., 1999).

Recently an automated procedure for measuring the volume and the CSA of the spinal cord has been developed (Coulon et al., 2002) and applied to the study of atrophy in MS (Hickman et al., 2003). Active B-spline surface fitting is used to delineate the cord. Rather than identifying the cord edge by absolute intensity, the gradient of intensity is used. The algorithm optimizes the B-spline surface fit to the cord such that intensity gradient is maximized globally while maintaining a smooth tube-like shape to the detected cord edge. Imposing this shape constraint might make the algorithm more robust against acquisition noise. Using this technique, it is possible to automatically correct for alignment of the cord cross-section relative to the acquisition plane, and for curvature of the cord, which is assumed to be negligible in other methods. In a direct comparison with intensity based contouring (Losseff et al., 1996), the method provided less repeatable results, possibly due to difficulty in consistently defining the anatomical landmarks required by the algorithm. Furthermore, cross-sectional areas were approximately 33% smaller than those measured by contouring, since the procedure tended to ignore voxels affected by partial volume averaging.

An automated procedure that uses edge detection to measure the cord CSA has also been developed (Vaithianathar et al., 2003). In common with the intensity based contouring algorithm, voxels affected by partial volume averaging at the cord-CSF boundary are identified and used to define the cord cross-section. A Sobel filter (Sonka et al., 1993) first operates on an axial image that includes the section of cord (Fig 1A) to produce an image of intensity gradient magnitude (Fig 1B). Non-maximal suppression (Sonka et al., 1993) is then employed to automatically and precisely locate all edges from the Sobel image. Removing these edges from the original axial image isolates different structures, including the cord, from their surroundings (Fig 1C). On each slice the edge defined only by the cord is identified by the user (Fig 1D), and the CSA is computed. This method requires no inhomogeneity correction since the cord edge is defined by intensity change rather than intensity. Furthermore, the method is not sensitive to lesional pathology, which appears hyper- or hypointense on MRI and might reduce the sensitivity of intensity based contouring. The procedure has been used in a 48 month serial study of 38 MS patients (20RR, 18SP) recruited to the interferon β-1a (Rebif) trial (Lin et al., 2003b). A volume-acquired, magnetization-prepared, rapid acquisition gradient echo (MPRAGE) image of the brain that included the cervical spinal cord was used in the study. Significant reduction in cord area was detected over 12 months, and a consistent correlation between EDSS change and cord area change was observed at months 12, 18 and 48. For purposes of the study, repeat scanning of control subjects over a median period of 23 months was performed to guard against any systematic change in cord area due to scanner drift.

Limitations of Current Methods

Many of the limitations of using MRI to monitor spinal cord atrophy in MS have now been addressed. Rapid imaging techniques allow high-resolution acquisitions, with good signal to noise ratio (SNR) and contrast. Motion artifact is reduced by short scan times, and cardiac gating can minimize ghosting artifact from the heart (Lycklama et al., 2003). Furthermore, advances in image analysis methods have led to automatic or semi-automatic algorithms to detect the cord edge, requiring minimal subjective user input (Losseff et al., 1996; Vaithianathar et al., 2003). The identification of clear landmarks in the cervical cord—at a level where the cord is straight, of uniform area, and surrounded by CSF—has helped to make these methods highly reproducible. However, there remain serious theoretical limitations to the analysis methods currently available.

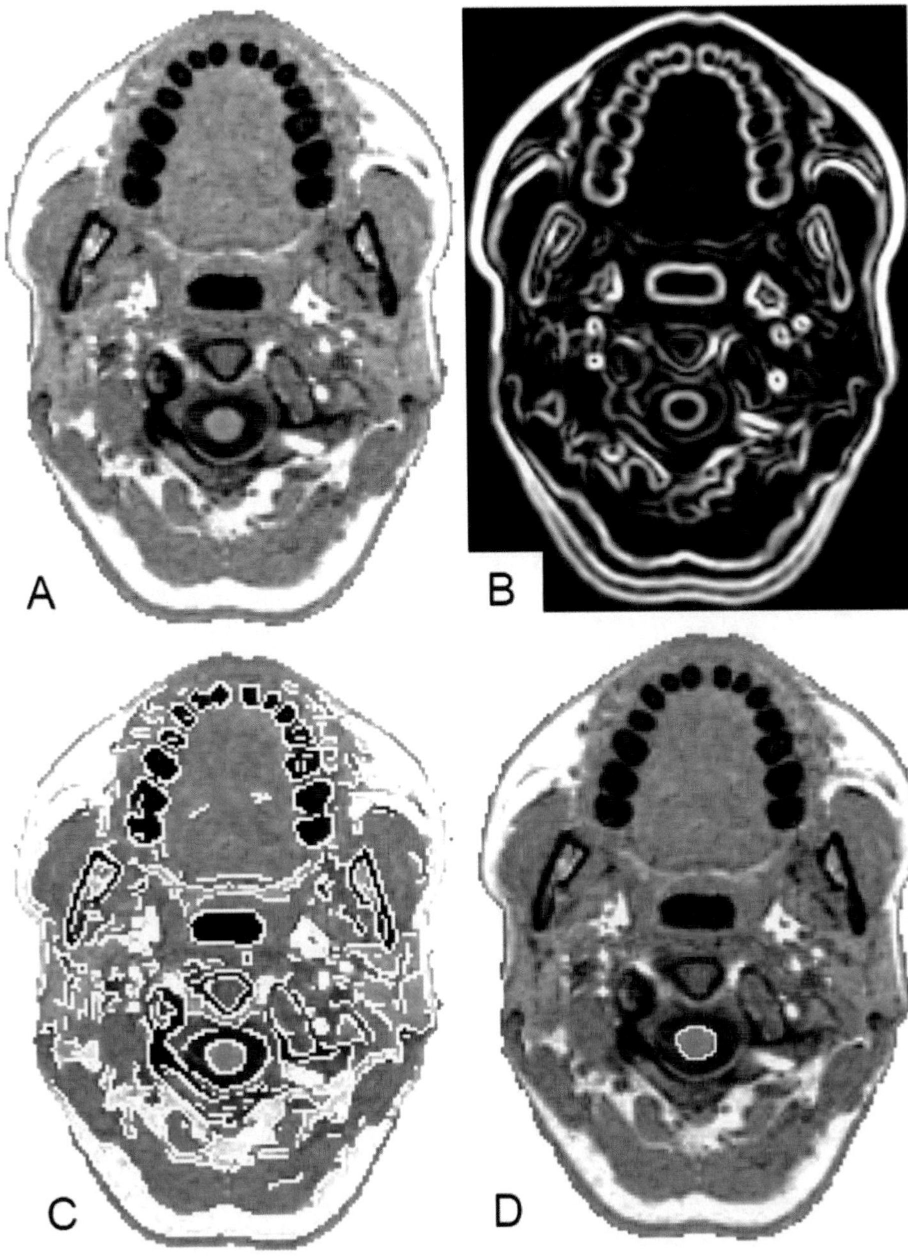

Fig 1. A) A single axial slice including a section of the cervical spinal cord. B) The same axial slice after using the Sobel filter. C) All edges detected using non-maximal suppression are removed from the original axial image to separate the different structures, including the cord, from their surroundings. D) The edge at the cord-CSF interface is manually identified and forms a region of interest encompassing only the cord.

Since typical cord diameter is only around ten times the voxel width in high resolution MRI, a substantial portion of the cord area lies at the edge, where it is susceptible to partial volume averaging with the surrounding CSF. This has been shown to result in significant over- or underestimation of CSA, depending on whether edge voxels are included (Losseff et al., 1996) or excluded (Hickman et al., 2003) from the computed area. The accuracy of the measurements is therefore limited. More serious is the theoretical limitation of the methods to detect small longitudinal changes in CSA, since even a single voxel represents more than 1% of the area. This might reduce the sensitivity of CSA measurement. Higher resolution MRI would directly improve our ability to accurately measure the CSA, providing SNR and contrast can be maintained.

Discussion

The spinal cord and, in particular, the cervical spinal cord, is a common site of involvement in MS and is thought to be of particular importance in the development of disability (Oppenheimer, 1978). Recent improvements in MRI have made routine acquisition of cord images practical (Lycklama et al., 2003). Furthermore, high resolution MRI and the introduction of automated image analysis procedures have made possible the accurate measurement of spinal cord CSA (Losseff et al., 1996; Vaithianathar et al., 2003). While conventional T2 lesion load measures in the cord lack specificity, the cord CSA may indirectly measure axonal loss. This is indicated by correlations between cord CSA and quantitative MRI parameters such as T1 relaxation time (Vaithianathar et al., 2003), which are thought to have greater specificity for axonal loss than T2 lesion assessments. More directly, the cervical cord CSA has shown significant correlation with physical disability measured by EDSS. The fact that pathology in such a small fraction of the CNS reflects disability emphasizes the importance of this site in MS.

Evidence that spinal cord atrophy contributes to disability in MS has come from several studies. Patients with cord atrophy detectible by manual outlining at one or more of four vertebral levels (C5, T2, T7 and T11) have been found to have more advanced disability reflected in higher EDSS scores (Kidd et al., 1993). Significant correlations between cord CSA and disability have also been observed using the more sensitive automated or semi-automated measurement techniques. Even in a small cohort of RR and SP patients, the use of automatic edge detection has revealed significant correlation between cord CSA and the EDSS (Vaithianathar et al., 2003). A similar correlation with the EDSS was observed using semi-automated, intensity-based contouring at the C2/C3 level in a study of 60 patients (15 in each subgroup: RR, benign, SP, PP) (Losseff et al., 1996). While the findings of these cross-sectional studies are of major importance, the inherent variability of the cord between genders and within the normal population means that between-subject differences can limit their power. This may partly explain the apparent normal cord CSA in RR MS patients, a finding common to several studies (Lin et al., 2003a; Lin et al., 2003b; Losseff et al., 1996; Stevenson et al., 1998), despite the high rate of cord atrophy in this subgroup (Stevenson et al., 1998).

Longitudinal studies measure within-subject differences and can overcome the limitations of group comparisons, although for such studies the possibility of systematic change due to scanner changes should ideally be monitored by scanning a known standard phantom (Leary et al., 1999). Using manual outlining on a single axial slice located at the mid C5 vertebral level, significant reduction in cord CSA was detected over 18 months in 14 SP patients, and this reduction correlated with increased EDSS (Paolillo et al., 1999). However, a 1-year study of 19 MS patients (10 PP, 9 SP) using a similar technique failed to replicate this correlation, although significant reduction in CSA was observed at C5 (Kidd et al., 1996). Using the more reproducible intensity contouring technique (Losseff et al., 1996), a 1-year study of 28 patients (4 benign, 6 RR, 6 SP, 12 PP) detected a significant reduction in CSA at the C2/C3 level, but this did not correlate with change in the EDSS score (Stevenson et al., 1998). Automatic edge detection has also been employed in a 4-year study of 38 MS patients (20RR, 18SP) and a consistent, significant correlation was seen between change in CSA and change in EDSS score at months 12, 18 and 48 (Lin et al., 2003b). While these results are to some extent contradictory, they are at least intriguing and the lack of consistency may be due to the general nature of the EDSS score, which represents an evaluation of neurologic impairment in eight functional systems (Sharrack and Hughes, 1996).

The sensitivity of automated and semi-automated methods in detecting change in cord CSA in MS has led directly to their use in evaluating cord atrophy in patients receiving treatment. Treatment with interferon-β showed no effect on cord atrophy in patients with PP MS in a 2-year study (Leary et al., 2003). Similarly, a 4-year study of patients with RR MS and SP MS showed no reduction in cord atrophy rate in patients treated with interferon-β (Lin et al., 2003b).

Conclusions

Improvements in MRI mean that acquisition of suitable images for measuring cord CSA is no longer a major technical challenge. The importance of atrophy in the cervical spinal cord in relation to disability in MS has been convincingly demonstrated in MRI studies using recently developed sensitive, yet relatively simple to implement, methods of measuring the CSA. This suggests a role for such methods in monitoring the progression of MS, and for exploring the efficacy of treatments aimed at preventing disability in MS. However, further development is needed to improve measurement accuracy, especially in handling partial volume effects.

References

Barnes D, Munro PM, Youl BD, Prineas JW, McDonald WI. The longstanding MS lesion. A quantitative MRI and electron microscopic study. *Brain* 1991; 114: 1271-80.

Coulon O, Hickman SJ, Parker GJ, Barker GJ, Miller DH, Arridge SR. Quantification of spinal cord atrophy from magnetic resonance images via a B-spline active surface model. *Magn Reson Med* 2002; 47: 1176-85.

Evangelou N, Konz D, Esiri MM, Smith S, Palace J, Matthews PM. Regional axonal loss in the corpus callosum correlates with cerebral white matter lesion volume and distribution in multiple sclerosis. *Brain* 2000; 123: 1845-9.

Ganter P, Prince C, Esiri MM. Spinal cord axonal loss in multiple sclerosis: a post-mortem study. *Neuropathol Appl Neurobiol* 1999; 25: 459-67.

Hickman SJ, Coulon O, Parker GJ, Barker GJ, Stevenson VL, Chard DT, et al. Application of a B-spline active surface technique to the measurement of cervical cord volume in multiple sclerosis from three-dimensional MR images. *J Magn Reson Imaging* 2003; 18: 368-71.

Kidd D, Thorpe JW, Kendall BE, Barker GJ, Miller DH, McDonald WI, et al. MRI dynamics of brain and spinal cord in progressive multiple sclerosis. *J Neurol Neurosurg Psychiatry* 1996; 60: 15-9.

Kidd D, Thorpe JW, Thompson AJ, Kendall BE, Moseley IF, MacManus DG, et al. Spinal cord MRI using multi-array coils and fast spin echo. II. Findings in multiple sclerosis. *Neurology* 1993; 43: 2632-7.

Kurtzke JF. Rating neurologic impairment in multiple sclerosis: an expanded disability status scale (EDSS). *Neurology* 1983; 33: 1444-52.

Leary SM, Miller DH, Stevenson VL, Brex PA, Chard DT, Thompson AJ. Interferon beta-1a in primary progressive MS: an exploratory, randomized, controlled trial. *Neurology* 2003; 60: 44-51.

Leary SM, Parker GJ, Stevenson VL, Barker GJ, Miller DH, Thompson AJ. Reproducibility of magnetic resonance imaging measurements of spinal cord atrophy: the role of quality assurance. *Magn Reson Imaging* 1999; 17: 773-6.

Lin X, Blumhardt LD, Constantinescu CS. The relationship of brain and cervical cord volume to disability in clinical subtypes of multiple sclerosis: a three-dimensional MRI study. *Acta Neurol Scand* 2003a; 108: 401-6.

Lin X, Tench CR, Turner B, Blumhardt LD, Constantinescu CS. Spinal cord atrophy and disability in multiple sclerosis over four years: application of a reproducible automated technique in monitoring disease progression in a cohort of the interferon beta-1a (Rebif) treatment trial. *J Neurol Neurosurg Psychiatry* 2003b; 74: 1090-4.

Liu C, Edwards S, Gong Q, Roberts N, Blumhardt LD. Three dimensional MRI estimates of brain and spinal cord atrophy in multiple sclerosis. *J Neurol Neurosurg Psychiatry* 1999; 66: 323-30.

Losseff NA, Miller DH. Measures of brain and spinal cord atrophy in multiple sclerosis. *J Neurol Neurosurg Psychiatry* 1998; 64 Suppl 1: S102-5.

Losseff NA, Webb SL, O'Riordan JI, Page R, Wang L, Barker GJ, et al. Spinal cord atrophy and disability in multiple sclerosis. A new reproducible and sensitive MRI method with potential to monitor disease progression. *Brain* 1996; 119: 701-8.

Lovas G, Szilagyi N, Majtenyi K, Palkovits M, Komoly S. Axonal changes in chronic demyelinated cervical spinal cord plaques. *Brain* 2000; 123: 308-17.

Lycklama G, Thompson A, Filippi M, Miller D, Polman C, Fazekas F, et al. Spinal-cord MRI in multiple sclerosis. *Lancet Neurol* 2003; 2: 555-62.

Matthews PM, Arnold DL. Magnetic resonance imaging of multiple sclerosis: new insights linking pathology to clinical evolution. *Curr Opin Neurol* 2001; 14: 279-87.

Oppenheimer DR. The cervical cord in multiple sclerosis. *Neuropathol Appl Neurobiol* 1978; 4: 151-62.

Paolillo A, Coles AJ, Molyneux PD, Gawne-Cain M, MacManus D, Barker GJ, et al. Quantitative MRI in patients with secondary progressive MS treated with monoclonal antibody Campath 1H. *Neurology* 1999; 53: 751-7.

Roberts N, Puddephat MJ, McNulty V. The benefit of stereology for quantitative radiology. *Br J Radiol* 2000; 73: 679-97.

Rocca MA, Mastronardo G, Horsfield MA, Pereira C, Iannucci G, Colombo B, et al. Comparison of three MR sequences for the detection of cervical cord lesions in patients with multiple sclerosis. *AJNR Am J Neuroradiol* 1999; 20: 1710-6.

Sharrack B, Hughes RA. Clinical scales for multiple sclerosis. J Neurol Sci 1996; 135: 1-9.

Sonka M, Hlavac V, Boyle R. *Image Processing, Analysis and Machine Vision*. London, England: Chapman & Hall, 1993.

Stevenson VL, Leary SM, Losseff NA, Parker GJ, Barker GJ, Husmani Y, et al. Spinal cord atrophy and disability in MS: a longitudinal study. *Neurology* 1998; 51: 234-8.

Thorpe JW, Kidd D, Moseley IF, Thompson AJ, MacManus DG, Compston DA, et al. Spinal MRI in patients with suspected multiple sclerosis and negative brain MRI. *Brain* 1996; 119 (Pt 3): 709-14.

Vaithianathar L, Tench CR, Morgan PS, Constantinescu CS. Magnetic resonance imaging of the cervical spinal cord in multiple sclerosis--a quantitative T1 relaxation time mapping approach. *J Neurol* 2003; 250: 307-15.

Zivadinov R, Locatelli L, Stival B, Bratina A, Grop A, Nasuelli D, et al. Normalized regional brain atrophy measurements in multiple sclerosis. *Neuroradiology* 2003; 45: 793-8.

In: Brain and Spinal Cord Atrophy in Multiple Sclerosis
Editors: R. Zivadinov and R. Bakshi, pp. 73-112
ISBN 1-59454-160-4

Chapter VII

MRI Measures of Pathology and their Relationship to Central Nervous System Atrophy in Multiple Sclerosis

Dominik S. Meier*, Howard L. Weiner, Samia J. Khoury, and Charles R. G. Guttmann
Center for Neurological Imaging and Partners Multiple Sclerosis Center
Brigham & Women's Hospital, Harvard Medical School
Boston, Massachusetts, U.S.A

Introduction

In multiple sclerosis (MS), inflammation, degeneration and repair are co-existing contributors to the net change in brain bulk. Various magnetic resonance imaging (MRI) metrics are available to assess brain atrophy and the pathological processes leading to it. The two most common definitions of atrophy as captured from MRI morphometry are either a measure of reduced normalized brain bulk relative to an age-matched normal control population, or a net loss of brain bulk over time. This applies to both global and regional measures. With brain bulk we mean to denote the sum of parenchymal tissue, both white and gray matter, including lesions. However, lesions of both white and gray matter, to the extent that they represent irreversible tissue degeneration, also constitute a form of atrophy, although not captured by global measures of brain bulk. The same holds for all surrogates of diffuse disease-reflecting tissue degeneration. We therefore want to mention at the outset that a lack of direct correlations between MRI metrics and brain bulk measures does not imply that those metrics are not sensitive to tissue loss. It may be that the MRI parenchymal volumetry is not sensitive to this form of tissue loss, or the two relate to different stages of the degenerative process and hence are separated in time. In our overview of relations between atrophy and

* Corresponding Author: Dominik Meier, Ph.D., Center for Neurological Imaging, Brigham and Women's Hospital, 221 Longwood Avenue, RFB 396, Boston, MA 02115. Phone: (617) 278-0800; Fax: (617) 264-5154; Email: *meier@bwh.harvard.edu*

other surrogates, we will refer to these two principal definitions of atrophy and focus on their pathological specificity toward the principal pathogenic mechanisms of inflammation, demyelination and axonal loss.

In this chapter we will discuss different MRI metrics currently applied in MS and how they relate to atrophy and the assessment of atrophy, i.e., particularly their sensitivity toward individual pathological processes that participate in the neurodegenerative process leading to tissue loss (Fig 1).

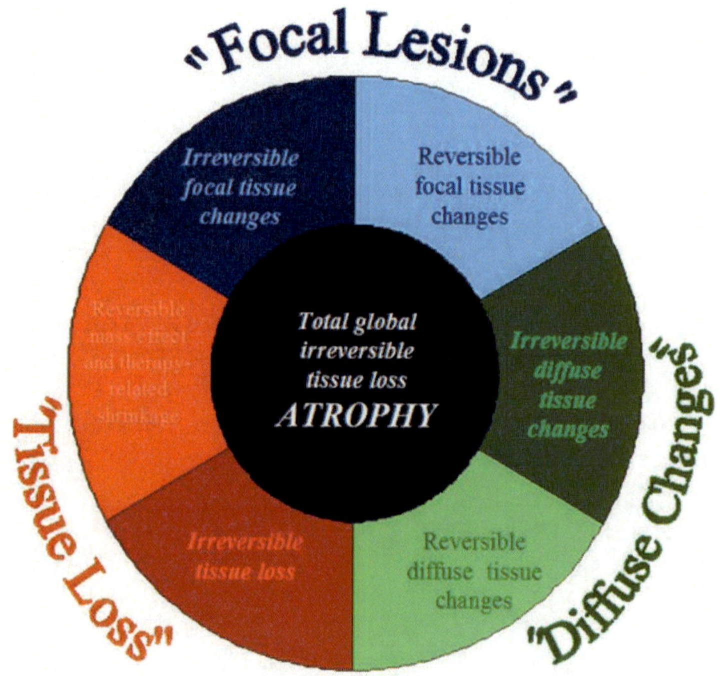

Fig 1. The sum of atrophy-related tissue changes comprises both reversible and irreversible, both focal and diffuse mechanisms. MRI morphometric variables exhibit different levels of sensitivity towards these mechanisms.

If it all comes down to atrophy in the end, why bother with other outcome measures? The additional value of other MRI metrics in terms of atrophy assessment would come from their being 1) more accurate with respect to degenerative processes (e.g., by being less subject to confounding factors like edematous volume changes), 2) more precise, i.e., more robust and reproducible in measurement, allowing detection of smaller changes, 3) more specific, distinguishing different components of atrophy (*e.g.* demyelination versus axonal loss), 4) more sensitive, i.e., capable of capturing disease earlier or in more subtle forms. For example, atrophy surrogates based on standard MRI structural morphometry will capture tissue loss to the extent that the lost parenchyma is replaced by cerebrospinal fluid (CSF), and this new CSF is correctly measured. Tissue density loss compensated by added intraparenchymal extracellular water will not be included in such atrophy measures, if it results only in MRI signal changes too subtle to affect the MRI tissue classification. This is where additional metrics capturing "diffuse" disease may provide a more comprehensive picture of the degenerative process. Several such measures with promising potential are discussed in the following sections.

There are also attributes that are not represented by specific MRI variables per se but are important parameters in the disease process. Two such aspects discussed below are the domains of time and space, relating to the dynamics and spatial prevalence of pathogenic mechanisms, respectively. Tools for their assessment are serial MRI and structure/anatomy-specific morphometry, respectively. To the extent that different MRI metrics capture different attributes of the underlying pathology, they will express different dynamics, which must be considered in analysis and comparison. MRI surrogates of atrophy are commonly considered to relate chiefly to irreversible tissue destruction, whereas lesion burden or spectroscopic measures have known transient components. To properly address this important domain of time, we distinguish here between disease activity, which we define as the current level of pathological process activity at the moment of evaluation, and disease severity, as the cumulative tissue damage resulting from past disease activity (Fig 2). In this context we must consider a single MRI exam as a snapshot in time and a global atrophy measure as integration in space. This places limitations on the validity of direct comparisons between different metrics, limitations which unfortunately are often ignored.

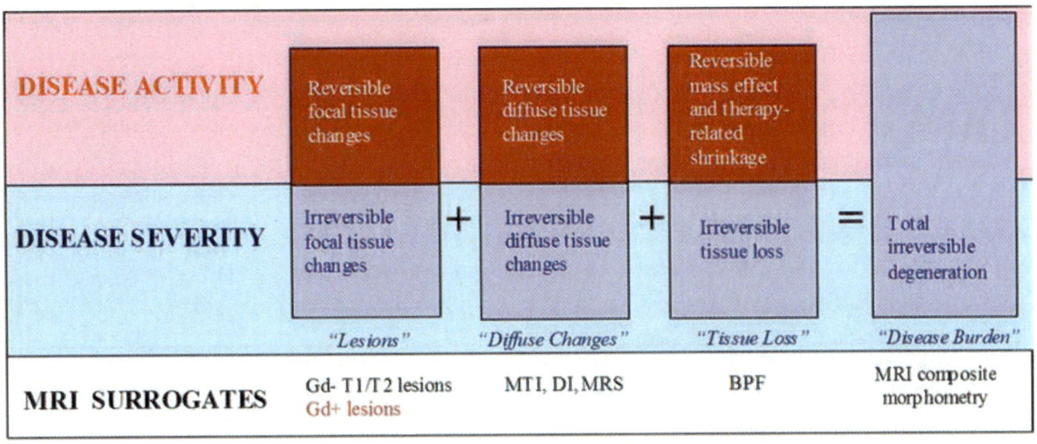

Fig 2. Breakdown of MS pathology into the two main groups of disease activity and severity. Each process in turn can be viewed as having a reversible and irreversible component. Putative MRI surrogates for individual processes are listed in the bottom row. Global brain volumetry only captures part of the total degenerative disease burden. Inflammation (e.g. edema) and regeneration reflect disease activity and are also confounders (dark gray) in the assessment of irreversible degeneration (disease severity, light gray).

Elucidating the relationship of MRI measures of pathology with atrophy will help assess their complementary value and position in the puzzle. For example, both MR spectroscopy and diffusion measures are collectively sensitive to axonal loss as well as subject to dilutive effects from inflammation. Similarly, magnetization transfer measures are sensitive to demyelination as well as axonal loss and dilutive edema. So the synergistic effect of these variables lies in exploiting their different sensitivities towards the same pathological process. This is where we stake our hopes on new levels of MRI specificity. At the current stage of knowledge, the result that a MS cohort differs in terms of a particular MRI metric from normal controls, or even that it differs between early relapsing-remitting (RR) and late secondary progressive (SP) disease is of limited additional value. To the extent that all parts of the central nervous system (CNS) are connected and mutually interrelate, they are all expected to be affected at some level. We know that MS brains are subject to pathological processes that eventually lead to loss of functional tissue and hence function. But to what degree this involves particular processes or merely mechanistic relationships, and the pathogenic sequence in which these processes occur, should be main focus of comprehensive MRI evaluation.

T2 Lesion Burden

White matter signal abnormalities (WMSA) on T2-weighted MRI images represent the most readily apparent tissue changes *in vivo*. Those hyperintense "T2 lesions" still represent the diagnostic hallmark of MS (McDonald et al., 2001). But despite their high sensitivity to tissue change, T2 WMSA lack pathological specificity and thus are of limited value for the assessment of disease progression and therapeutic response. T2-weighted MRI is collectively sensitive to different pathological processes, such as inflammation, edema, demyelination, axonal loss as well as repair processes, all of which may change the T2 signal in similar fashion (Guttmann et al., 1995a). Will then an understanding of how T2 lesions relate to atrophy provide reliable clues about the contributions of different pathological processes?

Studies of this relationship thus far arrived at discrepant/incongruent results. Several studies found no direct correlations between T2 lesion load and atrophy in either RR or SP MS (De Stefano et al., 2002; Ge et al., 2000; Sailer et al., 2001; van Walderveen et al., 1998), while other studies did observe such connections (Chard et al., 2003; Chard et al., 2002b; Lee et al., 1998; Liu et al., 1999; Rudick et al., 2000; Zivadinov et al., 2001a; Zivadinov et al., 2001b). The following will discuss a number of possible explanations for this discrepancy and apparently wavering connection.

Pathological Specificity

T2 prolongation is pathologically non-specific and thus significant portions of measured lesion load may represent non-destructive processes. The short T2 component (10 to 50 ms) of the T2 relaxation distribution appears to arise from myelin water and is absent in chronic demyelinated MS lesions (Moore et al., 2000), but the pathological proportions of demyelination are unknown, since inflammatory changes (edema and activated microglia) also raise the T2 signal, in absence of demyelination (De Groot et al., 2001). So individual lesions at different pathogenic stages will appear the same on T2-weighted MRI and their summation into a single lesion burden is confounding the measure of degenerated tissue with transient inflammatory changes and mass expansion from additional water. Common theories for the evolution from T2 lesions to atrophy lead via inflammation to demyelination and axonal transection as primary effects and via retrograde (affecting gray matter) and Wallerian (axonal loss) degeneration as secondary effects.

Spatial Variability

The prevalence of regional lesion distributions has not yet been researched extensively. T2 lesion burden appears to exhibit spatial propensities and, if measured locally, does correlate with specific disabilities (Pelletier et al., 2001; Sperling et al., 2001).

Temporal Variability

T2 lesion appearance fluctuates strongly over time (Guttmann et al., 1995a; Kikinis et al., 1999; Meier and Guttmann, 2003) and lesion burden obtained from a single MRI snapshot yields an imperfect picture of disease severity, confounded chiefly by inflammation. Interestingly, studies employing more differential methods of T2 lesion morphometry, such as difference imaging (Stevenson et al., 2002) have also not found better matches with atrophy. One problem related to longitudinal analysis of T2 lesion burden is the high level of spatio-temporal variability. A net global difference measure of T2 lesion burden significantly under-represents the total T2-weighted lesion activity, since new/enlarging and resolving lesions compensate each other, resulting in net changes appearing three times smaller than the actual T2-weighted lesion volume change (Lee et al., 1998). This transient nature would lead to the assumption that a measure of exclusively new T2 lesion volume would be a good surrogate or disease activity, which has indeed been observed in the form of greatly improved correlations with T1-gadolinium (Gd) volumes ($r = 0.72$, $P = 0.001$) compared to the net counterparts ($r = 0.45$, $P = 0.01$) and atrophy (Lee et al., 1998). It has been argued that substantially enhanced specificity towards the destructive disease components can be expected in quantitative serial MRI when distinguishing T2 WMSA into chronic, new/enlarging and resolving classes (Meier and Guttmann, 2003). Studies on relating such measures to subsequent atrophy are ongoing.

Hysteresis

With hysteresis we mean to denote that a measured value may lag behind its cause and also that its residual value differs based on whether this value was approached from above or below. Parenchymal volume loss may develop with a substantial time lag relative to the part of lesion burden relating to inflammation, but correlate directly with the portion representing demyelination or axonal loss. Studies incorporating a delayed effect did indeed find correlations of T2 lesion burden *change* with clinical disability (Weiner et al., 2000) and subsequent atrophy (Rudick et al., 2000). On a long enough timeline, the connection between lesion load and tissue destruction becomes very apparent. Long-term follow-up (14 years) showed 88% of patients with CIS and baseline T2 lesions developing clinically definite MS (Brex et al., 2002), as well as direct correlations of T2 lesions with disability (EDSS, $r=0.6$) and atrophy ($r=0.528$, $P = 0.004$) (Chard et al., 2003). The study of hysteresis effects may lead to better pathogenic models of degeneration in MS. This will require either extensive longitudinal studies or large cross-sectional studies with age and disease duration as the controlling variables.

MRI Sensitivity and Diffuse Disease

The sensitivity of T2-weighted MRI towards abnormal WM is commonly regarded as excellent. Yet the inconsistent correlations between WM lesions and other variables suggest that processes other than the focal lesions may contribute. Studies with comparable higher resolution MRI ($1.2\times1.2\times1.5$ mm^3 voxels) did find T2 lesion load directly correlated with both BPF ($r = -0.78$, $P < 0.001$) and GM loss ($r = -0.73$, $P < 0.001$) (Chard et al., 2002c). The term "normal appearing white matter" (NAWM) arose from the macroscopically normal appearance of MS tissue despite prevalent microscopic pathology (Allen et al., 2001). The radiological definition of NAWM refers chiefly to areas without focal T2 lesions and differs from a neuropathologic definition in that up to half of the lesions are macroscopically not visible (De Groot et al., 2001). In practice, focal lesions are often operator–defined, with arbitrary lesion size thresholds that indirectly force the definition of NAWM to include sub-threshold lesions. Hence, the MRI capture of diffuse disease becomes a highly significant issue, fueled by the fact that many forms of quantitative MRI [magnetization transfer ratio (MTR), magnetic resonance spectroscopy (MRS) and diffusion tensor imaging (DTI)] have found differences in otherwise radiologically NAWM and thus claim some sensitivity toward diffuse disease.

Atrophy Confounders

MRI surrogates of atrophy may themselves contain elements of transient volume changes, such as edema or therapy-induced shrinking (steroids). Those changes may obscure the true amount and rate of tissue degeneration. Hence, a large edematous T2 lesion not only adds a large non-destructive component to the global T2-lesion burden, but additionally increases apparent parenchymal volume. Good correlations of T2 lesion burden with GM loss were found, for example ($r = -0.73$, $P < 0.001$) (Chard et al., 2002c).

Spatial Sensitivity of Global Atrophy

Regional atrophy measures (see also chapter on regional atrophy) (Simon et al., 2004) have reported substantially higher sensitivity to change than global metrics. For example, associations of T2 lesion load with ventricular enlargement and corpus callosum thinning have been observed ($r= +0.50$ and -0.55, respectively, $P = 0.0003$-0.0012), indicating that at least a proportion of the T2 lesion burden indeed represents degenerative processes leading to brain atrophy (Liu et al., 1999). A regional atrophy measure such as ventricular enlargement may have sufficient sensitivity to capture the destructive components of those lesions, whereas a global atrophy measure may not.

Disease Phenotype

The brain is a moving target. It represents a complex regulatory system, both in function and underlying physiology, where the balance between neurodegenerative and reparatory processes can be tipped differently in different forms and phases of MS. From a quantitative

MRI perspective, these complexities appear as strong idiosyncrasies towards most morphometric variables. For clinically isolated syndromes (CIS), T2 lesions have proven high diagnostic power for conversion to clinically definite MS (Chard et al., 2003). For relapsing-remitting MS, results vary, indicating that further subtypes may await discovery. A separate case again is primary progressive (PP) MS, where T2 lesions alone explain neither observed brain atrophy nor the observed decrease in spectroscopic surrogates of axonal density (Pelletier et al., 2003). At least in this subtype, there seems to be a separate mechanism capable of creating detectable atrophy without exhibiting a significant corresponding level of T2 lesions.

Technical Artifacts

T2-weighted images have minimal to no contrast between CSF and WM lesions. In conjunction with partial volume effects, periventricular and cortical lesions become harder to detect reliably and may raise the number of false positives as well as obscure actual periventricular damage, leading to false negatives. Special sequences suppressing the CSF signal, such as FLAIR (fluid attenuated inversion recovery) have been successfully applied in MS lesion morphometry (Zivadinov and Bakshi, 2004). However, FLAIR images appear to yield fewer lesion counts in the posterior fossa and spinal cord, despite overall better sensitivity, which has been attributed to T1 relaxation time differences in those areas. Spatial variations of both lesion and NAWM relaxation times have been observed, leading to different contrast and lesion conspicuity in sequences such as FLAIR (Stevenson et al., 2000).

With all these factors in mind, we should hasten to add that the information value and specificity of the absence of T2 lesions (negative predictive value) is different from the added value of their presence. The high sensitivity of T2-weighted MRI makes it the method of choice for initial diagnosis and early follow-up. One may argue that neurodegenerative processes will become more apparent as time progresses, and that observed long-term correlations merely represent this same diagnostic value of early T2 lesions and CIS. We will discuss this issue of capturing disease dynamics in more detail below (see Temporal Relationships).

Studies with long-term follow-up suggest that earlier T2 lesion changes hold more predictive power of subsequent atrophy than later changes (Chard et al., 2003). A progressive interpretation of this finding is that early changes are more specific surrogates for basic degenerative disease activity, and that late stage lesion volumetry may be more confounded by the complex dynamics of the MS and the cumulative nature of T2 lesions. In other words, the transient component and collective T2 sensitivity renders T2 lesion burden partially sensitive to disease activity, which in due time will, directly or indirectly, lead to measurable atrophy. This would mean that disease activity surrogates from T2 lesion morphometry are most reliable in early disease, and that it would be more accurate to say that early T2 lesion load is representative of a disease activity level that eventually leads to atrophy than to claim a direct cause and effect relation to atrophy. In other words, we may mistake the more readily visible smoke for the fire. However, correlations across such long follow-up also indicate that there may be sustained and stable differences in disease activity, i.e., that patients with higher early activity also have *a* higher susceptibility to neurodegenerative processes, which would have important implications on decisions for early treatment.

Cortical Lesions and Gray Matter Damage

MS is still largely considered a WM disease. Yet pathological as well as MRI findings demonstrate a significant GM involvement (Bakshi et al., 2001a; Bakshi et al., 2002; Bo et al., 2003; Peterson et al., 2001; Sailer et al., 2003). Whether this involvement is secondary degeneration or a reflection of a distinct primary pathological mechanism is yet unknown. Pathological evaluation revealed one out of four active lesions arising within or adjacent to the cortex, suggesting that small cortical lesions are more common in MS than currently suggested by standard MRI protocols (Kidd et al., 1999). New high-resolution MRI protocols (Mugler et al., 2000) may raise sensitivity sufficiently to perform quantitative studies of cortical lesions, their topography (Fig 3), and their relation to atrophy, particularly cortical thinning, which has recently been established as substantial in early MS (Sailer et al., 2003).

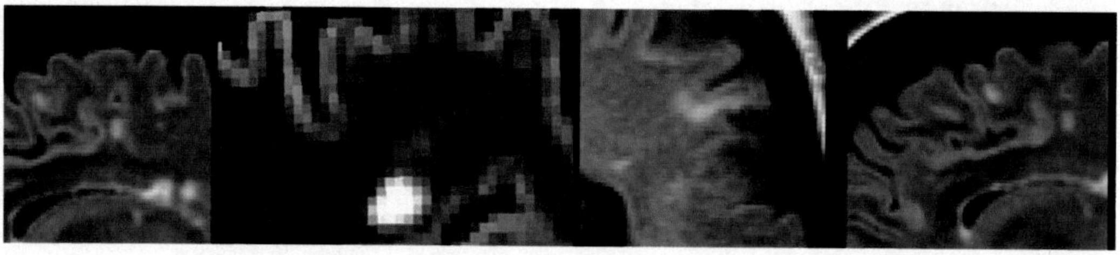

Fig 3. Examples of cortical lesions captured by a high-resolution FLAIR protocol. Cortical lesions as well as their position relative to the topography of the cortical band are clearly apparent. The CSF suppression inherent to FLAIR is especially beneficial in the cortical manifold, where partial volume effects may easily obscure cortical lesions. These lesions, albeit small compared to WM lesions, may express a different etiology, i.e. they may arise from primary pathogenic mechanism rather than secondary degeneration.

Subcortical GM assessment is less dependent on high-resolution, but GM lesions, whether cortical or subcortical, are technically challenging to detect reliably (Bakshi et al., 2001a). Strategies for detecting diffuse GM involvement (*e.g.* via MRS) (Kapeller et al., 2001; Sharma et al., 2001) will be discussed in the sections below.

A promising new avenue for the assessment of diffuse GM disease is MRI T2 hypointensity. This interesting measure was hypothesized to be arising from increased iron deposition (Drayer et al., 1987) and has been associated with a number of neurodegenerative conditions (Qian and Shen, 2001). T2 GM hypointensity is suspected to be predominantly due to pathological iron deposition (Drayer et al., 1987), which may be a primary or secondary process. Iron deposition has potentially neurotoxic effects and has been observed in other neurodegenerative diseases (Qian and Shen, 2001; Vymazal et al., 1999).

T2 shortening was observed in MS within cortical GM (Bakshi et al., 2000; Russo et al., 1997) as well as multiple deep gray matter structures (caudate, putamen, globus pallidus, thalamus, red nucleus) (Bakshi et al., 2001c, Bakshi et al., 2002). It has shown correlations with atrophy in the form of 3rd ventricle enlargement (Bakshi et al., 2001c) and, was found to be an independent predictor of whole brain atrophy (Bermel et al., 2003). GM hypointensity therefore appears to have potential as a marker for diffuse GM disease and subsequent tissue loss. It is also interesting as a complementary measure to other MRI morphometrics listed in this chapter, and may have dissociative qualities useful in defining disease phenotypes. The time course/evolution of GM abnormalities will provide valuable insights as to whether GM degeneration is a process secondary to WM damage, or if it is an etiologically separate event, and also the extent to which it represents irreversible tissue damage.

T1 Hypointense Lesions ("Black Holes")

The T1 longitudinal relaxation time of water differs measurably from one tissue to another and therefore can provide tissue contrast different from T2-weighted MRI. In purely physical terms T1 and T2 weighting form complements in exploiting the possible proton MR spectrum. How this physically orthogonal relation translates to differences in pathological specificity, however, should be approached with caution (Guttmann et al., 1995a). Many studies suggest the pathological specificity of hypointense lesions on T1-weighted spin-echo magnetic resonance images (T1 lesions) to be different than that of T2 lesions. This has led to the prevalent view that T1 lesions represent more serious tissue damage. As mentioned with T2 lesions above, we recommend considering the time factor in this distinction: Histopathologic analysis revealed that chronic T1 hypointense lesions chiefly represent extensive tissue destruction and axonal loss (van Walderveen et al., 1998), and the return to T1 isointensity has been proposed as an indicator for remyelination (Bitsch et al., 2001). Along the same line of thought, the appearance of hypointense lesions has been proposed as the MRI equivalent of a failure of remission (Truyen et al., 1996).

Several of the studies that did not find correlations of T2 lesions with atrophy did so for T1 lesions (Barkhof et al., 2001; Paolillo et al., 2000; Sailer et al., 2001). T1 lesion burden correlated with supratentorial brain volume ($r=0.48$; $P<0.01$) (Paolillo et al., 2000), cerebral volume (Sailer et al., 2001), cortical thinning ($r=0.54$, $P = 0.01$) (Sailer et al., 2003), global BPF ($r = -0.59$, $P = 0.002$) (Chard et al., 2002c) and global brain volume ($r = 0.53$, $P<0.01$). (Paolillo et al., 1999).

However, the same transient signal changes seen with T2-lesions (Fig 4) appear on T1 images (Guttmann et al., 1995a; Meier and Guttmann, 2003). Thus the level of pathological specificity of acute T1 lesions is yet unknown. In consequence, diagnostic and evaluative criteria have been revised from all T1-lesions to chronic T1-lesions, i.e., persistent T1 hypointensities that do not enhance on contrast-administered scans. T1 hypointensities can also arise from edematous water accumulation, just as with T2 hyperintensity. It should therefore be stressed that the physical specificity of T1-weighted MRI does not translate directly to pathological specificity, and that some of the observed differences between T1 and T2-lesions may arise from different sensitivities, i.e., different dynamic ranges that enhance conspicuity of destructive disease on T1 (Fig 5). The T1 signal per se is unlikely to distinguish between edema and demyelination any more than the T2 signal. If there are in fact dissociations in the relations of T1 and T2 lesions to atrophy, their evaluation in parallel may shed further light on the underlying pathogenic stages they capture or are most sensitive to (Leist et al., 2001; Sailer et al., 2001). T1 lesions are currently being employed as a secondary outcome measure in phase III clinical trials, and treatment effects have been demonstrated by reduced T1 lesion increase (Barkhof et al., 2001; Simon et al., 2000).

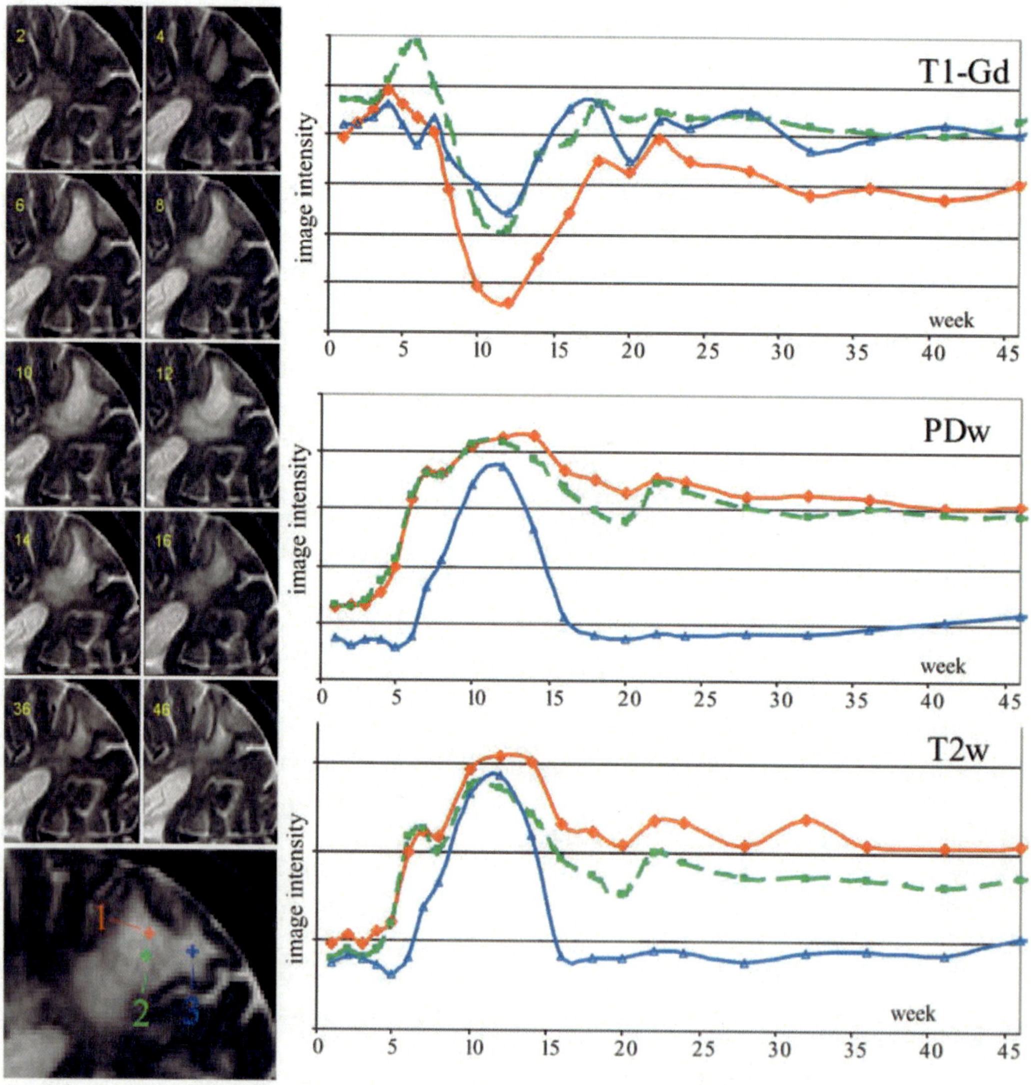

Fig 4. Example temporal intensity profiles extracted from a small point sample regions within an active lesion. Three channels of T1-Gd enhancement, proton-density weighting (PDw) and T2weighting T2w). Follow up occurred in weekly to monthly exams over a 1-year period. Note that the T1-Gd signal recovers to almost baseline, whereas lesion center portions of the dual echo signal remains hyperintense. Spatiotemporal propagation pattern of this lesion (see small thumbnails) further suggests that the majority of the signal change is coming from edematous water, rather than destructive tissue damage.

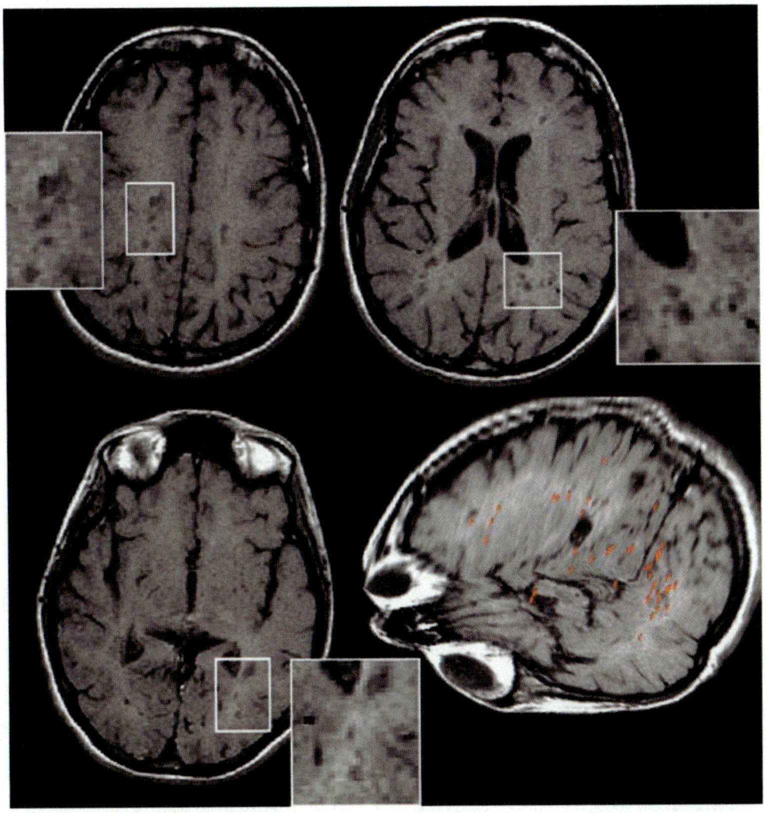

Fig 5. Example of a single MS patient with more than 60 individual black holes identified by a radiologist (rendered in red in the 3D view). Tighter correlations with atrophy are observed than for T2 lesions, supporting the theory that T1 hypointense lesions represent more severe and irreversible tissue destruction.

Do T1 lesions dissociate with clinical MS phenotypes? SP MS showed a very close relation between T1 lesion burden and clinical progression rate ($r = 0.81$, $P < 0.0001$) (Truyen et al., 1996). This would support the model of exhausted redundancy and repair capacity in SP, where any new tissue destruction translates directly to increased disability. Black holes were most prevalently observed in SPMS together with higher strata of disability (van Walderveen et al., 2001).

Contrast-Enhanced Lesions

A MRI exam prominent in MS involves the application of paramagnetic contrast agents such as Gd-DTPA, commonly in combinations with short TR and short TE (T1-weighted) spin-echo sequences. The intravenously administered contrast agent causes a change of local magnetization, leading to T1 hyperintensities (Gd+ lesions) in regions of blood-brain-barrier leakage. Because this leakage, in MS, has been linked to inflammation (Bruck et al., 1997), this contrast agent provides unique pathological specificity and consequently plays a substantial role in both diagnosis and treatment assessment. Since, in the currently predominant model, inflammation stands at the beginning of the pathogenic chain of MS, the assessment of Gd+ lesions is considered an effective and specific MRI surrogate of disease activity and hence a good outcome measure for therapy assessment. The lion's share of currently applied therapies (corticosteroids, beta-interferon, glatiramer acetate, immunoglobulins and immunosuppressive agents) impact the acute inflammatory aspect of MS activity, and Gd+ lesions are the principal MRI surrogate variable in evaluating the effect.

Direct correlations between Gd+ lesion burden and subsequent atrophy would therefore postulate that inflammation does play a significant role in the neurodegenerative cascade leading to tissue destruction. Baseline number of enhancing Gd+ lesions was a predictor for accumulation of T1 hypointense lesions (model $R^2 = 0.554$) (Simon et al., 2000). The account rendered by correlation studies between Gd+ lesions and atrophy is less contradictory than that of T2 lesions, but still some studies did find relations (Fisher et al., 2002; Leist et al., 2001; Lin and Blumhardt, 2001; Paolillo et al., 1999; Simon, 1999; Simon et al., 1999), while others did not (Chard et al., 2002c; Rovaris et al., 2001; Saindane et al., 2000). A possible explanation lies in the temporal sampling constraints. Since Gd+ lesions enhance only briefly for a period of 4 to 8 weeks (Cotton et al., 2003), a significant amount of hidden activity may contribute to the observed ambiguous relations. A recent review specifically on the relationship between Gd-enhanced MRI and progression of brain atrophy can be found in (Zivadinov and Zorzon, 2002).

The diagnostic and predictive power for parenchymal loss appears to be better in general for T1Gd-lesions than for T2 lesions or T1 black holes. Gd+ volume was found to be predictive of subsequent brain volume reduction in both RR (Fisher et al., 2002), and SP MS ($r = 0.77$, $p = 0.002$) (Paolillo et al., 1999). Additional pathological specificity may arise from the textural appearance of T1 lesions. Correlations between lesion load and atrophy were strongest in patients with the most ring enhancing lesions (Fig. 6). Such contrast pallors are considered to represent sustained tissue damage by glial scars and angiogenesis and would then indicate more aggressive/progressive pathology (Leist et al., 2001).

There are some technical challenges specific to the evaluation of the influence of T1Gd-lesions upon atrophy. One caveat is the potential swelling associated with inflammation, which would cause an initial overestimation of parenchymal volume and upon resolution look like atrophy. There are, however, several observations suggesting that the confounding contribution of edema is small and below the inferred parenchymal tissue loss. First, the Gd-lesion volume and associated edema are generally only a small fraction of the observed atrophy; second, parenchymal surrogates obtained distal from observed lesions with regional atrophy measures such as ventricular width did also reveal atrophy (Simon et al., 1999). One yet unaddressed confounder is that of diffuse inflammation below MRI sensitivity. Widespread (diffuse) inflammation has been suggested to set off a cascade of immune responses leading to axonal damage and hence atrophy (Brex et al., 2002). The detection of such low-level inflammation depends on MRI image resolution as well as dose and efficacy of administered contrast agent.

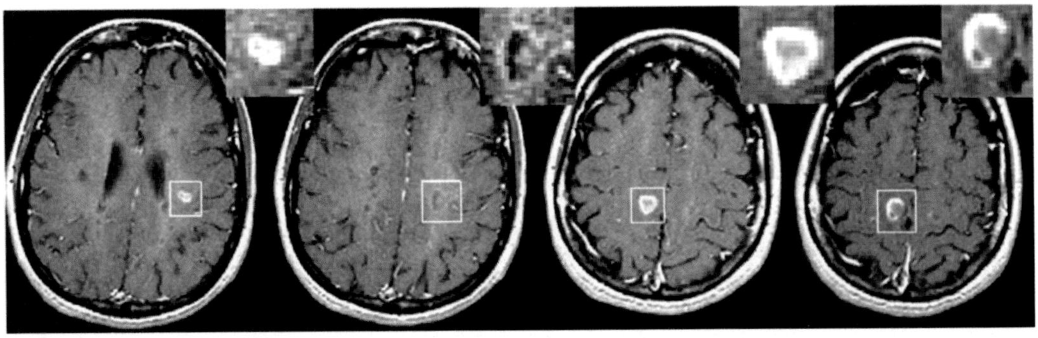

Fig 6. Example of Gd-enhancing lesions, for the same patient shown in Fig 4. A characteristic ring-enhancing pattern is visible, suspected to represent more destructive form of inflammation (Leist et al., 2001).

The other issue is that T1Gd-lesions represent disease activity and are transient in nature, i.e., apparent for weeks only (Cotton et al., 2003), whereas MRI metrics of atrophy are considered surrogates of irreversible tissue damage, or disease severity. Direct comparison will therefore be hampered by the fact that one is a differential of the other. Rather, integrated or cumulative Gd+ lesion load should be compared with other disease severity measures. High correlations of the cumulative number of new T1Gd-lesions with ventricular volume and ventricular diameter increase were indeed observed (linear regression, R^2=0.65, P = 0.007), and maintained after controlling for corticosteroid treatment (Leist et al., 2001).

Magnetization Transfer Imaging

Magnetization transfer (MT) is a principle applied to make the MRI signal partially dependent on otherwise invisible macromolecular structure. Macromolecules are invisible under normal MRI conditions, because the T2 relaxation times of their protons (less than 200 μs) are orders of magnitude below that of free water. Magnetization transfer imaging (MTI) applies an extra off-resonance saturation pulse intended to resonate with the bound protons in macromolecules. When this extra longitudinal magnetization is transferred from the bound protons to the surrounding free water, it there results in a signal change. This exchange is related to the number of hydrogen bonds and the diffusion of adjacent hydration layer protons into the free water. MTI is thus thought to correspond to protons in macromolecules of cell membranes, such as the cholesterol and galactocerebroside found in myelin (Kucharczyk et al., 1994). The MT signal is reduced in proportion to the density of macromolecules and thus would provide a potential surrogate for levels of axonal and myelin density, which was indeed observed in post-mortem studies (van Waesberghe et al., 1999). MTI has been successfully applied for clinical assessment in MS (Cercignani et al., 2000; Comi et al., 1999; Grossman, 1994; Grossman et al., 1994; Hiehle et al., 1995; Hiehle et al., 1994; Leary et al., 1999; Ropele et al., 2000; Rovaris and Filippi, 2000; Santos et al., 2002) and other conditions (HIV, Wallerian degeneration, optic neuritis, cerebral hemorrhage) (Grossman, 1994).

Like all the other MRI metrics discussed so far, the MT signal change in new MS lesions is transient (Dousset et al., 1998; Silver et al., 1998). Longitudinal studies suggest that MTI may nevertheless provide some specificity in assessing myelin and thereby distinguish progressive tissue destruction and remyelination (Rovira et al., 1999; van Waesberghe et al., 1998). MT recovery is therefore thought to indicate not only resolving inflammation, but also reparatory processes such as remyelination.

One potential confounder to MTI is the dilutive effect of edema, where the additional water also causes an MT reduction. Yet, MT reductions due to demyelinated lesions have been reported to be greater than those of edematous lesions but lower than the reduction observed in ischemic lesions (Mehta et al., 1996), which would point at a certain specificity of MT towards tissue destruction, particularly demyelination. This is supported by the transient MT drop observed in acute lesions (Dousset et al., 1998; Silver et al., 1998), which would exclude axonal loss as a significant contributor (which is likely irreversible), but instead points at gliosis and remyelination and resolving edema. Additional measures such as longitudinal trends of MT drops and water content have also been suggested as complements to help distinguishing edema and different lesion types (Ropele et al., 2000). So it appears that MTI is indeed predominantly sensitive to tissue destruction (Kimura et al., 1996), supporting the model of inflammation (and associated blood-brain-barrier opening) as the first stage of new acute lesions.

The chief contribution of MTI is its potential specificity to demyelination and its alleged sensitivity to detecting diffuse disease, both of which would make excellent complements to both global and local atrophy measures. There are several findings that indicate sensitivity towards damage of normal appearing white matter (NAWM). First, MT drops were frequently observed even before the appearance of a visible lesion (Kalkers et al., 2001; Lycklama a Nijeholt et al., 2000; Silver et al., 1998), and second, the magentization transfer ratio (MTR) of NAWM appears to differ between MS phenotypes and, more interestingly, shows different rates of progression (Filippi et al., 2000). Fig. 7 shows an example of MTR images alongside their T1 counterparts. A marked drop in MT signal is apparent in periventricular regions, not only those of black holes, but also in regions of apparent white matter isointensity, i.e., in NAWM. Results on the predictive value of MTR with regard to the clinical evolution of MS are still controversial. For RR and SP, the MTR of NAWM appears to be predictive of clinical evolution (Santos et al., 2002), whereas for early disease, i.e., conversion from CIS to clinically definite MS, results differ (Brex et al., 2001; Iannucci et al., 2000).

A technical difficulty in MTI is the calibration of the off-resonance pulse, which varies between scanners and therefore makes comparisons and multi-center trials difficult. Given the potential specificity of this measure towards capturing the myelin and axonal components of tissue loss, efforts towards standardization and calibration of the MT pulse would bring it closer to a valuable routine clinical outcome measure.

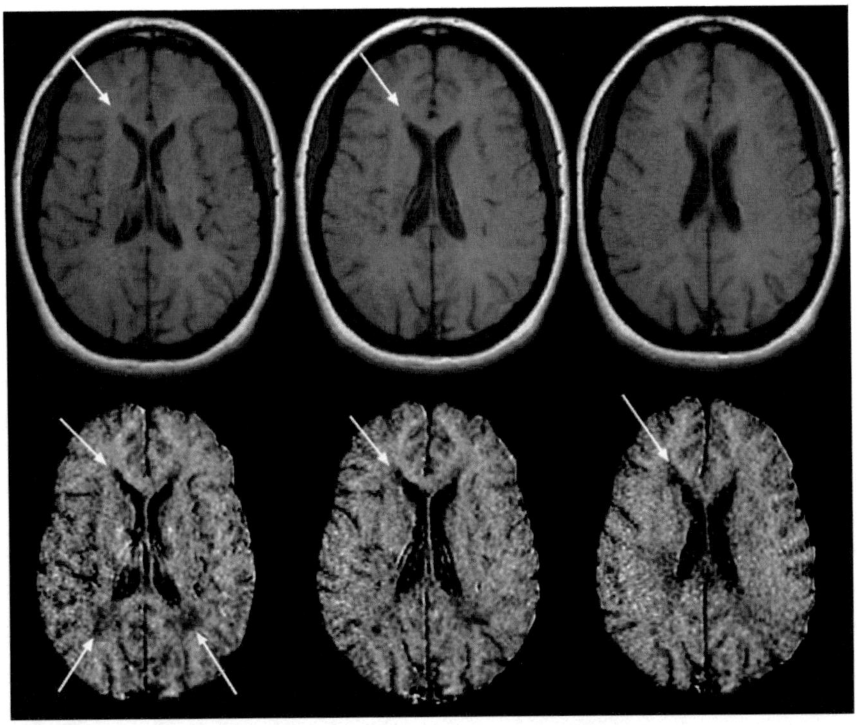

Fig 7. Three adjacent example slices from an MS patient. The T1-weighted series (top row) shows normal appearing white matter (NAWM) and periventricular chronic black holes (T1 hypointensity). The corresponding magnetization transfer ratio image (MTR) (bottom row) reveals significant drops of MT value for both the lesion as well as periventricular NAWM (arrows).

Diffusion Imaging

Diffusion describes random molecular motion in a gas or fluid. Although random, it is fast enough over short distances to support some of the fastest physiological mechanisms, namely those of synaptic transmission. Diffusion imaging (DI) sequences exploit the directionality of this process enforced by the anisotropic tissue structure. Strong additional gradients are applied to capture magnitude and directionality of water diffusion and from these values arrive at measures of structural tissue anisotropy. This provides an additional level of specificity that hitherto eluded the common "water" MR image. A common metric derived from DI imaging is the apparent diffusion coefficient (ADC). It is termed "apparent" because it is the main parameter in the diffusion equation for an isotropic fluid, which of course does not apply to biological tissue. Tissue membranes and other structural components limit diffusion along their principal axes and hence make it directional. This constrained directionality of free water diffusion thus becomes an elegant way to indirectly capture the orientation of biological structures. Tissue damage would reduce this anisotropy and thus raise ADC values.

DI is still largely experimental due to its technical difficulties (long scan times, motion artifacts, gradient limitations). But new DI sequences no longer acquire merely the magnitude of diffusion but also its directionality. Diffusion Tensor Imaging (DTI) applies multiple gradients to encode the principal directions of diffusion at each point. This has led to a renaissance of DI in MS, with stunning new structural assessment, such as fiber tracking and mapping (Fig. 8), which would find immediate use in studying the evolution of WM lesions. However, the interpretation of DTI images and mapping of degenerated pathways is difficult without a priori information about the anatomy under study.

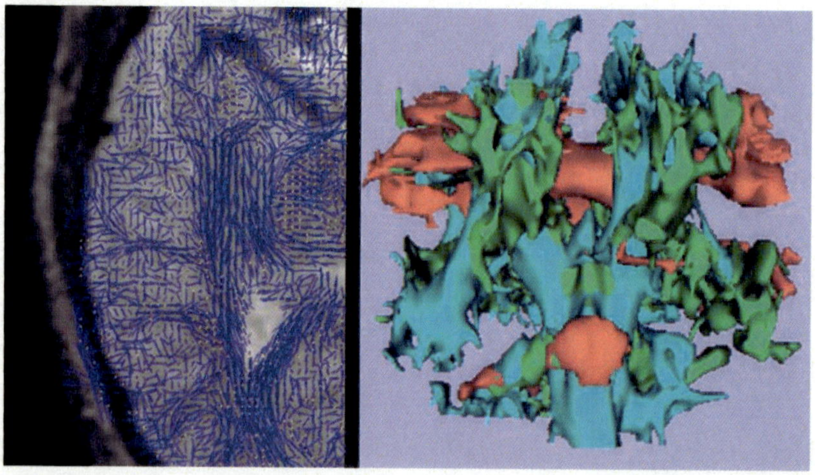

Fig 8. Examples of fiber anatomy captured by diffusion tensor imaging (images provided by Svetlana Egorova, MD). The directionality of diffusion is exploited to assess tissue anisotropy, which is most pronounced along the axis of a white matter fiber. This shows estimated tracks around an MS lesion as well as color-coded renderings of WM based on fiber direction (red=left-right, green=anterior-superior, blue=inferior-superior).

In isolated bundles of parallel fibers, secondary white matter degeneration (Wallerian) has been established conclusively with DTI, and a distinction between secondary and primary fiber loss also seems possible (Pierpaoli et al., 2001). DI's specificity toward the detection of demyelination or axonal loss in MS still has to be established clinically, but it is a definite candidate for a potential surrogate for diffuse disease. In well-defined tracts, such as the genu of the internal capsule, DTI revealed significant decreases in fractional anisotropy of NAWM in MS. Different types of focal lesions did also exhibit substantial DTI differences (Bammer et al., 2000), as did DTI measures between enhancing and non-enhancing lesions ($p<0.001$) (Werring et al., 2000) (Fig. 9). However, the same theoretical dilutive effects of edema apply here as they do for the previously discussed magnetization transfer and MR spectroscopy to be discussed next.

DTI studies further supported the suggestion of T1 hypointense areas as prominent sites of tissue destruction, in that T1 black holes coincided with sites of greatest loss of tissue anisotropy (indicating either fiber disruption or water dilution) (Filippi et al., 2001). To the extent that DI is in fact specific to local tissue degeneration, direct associations with global and regional atrophy can be expected. Some direct correlations between atrophy and mean diffusivity ($r=-0.58$, $p=0.007$) have indeed already been described (De Stefano et al., 2002).

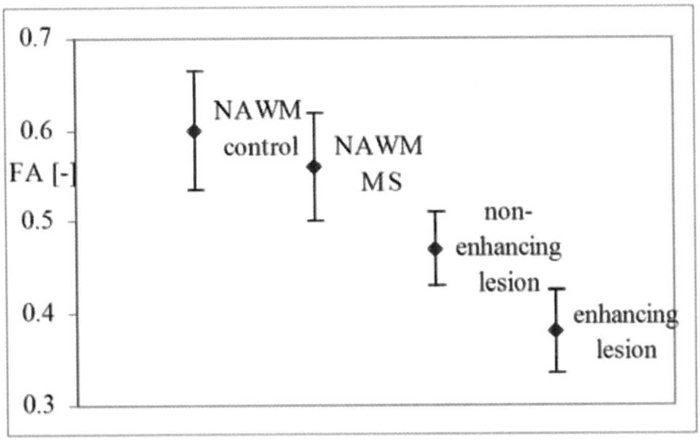

Fig 9. Fractional anisotropy (FA) measures of local tissue regions comprised of normal appearing WM (NAWM) in both healthy volunteers (control) and MS patients (MS), as well as in enhancing and non-enhancing lesions. Differences in FA among all groups is statistically significant ($P < 0.01$). Data from (Werring et al., 2000).

Magnetic Resonance Spectroscopy

MRS is a powerful noninvasive tool for biochemical characterization of brain tissue and metabolic investigation. It builds from the same phenomena as MRI, but measures resonances from substances other than water. The most prominent form is proton (H+) MRS, but spectra involving other nuclei, such as phosphorus (^{31}P) or sodium (^{23}NA) can also be interrogated at appropriate field strengths.

Neurophysiologic key markers include N-acetylated groups, dominated by N-acetyl aspartate (NAA, 2.0 ppm), creatine and phosphocreatine (Cr, 3.0 ppm), choline-compounds (Cho, 3.2 ppm), myo-inositol (Ins, 3.54 ppm), as well as amino acids, such as glutamate (Glx) and γ-aminobutyric acid (GABA) and sugars (glucose, inositol) (Fig. 10, Table 1).

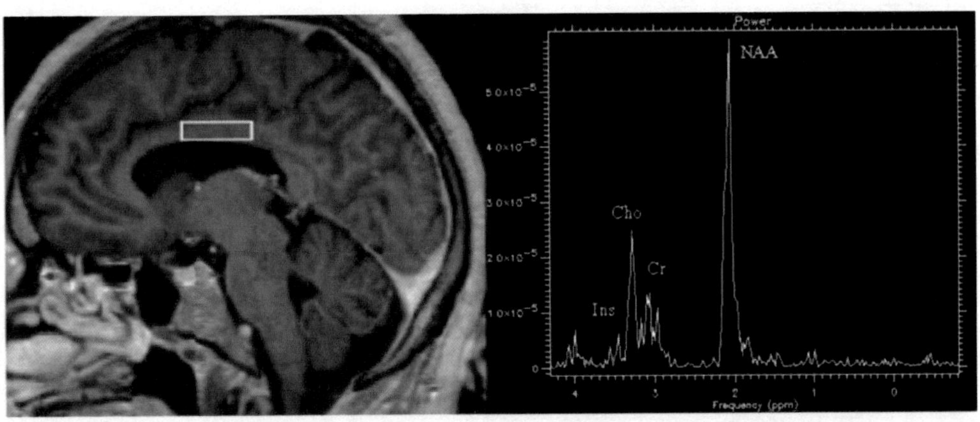

Fig 10. Example of an MRS spectrum (right) for a rectangular region prescribed in the corpus callosum (box, left) of a normal volunteer. Cho, Cr and NAA peaks are readily resolved. Metabolites such as lactate and macromolecules require different sequences.

Table 1. Overview of MRS metabolites and their relation to MS pathology and atrophy, "Q" indicates the putative quality of the signal, mostly determined by signal-to-noise ratio and ease of peak separation.

Compound / Molecule	Peak ppm	Putative Surrogate & Relevance	Q	Confounders	Refs
NAA, N-aspartyl-glutamate	2.0	axonal density & axonal function	****	includes reversible axonal dysfunction, *i.e.* not 100% a marker of structural axonal integrity	(Fu et al., 1998; Husted et al., 1994; Kapeller et al., 2001)
Cr, P-Cr	3.0	energy flux, evenly distributed and therefore used for normalization (NAA/Cr, Cho/Cr)	**	Present in all cells, therefore often used as normalizing reference , possibly not constant across pathology	(Brex et al., 1999; Urenjak et al., 1993; van Walderveen et al., 1999)
Cho	3.2	biomembranes, gliosis, raised in acute MS plaques	***		(Arnold et al., 1992; Narayana et al., 1998; Tartaglia et al., 2002)
Myo-Ins	3.54	glial cells & gliosis	**	confounded by water peak	(Chard et al., 2002a; Kapeller et al., 2001)
Lactate	1.3	inflammation	*	confounded by mobile lipids and macromolecules, low SNR	(Arnold et al., 1992)
Glutamate, Glutamine, GABA	~3.8	neuromodulation, excitotoxicity	*	close and crowded peaks, substantially higher concentrations in GM	(Chard et al., 2002a; Helms, 2001)
lipids & macromolecules	0.9-2.1, 3.0	myelin breakdown products, dissociates active versus chronic lesions	*	require short TE, reducing spectral separation, also need additional metabolite nulling scan	(Mader et al., 2000; Mader et al., 2001)

NAA is found predominantly in neurons and is therefore considered a marker of axonal function and/or density, i.e., NAA reductions are thought to represent either axonal loss or dysfunction. NAA reductions can in theory be caused by edematous dilution effects as well as inflammation and induced metabolic impairment. The value of NAA as a structural marker is reduced to the extent that its dependence on physiological fluctuations remains unknown. In our current understanding, NAA reductions caused by inflammation and metabolic impairment are reversible, whereas axonal transection and Wallerian degeneration are not (De Stefano et al., 1995). Observed NAA decreases reached up to 50% in NAWM (Fu et al., 1998) and up to 80% in lesions (Bitsch et al., 1999; Brex et al., 1999; De Stefano et al., 1995; Husted et al., 1994; Mader et al., 2001). Both percentages contain unknown proportions of reversible NAA reduction, i.e., the same caveat to transient signal changes mentioned with all the other MRI markers above applies here. But there are several indicators that speak for NAA as a predominantly structural rather than physiological marker. First, the observed NAA reduction in MS lesions is greater in proportion than the volume change in those lesions, indicating that reversible NAA change is unlikely to merely herald from edematous dilution effects (Helms, 2001). Second, direct correlations between NAA and atrophy have been observed (Davie et al., 1995; De Stefano et al., 2002). Finally, a direct relationship between NAA reduction and axonal density reduction has been established (Bitsch et al., 1999; Bjartmar et al., 2000). Hence, it would seem that significant NAA level drops indeed indicate a loss of neuronal integrity rather than solely transient dysfunction. In this light, the observed direct correlations between atrophy and NAA/Cr levels (De Stefano et al., 2002) would suggest that axonal loss is a substantial contributor to atrophy and that its contribution can be assessed by MRS, even in very early stages of disease (De Stefano et al., 2001).

The ability of MRS to capture the metabolic signature of a pathological process is very promising for applications in MS (Table 1). NAA levels, for example, were significantly reduced in demyelinated axons (42%) and in myelinated axons in NAWM (30%) (Bjartmar et al., 2000). Also, active (Gd-enhancing) lesions of both benign and SPMS patients showed comparable drops in NAA levels, but significantly higher residual NAA levels were found in chronic lesions of benign MS compared to SPMS (Falini et al., 1998), indicating better functional recovery and potentially different levels of structural repair. In CIS, reduced NAA concentrations were found in lesions but not in NAWM, whereas in SPMS, NAWM also showed significantly lower NAA than that of RRMS (Fu et al., 1998). Direct correlations between cerebral volume and NAA levels were observed in RR ($r=0.67$, $P<0.001$) (De Stefano et al., 2002) as well as SPMS ($r=0.73$, $P<0.01$) (Coles et al., 1999). This specificity is likely to be enhanced by monitoring other metabolites. For example, choline compounds and myo-inositol levels were also raised in lesions (Brex et al., 1999). Such changes in Cho levels have been suggested to be associated with early inflammatory cytokines in NAWM, even before a visible lesion develops (Tartaglia et al., 2002). Raised levels of myo-inositol compared to controls were also observed in cortical GM (Kapeller et al., 2001). Increases of choline and myo-inositol were found in sites of glial proliferation and elevated lactate was associated with inflammation (Bitsch et al., 1999). New MRS protocols have also achieved spectral separation between the lactate peak and macromolecules (Mader et al., 2001).

MRS has also been suggested as a marker for diffuse disease: NAA reductions in NAWM were observed in some studies (Fu et al., 1998; Husted et al., 1994; Kapeller et al., 2001) and not in others (Bitsch et al., 1999; Brex et al., 1999). A reliable MRS surrogate of diffuse disease would be especially helpful in longitudinal studies to elucidate how and when

NAWM degenerates and to what extent the observed drops in NAA are transient. Cortical GM also showed reduced NAA and raised Ins compared to controls (Kapeller et al., 2001), and persistently reduced cerebellar WM NAA levels coinciding with cerebellar atrophy were found in MS patients with ataxia compared to patients with no cerebellar symptoms (Davie et al., 1995).

The main technical challenges in MRS are spatial resolution limits due to rapid loss of SNR with smaller FOV, i.e., fairly large quantities of tissue are required for a reliable signal, which limits studies to the most abundant metabolites and relatively large anatomical regions of interest. Also, the determination of absolute concentration measures from the observed spectra requires careful calibration and complex spectral fitting algorithms. Self-normalizing ratios, such as NAA/Cr have therefore often been used as surrogates of absolute NAA concentrations. The rationale is that Cr is a principal energy metabolite and therefore assumed to be evenly and constantly distributed throughout the brain. There are concerns, however, that fluctuations of Cr, as in fact observed in MS lesions (Brex et al., 1999), would render it unfit as a variable for normalization. Astrocytes also have higher Cr levels than neurons, which could explain Cr rises in gliosis (Urenjak et al., 1993; van Walderveen et al., 1999). Since glial cell proliferation is a possible pathological factor in MS, the use of Cr as a variable for normalization becomes problematic. Cr and Cho levels also correlate with age (Leary et al., 2000), requiring proper normalization and control in longitudinal and cross-sectional studies.

Spatial Relationships

Global atrophy measures have moved into the limelight recently because they have been linked to disability and demonstrate treatment effects. However, in light of the view that MS is a complex superposition of multiple inflammatory, degenerative and repair processes, MRI markers that are collectively sensitive become difficult to interpret in terms of pathology. This makes an unequivocal statement in favor of both regional morphometric measures and short-term follow-up. If different pathological processes exhibit prevalences that differ in either space or time, then the specificity of MRI markers that integrate over large areas or long time-periods is likely to be reduced. As outlined in the introduction, atrophy defined as loss of functional tissue is not equivalent to atrophy defined as loss of parenchymal bulk. The former includes all transient and irreversible changes in tissue impeding function, as well as density loss below MRI sensitivity, such as focal degeneration in lesions replaced with extracellular water (Fig 1). The latter may arise as a result from shrinkage and tissue collapse due to diffuse parenchymal density loss as well as focal tissue degeneration, affecting both gray and white matter and neuronal components as well as myelin or axons. Hence, accurate interpretation of WM volume loss requires knowledge of volumetric WM composition, and how it is affected by pathology. Half of WM volume is estimated to be comprised of axons, a quarter of myelin and the remainder of glial cells, vasculature and extracellular fluid (Fig. 11) (Adams, 1989; Miller et al., 2002). Hence, both demyelination and axonal loss, to the extent that the replacing CSF is excluded in the measure, would contribute at different levels to the chosen atrophy surrogate. To the extent that axonal loss results in mere reduction of axonal density (Evangelou et al., 2000), atrophy measure may not capture this portion and therefore underestimate. Regional atrophy measures such as ventricular enlargement, on the other hand, may be susceptible to tissue shifts caused by regional reduction of axonal density and therefore be more sensitive. This difference in sensitivity between regional and global atrophy measures also arises in part from nonlinearities in normalization (volume %). Hence, small structures exhibit larger relative atrophy rates than larger ones and may therefore be better suited for longitudinal studies with brief follow-up (less than 1-2 years). Reproducibility of small structure measurement becomes an issue, however, because repositioning and partial volume effects significantly reduce precision, especially for smaller and complexly shaped structures (Kikinis et al., 1992).

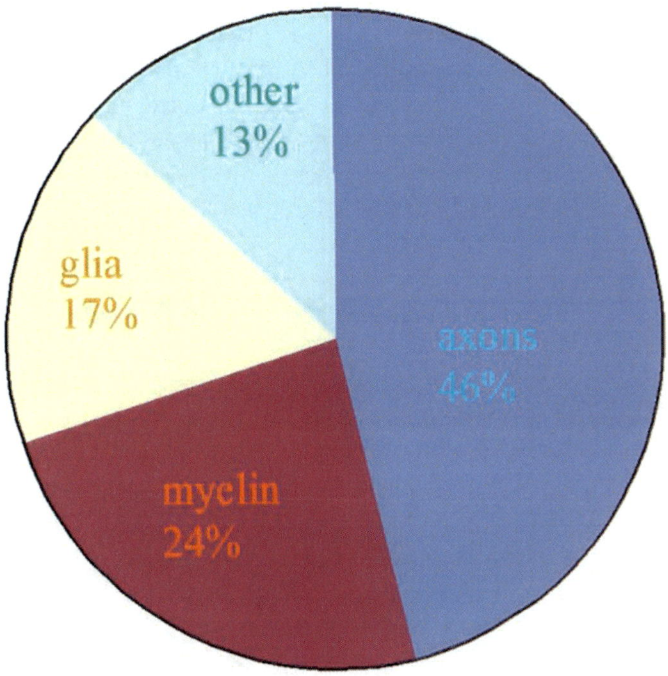

Fig 11. Estimates of white matter composition [data from (Adams, 1989; Miller et al., 2002)]. Half the WM volume is estimated to be comprised of axons, a quarter of myelin and the remainder glial cells, vasculature and extracellular fluid.

High-resolution MRI and advanced image processing (Fischl and Dale, 2000) made possible the regional measure of lesion burden and cortical thickness. First studies observed a thinning more prevalent in frontal and temporal regions and also occurring soon after disease onset (Sailer et al., 2003). The distribution of white matter damage in these patients at least partly supports the theory of retrograde degeneration. This lets us assume that different brain regions exhibit different levels of plasticity, and therefore are more sensitive to damage of afferent or efferent pathways. Although both motor and somatosensory cortices have been shown to exhibit remarkable plasticity (Manger et al., 1996; Merzenich et al., 1984) and congruent sensitivity to axonal damage (Bonatz et al., 2000), the visual cortex does not seem to follow this trophic pattern to the same extent, showing little effect to common damage to optic nerve and lateral geniculi (Evangelou et al., 2001). Furthermore, observed relationships between atrophy and WM lesions in RR but not PP MS (De Stefano et al., 2003) raise questions about undetected diffuse disease. Regional atrophy measures can provide a very sensitive tool for isolating the individual substrates and pathological sequences of atrophy.

Ventricular enlargement is among the most commonly applied (Brex et al., 2000; Luks et al., 2000; Matthews et al., 1996; Rao et al., 1985; Redmond et al., 2000; Simon et al., 1999) and easily implemented measures of regional atrophy. It is an interesting measure, as it is probably sensitive to density loss of periventricular WM. Ventricular fraction, for example, as a marker for central atrophy, showed greater sensitivity to change (up to five times greater atrophy rates) than the whole-brain parenchymal fraction, and sufficient sensitivity to distinguish MS subtypes (Kalkers et al., 2002).

A critical issue in cross-sectional morphometry is dissociating normal variability in head and brain size from pathological degeneration. As lost tissue is replaced by extracellular water, CSF becomes an important complement to parenchymal volume measure in terms of normalization. Hence, the most reproducible atrophy surrogates measure CSF volume normalized by parenchymal volume or vice versa. The same holds for GM atrophy: fractional GM loss was observed with a corresponding increase in fractional CSF, i.e., a 4% GM loss was associated with a corresponding 4% CSF gain (Quarantelli et al., 2003).

Temporal Relationships

Comprehensive assessment of MS pathology requires measurement of both disease activity and severity, the former indicating current rate of progression, the latter as a surrogate for cumulative disease burden, i.e., the residual of past disease activity. Apart from MRI surrogates with a tight relation to pathophysiological processes such as Gd-enhancing lesions (see above), the only approach to capturing disease activity is from differential measures of serial MRI, i.e., by repeating the same MRI protocol and evaluating the changes. Atrophy in longitudinal studies is assessed in this fashion. This adds another level of complexity to quantitative MRI evaluation, as now the patterns studied become spatiotemporal (4-dimensional), and require high-precision registration and intensity normalization (Meier and Guttmann, 2003). An example of the importance of MRI disease activity is the established observation that Gd-lesions (and T2-lesions) fluctuate at much greater frequency than observed relapses, indicating that pathological activity is substantially higher than suggested from clinical outcome measures (Cotton et al., 2003; Guttmann et al., 1995b; Kikinis et al., 1999; Meier and Guttmann, 2003). This is not surprising considering the redundant and compensatory qualities of CNS circuitry. But especially for therapy choice and evaluation, this dissociation between pathological specificity and clinical specificity suggests an increasingly relevant role of MRI in the future. This is pertinent to the observation that MRI lesion dynamics may vary with MS disease stages and clinical phenotypes. New diagnostic criteria for MS now involve serial MRI to establish dissemination in space and time (McDonald et al., 2001).

Atrophy is a slow process and thus requires increased precision/sensitivity in measurement. Global atrophy rates in MS are estimated to ca. 0.5-1% per year (Fisher et al., 2002; Guttmann et al., 2000; Hardmeier et al., 2003; Horsfield et al., 2003). Hence, reliable detection of global atrophy requires either longer follow-up or larger sample sizes in the form of cross-sectional studies. For example, recent studies found evidence of atrophy as early as 3 months after onset (Hardmeier et al., 2003). Regional atrophy can provide a substantial boost in sensitivity (see above), and is therefore recommendable for studies with shorter follow-up.

The value of many of the associated MRI variables described above comes to bear in the longitudinal component of disease progression and pathogenesis. In other words, most MRI markers express collective sensitivity to multiple processes (such as edema, inflammation, demyelination, axonal loss), but are sensitive to different degrees and hence in combination carry additional dissociative quality. For example, direct analysis of serial MRI signal dynamics indicated that the site and extent of permanent damage relate to the nature and intensity of the initial insult (Fig 12) (Meier and Guttmann, 2003). Signal dynamics show that both T1 and T2 signals can recover partially or completely within weeks to months after the initial inflammatory insult.

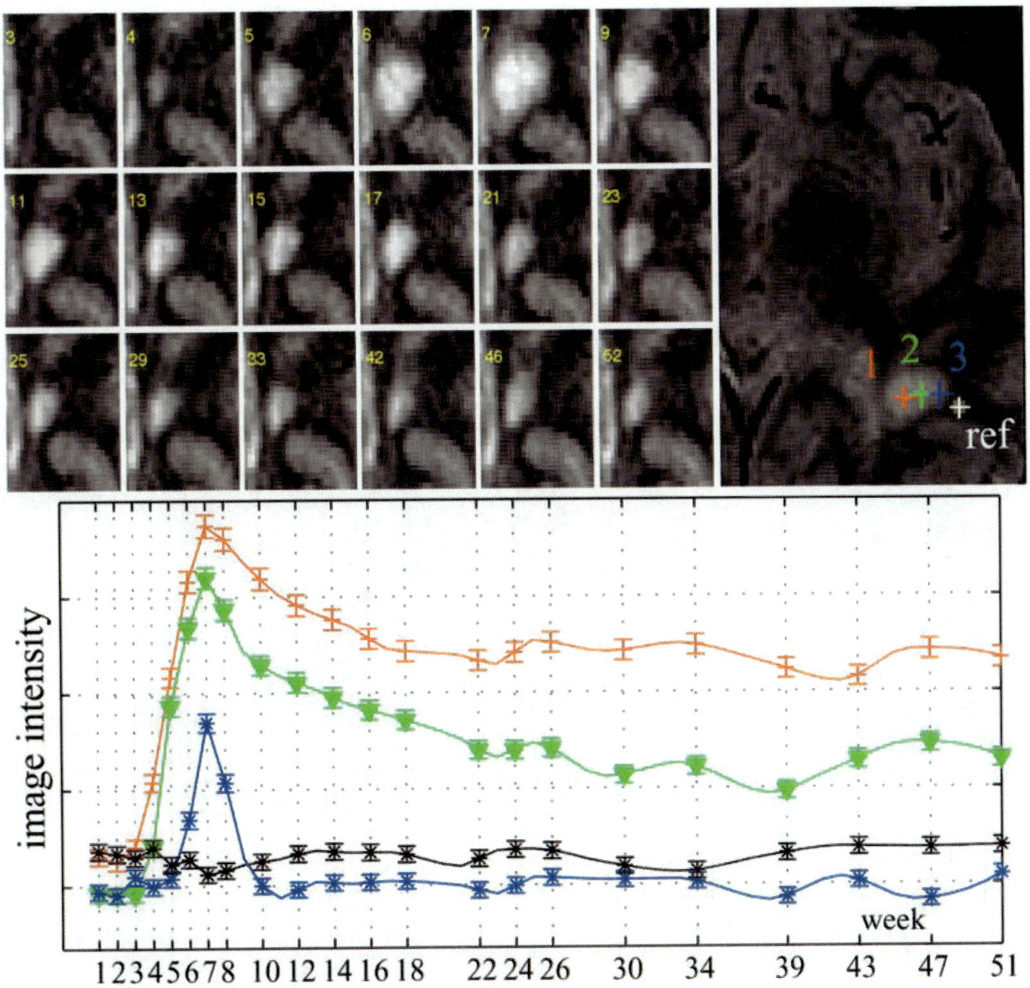

Fig 12. Example of lesion evolution over a 1-year follow-up, extracted from frequent MRI using methods of time series analysis (Meier and Guttmann, 2003). Lesion appearance and resolution are shown on a single slice of a proton-density weighted scan, with temporal profiles extracted for three regions of interest (ROI 1-3). Note the partial and full recovery in central and peripheral parts of the lesion, respectively.

Analogous suggestions arise from serial MTR studies, in that the balance between de- and regenerative processes appears to be tipped in the early stages of lesion formation. Global disease severity is therefore composed of lesions with different levels of destructive character. The poor correlation between T2 lesion load and atrophy is partly explained by these facts, i.e., (1) only a portion of the visible lesion is indeed responsible for tissue destruction, (2) tissue destruction is subject to hysteresis, and (3) diffuse disease (NAWM) also leads to atrophy by routes not captured in lesion burden metrics.

Histopathologic analysis identified about half of all T2 hyperintense WMSA as active lesions, including lesions without demyelination but with edema and gliosis (De Groot et al., 2001). This matches our own observations, that approximately half of T2 lesions in RR represent transient and potentially reversible WM changes (Fig. 13).

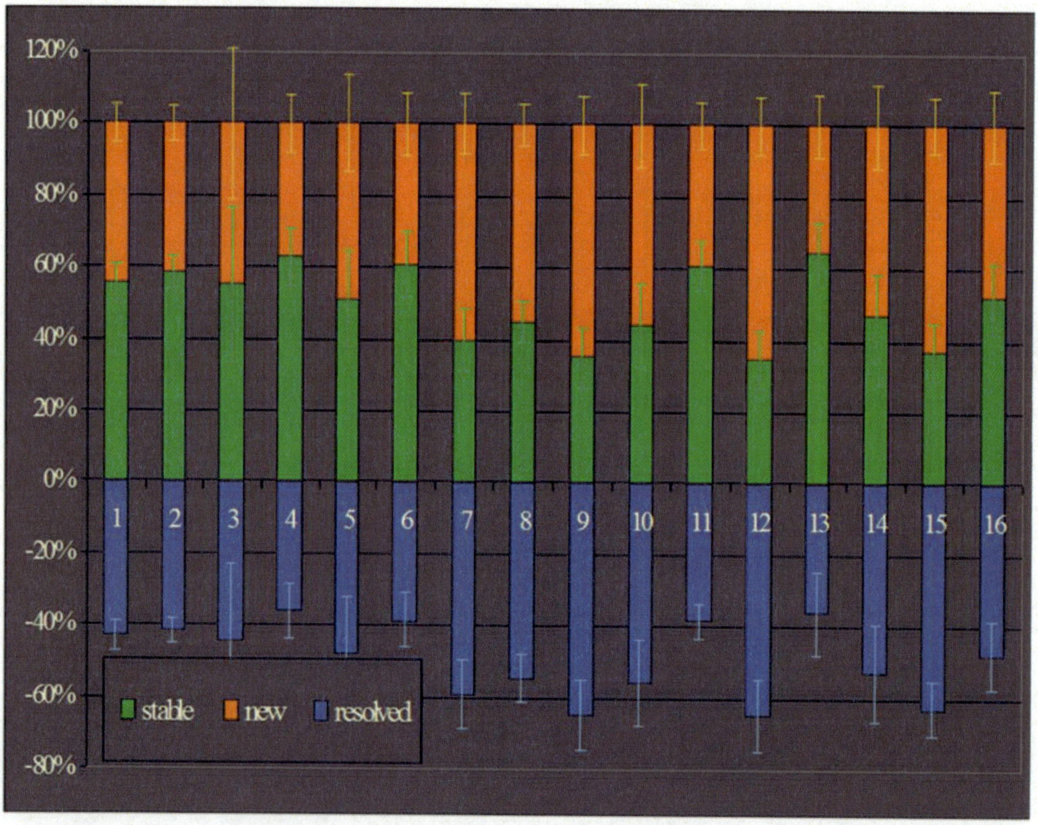

Fig 13. Examples of 'Differential Morphometry' applied to serial MRI of T2 lesion burden. Shown are average normalized volumes of lesion burden from 16 MS patients followed over a 1-year period. Total lesion burden in each successive image pair was classified as stable, new/enlarging or resolving. Results suggest that more than half of the total lesion burden captured at an individual time point can express transient "turnover" volume of either new/enlarging or resolving lesions. Global rates of lesion burden in longitudinal studies may obscure this fact and drastically underestimate the amount of disease activity.

Temporal dissociations therefore shed new light on alleged pathological specificity (Fig 14). If T2 lesions in early disease reflect mostly inflammation but in later stages shift to degeneration, then disease duration becomes a significant confounder, as age and disease duration are in global atrophy. In other words, T2 lesions at onset (CIS, RR) may be more of a surrogate for disease activity than for severity. Similar conclusions arise from the data of a large long-term follow-up study, where the development of clinically definite MS was tightly associated with the presence of any T2 lesion but not with the actual number or volume. The percentage of patients developing clinically definite MS with zero baseline T2 lesions was 19% vs. 88% for any >1, irrespective of how many (Brex et al., 2002). Similarly, the presence of any T1-Gd lesions was associated with comparatively smaller supratentorial (p=0.02) and infratentorial (p=0.002) brain volumes (Lin and Blumhardt, 2001).

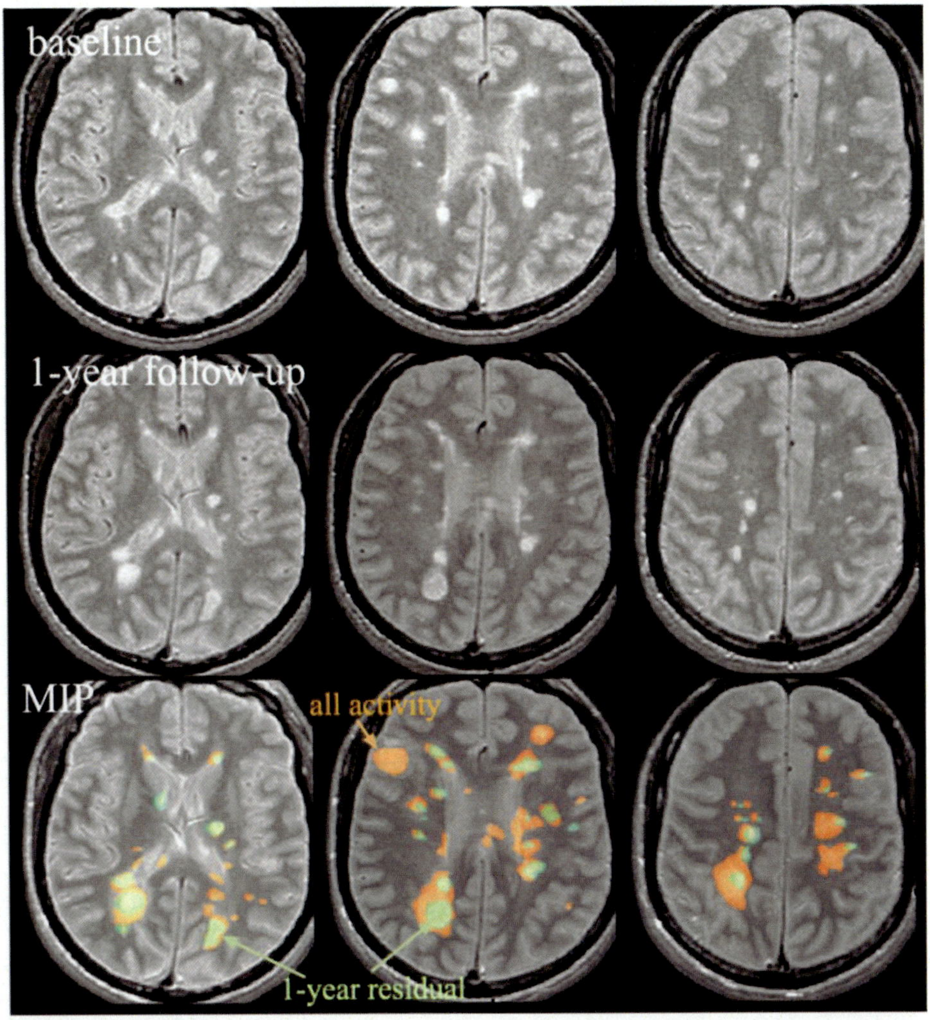

Fig 14. Example of integrated T2 lesion distribution by maximum intensity projection (MIP). top row: baseline exam, middle row: last exam after 1-year follow-up, bottom-row: MIP image showing all T2 activity over the follow-up period, integrated from 24 weekly to monthly MRIs. Residual lesion activity at 1-year is shown in green, integrated activity from past time points in orange. The MIP integrates all lesion accrual over the follow-up period to give direct view of the disease activity, thereby accounting for the transient nature of a T2 lesion.

Dissociations and the Clinico-Radiological Paradox

The lack of correlation of many MRI markers with clinical measures is also due, at least in part, to a substantial lack of specificity and sensitivity of many forms of clinical evaluations. The "targeted neurological deficit (TND)" is an outcome measure used in a few MS clinical trials. In contrast to standard batteries of assessing disability, the TND strategy first identifies a specific neurological deficit as relevant (e.g., a specific motor or sensory impairment, such as left leg weakness), and then serially evaluates this a priori defined feature in a longitudinal study. This focus on a specific deficit provides greatly enhanced sensitivity (Rudick et al., 1996; Rudick et al., 1997) and would be a good match with focal MRI morphometry such as regional atrophy (Bakshi et al., 2001b; Benedict et al., 2002; Sailer et al., 2003; Zivadinov et al., 2003) or regional lesion load (Feinstein et al., 2004; Sperling et al., 2001). Post-mortem studies further indicated smaller axons to be disproportionately more affected compared to larger ones (Ganter et al., 1999). This is one possible explanation for the clinico-radiological paradox (Barkhof, 2002), since small fibers may nevertheless be responsible for critical functions, and the validity of direct linear correlations between disability and atrophy is questioned further.

Global atrophy measures such as the BPF chiefly measure WM changes, which in turn are dominated by ventricular enlargement. Hence the contribution of global GM atrophy to the BPF is difficult to assess. It is important to realize that findings attributing brain parenchymal volume loss predominantly to white matter (Ge et al., 2001) are not to be equated with an analogous prevalence of disease activity. While GM involvement is more difficult to capture and normalize, it was conclusively demonstrated from post mortem histology (Peterson et al., 2001) (Kidd et al., 1999) and also recently identified from high-resolution MRI (Sailer et al., 2003). The latter showed cortical thinning only after 3 years disease duration, whereas WM atrophy (central) appears to occur early after onset (Chard et al., 2002c; De Stefano et al., 2003; Luks et al., 2000). This suggests that GM and WM atrophy occur at different rates, phases and relative amounts and hence require different approaches to measurement.

Effects on tissue volume may arise not only from axonal loss, but also from glial cell proliferation, inflammation and edema. Astrocytosis and edema have positive mass effects, whereas isomorphic gliosis may result in negative mass effect (Miller et al., 2002). Such confounders may be addressed directly by deformation analysis from short-term frequent MRI or indirectly by exploiting the fact that different morphological MRI variables express different levels of sensitivity to mass effects.

Normalization in brain volumetry is required to address both normal anatomical variance as well as normal aging effects. Different reference structures have been suggested, including the scalp (Freeborough and Fox, 1997), the smoothed outer brain contour (Rudick et al., 1999) , and the intracranial cavity (Chard et al., 2002c; Guttmann et al., 2000; Whitwell et al., 2001).

Normalization with time is not less complex, since atrophy rates, both normal and pathologically accelerated, likely are nonlinear. Different rates of infratentorial atrophy were observed in SP and RR (Liu et al., 1999). In the spinal cord, however, reversed rates were seen with SP atrophy less than with PP or benign MS (Stevenson et al., 1998). If we consider atrophy as a combination of primary and secondary processes, the dynamics and spatiotemporal idiosyncrasies of observed parenchymal loss can be expected to exhibit a highly complex pattern, complicating conclusions from cross-sectional studies. A slowing of atrophy rates was observed with progressing disease, which may be accounted for by de facto slowing of tissue destruction (due to either normal aging or MS pathology) or delayed treatment effects (Fisher et al., 2002). Discussion has reemerged regarding the different specificity of MRI metrics assessing diffuse and focal disease. One of the principal values of MRI's in vivo capability is to elucidate how the two processes relate to each other. Are both the same process and the observed dissociations merely a sensitivity issue? Is one a cause or consequence of the other? Do they represent different processes entirely? As we begin to understand that the dynamics of MS expressed in MRI as well as clinical variables are highly nonlinear and variable, it becomes apparent that the knowledge we gain from direct correlations between diffuse and focal disease surrogates can be marginal at best. More comprehensive models and longitudinal studies are required. Such nonlinear effects can become particularly perilous when trying to make conclusions about longitudinal relations from cross-sectional studies. For example, the estimated atrophy rates in normal aging and MS are derived from cross-sectional analysis and their accuracy is consequently reduced. This applies to the entire spectrum of quantitative MRI. Reported significant differences in morphometric variables from cross-sectional comparison do not necessarily translate to longitudinal models and individual assessment. The more complex the mechanism, the greater the danger of misinterpretation.

Conclusions

A summary of the discussed MRI variables and how they relate to atrophy is shown in Table 2. Although no single MRI variable reaches outstanding specificity to a particular pathological process involved in parenchymal degeneration, it appears that there is substantial information to be gained by exploiting their complementary nature and different sensitivities. A next generation of quantitative MRI assessment should therefore take advantage of the potential of MRI to provide multidimensional data. This includes multidimensional decision and classification systems that depart from the concept that tries to combine multiple parameters into a single index. The same applies to clinical evaluation, where the integration of multiple metrics into a single index, such as EDSS, is simplifying the analysis at the cost of specificity.

Selection and design of a multi-parametric MRI coverage/assessment would appear most effective if done with the target of maximizing dissociating qualities of different variables. Hence, the most complementary/synergistic MRI variables are likely those which cancel or isolate individual aspects of pathology that are most critical in disease monitoring and therapy evaluation, i.e., selecting the puzzle pieces leading to a more complete picture (Fig. 15). For example, reports claim that NAA is primarily sensitive to axonal loss, whereas MTI captures demyelination. It seems feasible that atrophy studies in synergy with such combined measures could further elucidate the principal contributors to parenchymal volume loss.

Table 2. Overview of discussed MRI metrics and their relation to atrophy. d/f = diffuse/focal measure.

Variable	f/d	MRI Mechanism	Atrophy Relation	*Pathological Significance*	*Clinical Significance*	*Reference*
T2 lesions	f	T2 prolongation by added water, tissue density loss or tissue composition change	indirect: chronic lesions indicate focal tissue matrix/density loss	non-specific (inflammation, demyelination, axonal loss, gliosis) enlarging T2 lesion associates with inflammation & active disease	significant predictor for diagnosis, less for evaluating disease progression or disability	(Chard et al., 2003; Chard et al., 2002b; Liu et al., 1999; Moore et al., 2000; Rudick et al., 2000; Sailer et al., 2001; Stevenson et al., 2000; van Walderveen et al., 1998)
T2 diffuse GM hypointensity	d	signal spoiling by iron deposition	diffuse tissue matrix/density loss, correlated with 3rd ventricle width	indicates cytotoxic environment, apoptosis precursor	predictor of clinical progression	(Bakshi et al., 2002; Bakshi et al., 2001c)
T1 black holes	f	T1 change by added water, tissue density loss or tissue composition change. T1 is more specific to tissue quality change than T2.	direct: demyelination, tissue matrix/density loss	focal tissue destruction by demyelination or axonal loss (except acute hypointense T1 may be edema associated with inflammation)	surrogate of irreversible neurodegeneration, used as secondary outcome in phase III trials,	(Barkhof et al., 2001; Bitsch et al., 2001; Chard et al., 2002c; Truyen et al., 1996; van Walderveen et al., 1998)
T1 Gd enhancing lesions	f	blood-brain-barrier breakdown, contrast-mediated spoiling of T1	indirect: transient swelling by edema, subsequent focal tissue loss, small volume	inflammation, active disease, beginning of degenerative cascade	indicates active disease, transient, some lesions recover w/o visible permanent damage; high clinical specificity and sensitivity to treatment with immuno-modulatory mechanisms	(Bruck et al., 1997; Cotton et al., 2003; Fisher et al., 2002; Paolillo et al., 1999; Simon et al., 2000)

Table 3. Continued.

Variable	f/d	MRI Mechanism	Atrophy Relation	*Pathological Significance*	*Clinical Significance*	*Reference*
MTI	d	saturation of proton-bound water, transfer of off-resonance saturation	direct: demyelination, tissue matrix/density loss	macromolecular density, demyelination and axonal loss	partly predictive of clinical evolution, and conversion from CIS to clinically definite MS.	(Cercignani et al., 2000; Comi et al., 1999; Dousset et al., 1998; Leary et al., 1999; Santos et al., 2002; Silver et al., 1998)
DTI	f,d	additional gradient-induced directional encoding of diffusion rates, relates to tissue anisotropy	direct: demyelination, axonal loss	WM fiber tracking, tissue density loss, replaced by water/CSF	correlations with disability and disease duration	(Bammer et al., 2000; De Stefano et al., 2002; Filippi et al., 2001)
MRS	d,f	metabolite concentration measure, chemical shift, low SNR	direct: axonal loss in lesions and NAWM, not purely structural, NAA levels correlate with brain volume	surrogate for axonal loss and/or dysfunction, chronic/transient changes in metabolic environment, other metabolites give access to study individual pathological mechanism components	compound of neuronal dysfunction and degeneration,	(Bitsch et al., 1999; Brex et al., 1999; De Stefano et al., 1995; Fu et al., 1998; Kapeller et al., 2001)

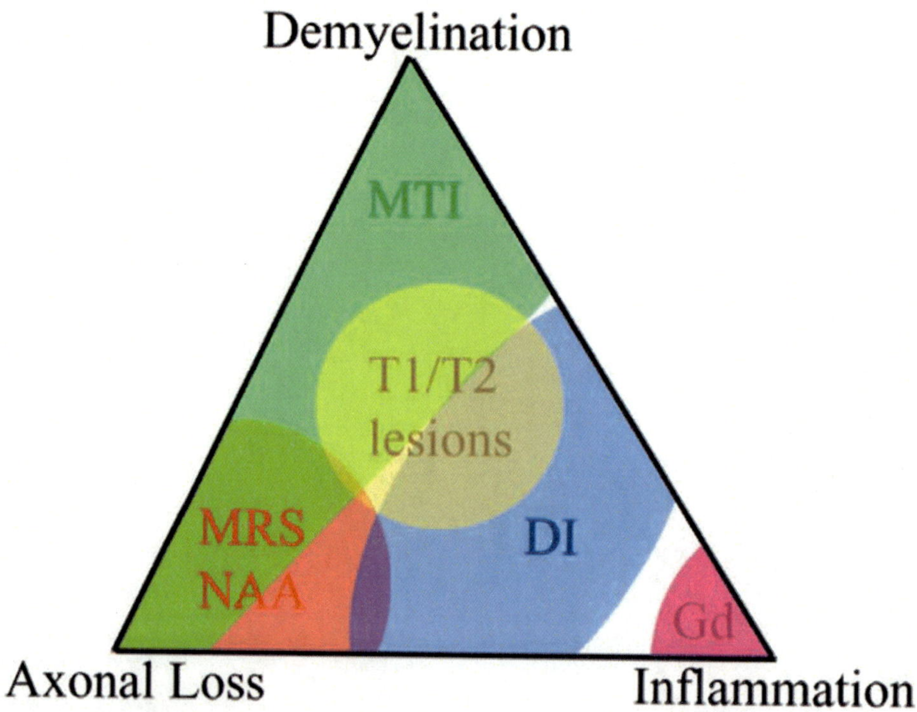

Fig 15. Triad of pathological processes and the overlapping and complementary MRI surrogates. Currently all available MRI surrogates express collective sensitivity to the principal underlying pathogenic mechanisms, but recent findings suggest that they nevertheless are more sensitive toward one process than another, which carries potential in their application as complementary and mutually dissociative measures (MRS:NAA Spectroscopy; MTI=magnetization transfer imaging, DI=diffusion imaging, Gd=Gd-contrast enhancing lesions).

The complexity of MS also calls for a dynamic assignment of relevance for different MRI surrogates. T1-Gd performs better than clinical disability as a primary outcome in early disease stages, whereas metrics pertaining to tissue damage and loss become more relevant in long-term evaluation or in later stages of MS. MRI is established as more sensitive and precise than clinical measures, apparent from smaller sample sizes for MRI trials (Sormani et al., 2001; Tubridy et al., 1998). MRI is also likely to establish better pathological specificity because it provides a direct look at structure without the distorting overlay of function.

Considering the highly dynamic and possibly nonlinear characteristic of this disease, direct correlations among different markers should also be interpreted carefully. How meaningful is a direct correlation of r=0.48 between T1 lesion burden and supratentorial brain volume? When comparing nonlinear systems by direct linear correlations, residual correlation will arise from the fact that the two variables compared depend at different levels on a third, which in MS is most predominantly time and disease duration.

References

Adams CWP. *A colour atlas of multiple sclerosis and other myelin disorders*. London: Wolfe, 1989.

Allen IV, McQuaid S, Mirakhur M, Nevin G. Pathological abnormalities in the normal-appearing white matter in multiple sclerosis. *Neurol Sci* 2001; 22: 141-4.

Arnold DL, Matthews PM, Francis GS, O'Connor J, Antel JP. Proton magnetic resonance spectroscopic imaging for metabolic characterization of demyelinating plaques. *Ann Neurol* 1992; 31: 235-41.

Bakshi R, Ariyaratana S, Benedict RH, Jacobs L. Fluid-attenuated inversion recovery magnetic resonance imaging detects cortical and juxtacortical multiple sclerosis lesions. *Arch Neurol* 2001a; 58: 742-8.

Bakshi R, Benedict RH, Bermel RA, Caruthers SD, Puli SR, Tjoa CW, et al. T2 hypointensity in the deep gray matter of patients with multiple sclerosis: a quantitative magnetic resonance imaging study. *Arch Neurol* 2002; 59: 62-8.

Bakshi R, Benedict RH, Bermel RA, Jacobs L. Regional brain atrophy is associated with physical disability in multiple sclerosis: semiquantitative magnetic resonance imaging and relationship to clinical findings. *J Neuroimaging* 2001b; 11: 129-36.

Bakshi R, Dmochowski J, Shaikh ZA, Jacobs L. Gray matter T2 hypointensity is related to plaques and atrophy in the brains of multiple sclerosis patients. *J Neurol Sci* 2001c; 185: 19-26.

Bakshi R, Shaikh ZA, Janardhan V. MRI T2 shortening ('black T2') in multiple sclerosis: frequency, location, and clinical correlation. *Neuroreport* 2000; 11: 15-21.

Bammer R, Augustin M, Strasser-Fuchs S, Seifert T, Kapeller P, Stollberger R, et al. Magnetic resonance diffusion tensor imaging for characterizing diffuse and focal white matter abnormalities in multiple sclerosis. *Magn Reson Med* 2000; 44: 583-91.

Barkhof F. The clinico-radiological paradox in multiple sclerosis revisited. *Curr Opin Neurol* 2002; 15: 239-45.

Barkhof F, van Waesberghe JH, Filippi M, Yousry T, Miller DH, Hahn D, et al. T(1) hypointense lesions in secondary progressive multiple sclerosis: effect of interferon beta-1b treatment. *Brain* 2001; 124: 1396-402.

Benedict RH, Bakshi R, Simon JH, Priore R, Miller C, Munschauer F. Frontal cortex atrophy predicts cognitive impairment in multiple sclerosis. *J Neuropsychiatry Clin Neurosci* 2002; 14: 44-51.

Bermel RA, Puli SR, Fabiano AJ, Fisher E, Rudick RA, Weinstock-Guttman B, Simon JH, Munschauer FE, Bakshi R. Gray matter T2 hypointensity predicts longitudinal brain atrophy in multiple sclerosis: effect of intramuscular interferon beta-1a treatment (abstract). 2003 annual meeting of the American Academy of Neurology - Honolulu, HI. *Neurology 2003; 60*(suppl. 1): A422.

Bitsch A, Bruhn H, Vougioukas V, Stringaris A, Lassmann H, Frahm J, et al. Inflammatory CNS demyelination: histopathologic correlation with in vivo quantitative proton MR spectroscopy. *AJNR Am J Neuroradiol* 1999; 20: 1619-27.

Bitsch A, Kuhlmann T, Stadelmann C, Lassmann H, Lucchinetti C, Bruck W. A longitudinal MRI study of histopathologically defined hypointense multiple sclerosis lesions. *Ann Neurol* 2001; 49: 793-6.

Bjartmar C, Kidd G, Mork S, Rudick R, Trapp BD. Neurological disability correlates with spinal cord axonal loss and reduced N-acetyl aspartate in chronic multiple sclerosis patients. *Ann Neurol* 2000; 48: 893-901.

Bo L, Vedeler CA, Nyland H, Trapp BD, Mork SJ. Intracortical multiple sclerosis lesions are not associated with increased lymphocyte infiltration. *Mult Scler* 2003; 9: 323-31.

Bonatz H, Rohrig S, Mestres P, Meyer M, Giehl KM. An axotomy model for the induction of death of rat and mouse corticospinal neurons in vivo. *J Neurosci Methods* 2000; 100: 105-15.

Brex PA, Ciccarelli O, O'Riordan JI, Sailer M, Thompson AJ, Miller DH. A longitudinal study of abnormalities on MRI and disability from multiple sclerosis. *N Engl J Med* 2002; 346: 158-64.

Brex PA, Gomez-Anson B, Parker GJ, Molyneux PD, Miszkiel KA, Barker GJ, et al. Proton MR spectroscopy in clinically isolated syndromes suggestive of multiple sclerosis. *J Neurol Sci* 1999; 166: 16-22.

Brex PA, Jenkins R, Fox NC, Crum WR, O'Riordan JI, Plant GT, et al. Detection of ventricular enlargement in patients at the earliest clinical stage of MS. *Neurology* 2000; 54: 1689-91.

Brex PA, Leary SM, Plant GT, Thompson AJ, Miller DH. Magnetization transfer imaging in patients with clinically isolated syndromes suggestive of multiple sclerosis. *AJNR Am J Neuroradiol* 2001; 22: 947-51.

Bruck W, Bitsch A, Kolenda H, Bruck Y, Stiefel M, Lassmann H. Inflammatory central nervous system demyelination: correlation of magnetic resonance imaging findings with lesion pathology. *Ann Neurol* 1997; 42: 783-93.

Cercignani M, Iannucci G, Rocca MA, Comi G, Horsfield MA, Filippi M. Pathologic damage in MS assessed by diffusion-weighted and magnetization transfer MRI. *Neurology* 2000; 54: 1139-44.

Chard DT, Brex PA, Ciccarelli O, Griffin CM, Parker GJ, Dalton C, et al. The longitudinal relation between brain lesion load and atrophy in multiple sclerosis: a 14 year follow up study. *J Neurol Neurosurg Psychiatry* 2003; 74: 1551-4.

Chard DT, Griffin CM, McLean MA, Kapeller P, Kapoor R, Thompson AJ, et al. Brain metabolite changes in cortical grey and normal-appearing white matter in clinically early relapsing-remitting multiple sclerosis. *Brain* 2002a; 125: 2342-52.

Chard DT, Griffin CM, Parker GJ, Kapoor R, Thompson AJ, Miller DH. Brain atrophy in clinically early relapsing-remitting multiple sclerosis. *Brain* 2002b; 125: 327-37.

Chard DT, Griffin CM, Parker GJ, Kapoor R, Thompson AJ, Miller DH. Brain atrophy in clinically early relapsing-remitting multiple sclerosis. *Brain* 2002c; 125: 327-37.

Coles AJ, Wing MG, Molyneux P, Paolillo A, Davie CM, Hale G, et al. Monoclonal antibody treatment exposes three mechanisms underlying the clinical course of multiple sclerosis. *Ann Neurol* 1999; 46: 296-304.

Comi G, Rovaris M, Falautano M, Santuccio G, Martinelli V, Rocca MA, et al. A multiparametric MRI study of frontal lobe dementia in multiple sclerosis. *J Neurol Sci* 1999; 171: 135-44.

Cotton F, Weiner HL, Jolesz FA, Guttmann CR. MRI contrast uptake in new lesions in relapsing-remitting MS followed at weekly intervals. *Neurology* 2003; 60: 640-6.

Davie CA, Barker GJ, Webb S, Tofts PS, Thompson AJ, Harding AE, et al. Persistent functional deficit in multiple sclerosis and autosomal dominant cerebellar ataxia is associated with axon loss. *Brain* 1995; 118: 1583-92.

De Groot CJ, Bergers E, Kamphorst W, Ravid R, Polman CH, Barkhof F, et al. Post-mortem MRI-guided sampling of multiple sclerosis brain lesions: increased yield of active demyelinating and (p)reactive lesions. *Brain* 2001; 124: 1635-45.

De Stefano N, Iannucci G, Sormani MP, Guidi L, Bartolozzi ML, Comi G, et al. MR correlates of cerebral atrophy in patients with multiple sclerosis. *J Neurol* 2002; 249: 1072-7.

De Stefano N, Matthews PM, Arnold DL. Reversible decreases in N-acetylaspartate after acute brain injury. *Magn Reson Med* 1995; 34: 721-7.

De Stefano N, Matthews PM, Filippi M, Agosta F, De Luca M, Bartolozzi ML, et al. Evidence of early cortical atrophy in MS: relevance to white matter changes and disability. *Neurology* 2003; 60: 1157-62.

De Stefano N, Narayanan S, Francis GS, Arnaoutelis R, Tartaglia MC, Antel JP, et al. Evidence of axonal damage in the early stages of multiple sclerosis and its relevance to disability. *Arch Neurol* 2001; 58: 65-70.

Dousset V, Gayou A, Brochet B, Caille JM. Early structural changes in acute MS lesions assessed by serial magnetization transfer studies. *Neurology* 1998; 51: 1150-5.

Drayer B, Burger P, Hurwitz B, Dawson D, Cain J. Reduced signal intensity on MR images of thalamus and putamen in multiple sclerosis: increased iron content? *AJR Am J Roentgenol* 1987; 149: 357-63.

Evangelou N, Esiri MM, Smith S, Palace J, Matthews PM. Quantitative pathological evidence for axonal loss in normal appearing white matter in multiple sclerosis. *Ann Neurol* 2000; 47: 391-5.

Evangelou N, Konz D, Esiri MM, Smith S, Palace J, Matthews PM. Size-selective neuronal changes in the anterior optic pathways suggest a differential susceptibility to injury in multiple sclerosis. *Brain* 2001; 124: 1813-20.

Falini A, Calabrese G, Filippi M, Origgi D, Lipari S, Colombo B, et al. Benign versus secondary-progressive multiple sclerosis: the potential role of proton MR spectroscopy in defining the nature of disability. *AJNR Am J Neuroradiol* 1998; 19: 223-9.

Feinstein A, Roy P, Lobaugh N, Feinstein K, O'Connor P, Black S. Structural brain abnormalities in multiple sclerosis patients with major depression. *Neurology* 2004; 62: 586-90.

Filippi M, Cercignani M, Inglese M, Horsfield MA, Comi G. Diffusion tensor magnetic resonance imaging in multiple sclerosis. *Neurology* 2001; 56: 304-11.

Filippi M, Inglese M, Rovaris M, Sormani MP, Horsfield P, Iannucci PG, et al. Magnetization transfer imaging to monitor the evolution of MS: a 1-year follow-up study. *Neurology* 2000; 55: 940-6.

Fischl B, Dale AM. Measuring the thickness of the human cerebral cortex from magnetic resonance images. *Proc Natl Acad Sci USA* 2000; 97: 11050-5.

Fisher E, Rudick RA, Simon JH, Cutter G, Baier M, Lee JC, et al. Eight-year follow-up study of brain atrophy in patients with MS. *Neurology* 2002; 59: 1412-20.

Freeborough PA, Fox NC. The boundary shift integral: an accurate and robust measure of cerebral volume changes from registered repeat MRI. *IEEE Trans Med Imaging* 1997; 16: 623-9.

Fu L, Matthews PM, De Stefano N, Worsley KJ, Narayanan S, Francis GS, et al. Imaging axonal damage of normal-appearing white matter in multiple sclerosis. *Brain* 1998; 121: 103-13.

Ganter P, Prince C, Esiri MM. Spinal cord axonal loss in multiple sclerosis: a post-mortem study. *Neuropathol Appl Neurobiol* 1999; 25: 459-67.

Ge Y, Grossman RI, Udupa JK, Babb JS, Nyul LG, Kolson DL. Brain atrophy in relapsing-remitting multiple sclerosis: fractional volumetric analysis of gray matter and white matter. *Radiology* 2001; 220: 606-10.

Ge Y, Grossman RI, Udupa JK, Wei L, Mannon LJ, Polansky M, et al. Brain atrophy in relapsing-remitting multiple sclerosis and secondary progressive multiple sclerosis: longitudinal quantitative analysis. *Radiology* 2000; 214: 665-70.

Grossman RI. Magnetization transfer in multiple sclerosis. *Ann Neurol* 1994; 36 Suppl: S97-9.

Grossman RI, Gomori JM, Ramer KN, Lexa FJ, Schnall MD. Magnetization transfer: theory and clinical applications in neuroradiology. *Radiographics* 1994; 14: 279-90.

Guttmann CR, Ahn SS, Hsu L, Kikinis R, Jolesz FA. The evolution of multiple sclerosis lesions on serial MR. *AJNR Am J Neuroradiol* 1995a; 16: 1481-91.

Guttmann CR, Ahn SS, Hsu L, Kikinis R, Jolesz FA. The evolution of multiple sclerosis lesions on serial MR. *AJNR Am J Neuroradiol* 1995b; 16: 1481-91.

Guttmann CR, Warfield SK, Guimond A, Kikinis R, Albert MS, Jolesz FA. Variability of brain atrophy estimates in multiple sclerosis (abstract). *Proc Int Soc Magn Reson Med* 2000; 8: 1188.

Hardmeier M, Wagenpfeil S, Freitag P, Fisher E, Rudick RA, Kooijmans-Coutinho M, et al. Atrophy is detectable within a 3-month period in untreated patients with active relapsing remitting multiple sclerosis. *Arch Neurol* 2003; 60: 1736-9.

Helms G. Volume correction for edema in single-volume proton MR spectroscopy of contrast-enhancing multiple sclerosis lesions. *Magn Reson Med* 2001; 46: 256-63.

Hiehle JF, Jr., Grossman RI, Ramer KN, Gonzalez-Scarano F, Cohen JA. Magnetization transfer effects in MR-detected multiple sclerosis lesions: comparison with gadolinium-enhanced spin-echo images and nonenhanced T1-weighted images. *AJNR Am J Neuroradiol* 1995; 16: 69-77.

Hiehle JF, Jr., Lenkinski RE, Grossman RI, Dousset V, Ramer KN, Schnall MD, et al. Correlation of spectroscopy and magnetization transfer imaging in the evaluation of demyelinating lesions and normal appearing white matter in multiple sclerosis. *Magn Reson Med* 1994; 32: 285-93.

Horsfield MA, Rovaris M, Rocca MA, Rossi P, Benedict RH, Filippi M, et al. Whole-brain atrophy in multiple sclerosis measured by two segmentation processes from various MRI sequences. *J Neurol Sci* 2003; 216: 169-77.

Husted CA, Goodin DS, Hugg JW, Maudsley AA, Tsuruda JS, de Bie SH, et al. Biochemical alterations in multiple sclerosis lesions and normal-appearing white matter detected by in vivo 31P and 1H spectroscopic imaging. *Ann Neurol* 1994; 36: 157-65.

Iannucci G, Tortorella C, Rovaris M, Sormani MP, Comi G, Filippi M. Prognostic value of MR and magnetization transfer imaging findings in patients with clinically isolated syndromes suggestive of multiple sclerosis at presentation. *AJNR Am J Neuroradiol* 2000; 21: 1034-8.

Kalkers NF, Ameziane N, Bot JC, Minneboo A, Polman CH, Barkhof F. Longitudinal brain volume measurement in multiple sclerosis: rate of brain atrophy is independent of the disease subtype. *Arch Neurol* 2002; 59: 1572-6.

Kalkers NF, Hintzen RQ, van Waesberghe JH, Lazeron RH, van Schijndel RA, Ader HJ, et al. Magnetization transfer histogram parameters reflect all dimensions of MS pathology, including atrophy. *J Neurol Sci* 2001; 184: 155-62.

Kapeller P, McLean MA, Griffin CM, Chard D, Parker GJ, Barker GJ, et al. Preliminary evidence for neuronal damage in cortical grey matter and normal appearing white matter in short duration relapsing-remitting multiple sclerosis: a quantitative MR spectroscopic imaging study. *J Neurol* 2001; 248: 131-8.

Kidd D, Barkhof F, McConnell R, Algra PR, Allen IV, Revesz T. Cortical lesions in multiple sclerosis. *Brain* 1999; 122: 17-26.

Kikinis R, Guttmann CR, Metcalf D, Wells WM, 3rd, Ettinger GJ, Weiner HL, et al. Quantitative follow-up of patients with multiple sclerosis using MRI: technical aspects. *J Magn Reson Imaging* 1999; 9: 519-30.

Kikinis R, Shenton ME, Gerig G, Martin J, Anderson M, Metcalf D, et al. Routine quantitative analysis of brain and cerebrospinal fluid spaces with MR imaging. *J Magn Reson Imaging* 1992; 2: 619-29.

Kimura H, Meaney DF, McGowan JC, Grossman RI, Lenkinski RE, Ross DT, et al. Magnetization transfer imaging of diffuse axonal injury following experimental brain injury in the pig: characterization by magnetization transfer ratio with histopathologic correlation. *J Comput Assist Tomogr* 1996; 20: 540-6.

Kucharczyk W, Macdonald PM, Stanisz GJ, Henkelman RM. Relaxivity and magnetization transfer of white matter lipids at MR imaging: importance of cerebrosides and pH. *Radiology* 1994; 192: 521-9.

Leary SM, Brex PA, MacManus DG, Parker GJ, Barker GJ, Miller DH, et al. A (1)H magnetic resonance spectroscopy study of aging in parietal white matter: implications for trials in multiple sclerosis. *Magn Reson Imaging* 2000; 18: 455-9.

Leary SM, Silver NC, Stevenson VL, Barker GJ, Miller DH, Thompson AJ. Magnetisation transfer of normal appearing white matter in primary progressive multiple sclerosis. *Mult Scler* 1999; 5: 313-6.

Lee MA, Smith S, Palace J, Matthews PM. Defining multiple sclerosis disease activity using MRI T2-weighted difference imaging. *Brain* 1998; 12: 2095-102.

Leist TP, Gobbini MI, Frank JA, McFarland HF. Enhancing magnetic resonance imaging lesions and cerebral atrophy in patients with relapsing multiple sclerosis. *Arch Neurol* 2001; 58: 57-60.

Lin X, Blumhardt LD. Inflammation and atrophy in multiple sclerosis: MRI associations with disease course. *J Neurol S*ci 2001; 189: 99-104.

Liu C, Edwards S, Gong Q, Roberts N, Blumhardt LD. Three dimensional MRI estimates of brain and spinal cord atrophy in multiple sclerosis. *J Neurol Neurosurg Psychiatry* 1999; 66: 323-30.

Luks TL, Goodkin DE, Nelson SJ, Majumdar S, Bacchetti P, Portnoy D, et al. A longitudinal study of ventricular volume in early relapsing-remitting multiple sclerosis. *Mult Scler* 2000; 6: 332-7.

Lycklama a Nijeholt GJ, Castelijns JA, Lazeron RH, van Waesberghe JH, Polman CH, Uitdehaag BM, et al. Magnetization transfer ratio of the spinal cord in multiple sclerosis: relationship to atrophy and neurologic disability. *J Neuroimaging* 2000; 10: 67-72.

Mader I, Roser W, Kappos L, Hagberg G, Seelig J, Radue EW, et al. Serial proton MR spectroscopy of contrast-enhancing multiple sclerosis plaques: absolute metabolic values over 2 years during a clinical pharmacological study. *AJNR Am J Neuroradiol* 2000; 21: 1220-7.

Mader I, Seeger U, Weissert R, Klose U, Naegele T, Melms A, et al. Proton MR spectroscopy with metabolite-nulling reveals elevated macromolecules in acute multiple sclerosis. *Brain* 2001; 124: 953-61.

Manger PR, Woods TM, Jones EG. Plasticity of the somatosensory cortical map in macaque monkeys after chronic partial amputation of a digit. *Proc R Soc Lond B Biol Sci* 1996; 263: 933-9.

Matthews PM, Pioro E, Narayanan S, De Stefano N, Fu L, Francis G, et al. Assessment of lesion pathology in multiple sclerosis using quantitative MRI morphometry and magnetic resonance spectroscopy. *Brain* 1996; 119: 715-22.

McDonald WI, Compston A, Edan G, Goodkin D, Hartung HP, Lublin FD, et al. Recommended diagnostic criteria for multiple sclerosis: guidelines from the International Panel on the diagnosis of multiple sclerosis. *Ann Neurol* 2001; 50: 121-7.

Mehta RC, Pike GB, Enzmann DR. Measure of magnetization transfer in multiple sclerosis demyelinating plaques, white matter ischemic lesions, and edema. *AJNR Am J Neuroradiol* 1996; 17: 1051-5.

Meier DS, Guttmann CR. Time-series analysis of MRI intensity patterns in multiple sclerosis. *Neuroimage* 2003; 20: 1193-209.

Merzenich MM, Nelson RJ, Stryker MP, Cynader MS, Schoppmann A, Zook JM. Somatosensory cortical map changes following digit amputation in adult monkeys. *J Comp Neurol* 1984; 224: 591-605.

Miller DH, Barkhof F, Frank JA, Parker GJ, Thompson AJ. Measurement of atrophy in multiple sclerosis: pathological basis, methodological aspects and clinical relevance. *Brain* 2002; 125: 1676-95.

Moore GR, Leung E, MacKay AL, Vavasour IM, Whittall KP, Cover KS, et al. A pathology-MRI study of the short-T2 component in formalin-fixed multiple sclerosis brain. *Neurology* 2000; 55: 1506-10.

Mugler JP, 3rd, Bao S, Mulkern RV, Guttmann CR, Robertson RL, Jolesz FA, et al. Optimized single-slab three-dimensional spin-echo MR imaging of the brain. *Radiology* 2000; 216: 891-9.

Narayana PA, Doyle TJ, Lai D, Wolinsky JS. Serial proton magnetic resonance spectroscopic imaging, contrast-enhanced magnetic resonance imaging, and quantitative lesion volumetry in multiple sclerosis. *Ann Neurol* 1998; 43: 56-71.

Paolillo A, Coles AJ, Molyneux PD, Gawne-Cain M, MacManus D, Barker GJ, et al. Quantitative MRI in patients with secondary progressive MS treated with monoclonal antibody Campath 1H. *Neurology* 1999; 53: 751-7.

Paolillo A, Pozzilli C, Gasperini C, Giugni E, Mainero C, Giuliani S, et al. Brain atrophy in relapsing-remitting multiple sclerosis: relationship with 'black holes', disease duration and clinical disability. *J Neurol Sci* 2000; 174: 85-91.

Pelletier D, Nelson SJ, Oh J, Antel JP, Kita M, Zamvil SS, et al. MRI lesion volume heterogeneity in primary progressive MS in relation with axonal damage and brain atrophy. *J Neurol Neurosurg Psychiatry* 2003; 74: 950-2.

Pelletier J, Suchet L, Witjas T, Habib M, Guttmann CR, Salamon G, et al. A longitudinal study of callosal atrophy and interhemispheric dysfunction in relapsing-remitting multiple sclerosis. *Arch Ne*urol 2001; 58: 105-11.

Peterson JW, Bo L, Mork S, Chang A, Trapp BD. Transected neurites, apoptotic neurons, and reduced inflammation in cortical multiple sclerosis lesions. *Ann Neurol* 2001; 50: 389-400.

Pierpaoli C, Barnett A, Pajevic S, Chen R, Penix LR, Virta A, et al. Water diffusion changes in Wallerian degeneration and their dependence on white matter architecture. *Neuroimage* 2001; 13: 1174-85.

Qian ZM, Shen X. Brain iron transport and neurodegeneration. *Trends Mol Med* 2001; 7: 103-8.

Quarantelli M, Ciarmiello A, Morra VB, Orefice G, Larobina M, Lanzillo R, et al. Brain tissue volume changes in relapsing-remitting multiple sclerosis: correlation with lesion load. *Neuroimage* 2003; 18: 360-6.

Rao SM, Glatt S, Hammeke TA, McQuillen MP, Khatri BO, Rhodes AM, et al. Chronic progressive multiple sclerosis. Relationship between cerebral ventricular size and neuropsychological impairment. *Arch Neurol* 1985; 42: 678-82.

Redmond IT, Barbosa S, Blumhardt LD, Roberts N. Short-term ventricular volume changes on serial MRI in multiple sclerosis. *Acta Neurol Scand* 2000; 102: 99-105.

Ropele S, Strasser-Fuchs S, Augustin M, Stollberger R, Enzinger C, Hartung HP, et al. A comparison of magnetization transfer ratio, magnetization transfer rate, and the native relaxation time of water protons related to relapsing-remitting multiple sclerosis. *AJNR Am J Neuroradiol* 2000; 21: 1885-91.

Rovaris M, Comi G, Rocca MA, Wolinsky JS, Filippi M. Short-term brain volume change in relapsing-remitting multiple sclerosis: effect of glatiramer acetate and implications. *Brain* 2001; 124: 1803-12.

Rovaris M, Filippi M. MRI correlates of cognitive dysfunction in multiple sclerosis patients. *J Neurovirol* 2000; 6 Suppl 2: S172-5.

Rovira A, Alonso J, Cucurella G, Nos C, Tintore M, Pedraza S, et al. Evolution of multiple sclerosis lesions on serial contrast-enhanced T1-weighted and magnetization-transfer MR images. *AJNR Am J Neuroradiol* 1999; 20: 1939-45.

Rudick R, Antel J, Confavreux C, Cutter G, Ellison G, Fischer J, et al. Clinical outcomes assessment in multiple sclerosis. *Ann Neurol* 1996; 40: 469-79.

Rudick R, Antel J, Confavreux C, Cutter G, Ellison G, Fischer J, et al. Recommendations from the National Multiple Sclerosis Society Clinical Outcomes Assessment Task Force. *Ann Neurol* 1997; 42: 379-82.

Rudick RA, Fisher E, Lee JC, Duda JT, Simon J. Brain atrophy in relapsing multiple sclerosis: relationship to relapses, EDSS, and treatment with interferon beta-1a. *Mult Scler* 2000; 6: 365-72.

Rudick RA, Fisher E, Lee JC, Simon J, Jacobs L. Use of the brain parenchymal fraction to measure whole brain atrophy in relapsing-remitting MS. Multiple Sclerosis Collaborative Research Group. *Neurology* 1999; 53: 1698-704.

Russo C, Smoker WR, Kubal W. Cortical and subcortical T2 shortening in multiple sclerosis. *AJNR Am J Neuroradiol* 1997; 18: 124-6.

Sailer M, Fischl B, Salat D, Tempelmann C, Schonfeld MA, Busa E, et al. Focal thinning of the cerebral cortex in multiple sclerosis. *Brain* 2003; 126: 1734-44.

Sailer M, Losseff NA, Wang L, Gawne-Cain ML, Thompson AJ, Miller DH. T1 lesion load and cerebral atrophy as a marker for clinical progression in patients with multiple sclerosis. A prospective 18 months follow-up study. *Eur J Neurol* 2001; 8: 37-42.

Saindane AM, Ge Y, Udupa JK, Babb JS, Mannon LJ, Grossman RI. The effect of gadolinium-enhancing lesions on whole brain atrophy in relapsing-remitting MS. *Neurology* 2000; 55: 61-5.

Santos AC, Narayanan S, de Stefano N, Tartaglia MC, Francis SJ, Arnaoutelis R, et al. Magnetization transfer can predict clinical evolution in patients with multiple sclerosis. *J Neurol* 2002; 249: 662-8.

Sharma R, Narayana PA, Wolinsky JS. Grey matter abnormalities in multiple sclerosis: proton magnetic resonance spectroscopic imaging. *Mult Scler* 2001; 7: 221-6.

Silver NC, Lai M, Symms MR, Barker GJ, McDonald WI, Miller DH. Serial magnetization transfer imaging to characterize the early evolution of new MS lesions. *Neurology* 1998; 51: 758-64.

Simon JH. From enhancing lesions to brain atrophy in relapsing MS. *J Neuroimmunol* 1999; 98: 7-15.

Simon JH, Jacobs LD, Campion MK, Rudick RA, Cookfair DL, Herndon RM, et al. A longitudinal study of brain atrophy in relapsing multiple sclerosis. The Multiple Sclerosis Collaborative Research Group (MSCRG). *Neurology* 1999; 53: 139-48.

Simon JH, Lull J, Jacobs LD, Rudick RA, Cookfair DL, Herndon RM, et al. A longitudinal study of T1 hypointense lesions in relapsing MS: MSCRG trial of interferon beta-1a. Multiple Sclerosis Collaborative Research Group. *Neurology* 2000; 55: 185-92.

Simon JH. In: Zivadinov R, Bakshi R, eds. *Brain and Spinal Cord Atrophy in Multiple Sclerosis. Linear and regional measures of brain atrophy in multiple sclerosis.* New York: Nova Science Publisher 2004 (in press).

Sormani MP, Miller DH, Comi G, Barkhof F, Rovaris M, Bruzzi P, et al. Clinical trials of multiple sclerosis monitored with enhanced MRI: new sample size calculations based on large data sets. *J Neurol Neurosurg Psychiatry* 2001; 70: 494-9.

Sperling RA, Guttmann CR, Hohol MJ, Warfield SK, Jakab M, Parente M, et al. Regional magnetic resonance imaging lesion burden and cognitive function in multiple sclerosis: a longitudinal study. *Arch Neurol* 2001; 58: 115-21.

Stevenson VL, Leary SM, Losseff NA, Parker GJ, Barker GJ, Husmani Y, et al. Spinal cord atrophy and disability in MS: a longitudinal study. *Neurology* 1998; 51: 234-8.

Stevenson VL, Parker GJ, Barker GJ, Birnie K, Tofts PS, Miller DH, et al. Variations in T1 and T2 relaxation times of normal appearing white matter and lesions in multiple sclerosis. *J Neurol Sci* 2000; 178: 81-7.

Stevenson VL, Smith SM, Matthews PM, Miller DH, Thompson AJ. Monitoring disease activity and progression in primary progressive multiple sclerosis using MRI: sub-voxel registration to identify lesion changes and to detect cerebral atrophy. *J Neurol* 2002; 249: 171-7.

Tartaglia MC, Narayanan S, De Stefano N, Arnaoutelis R, Antel SB, Francis SJ, et al. Choline is increased in pre-lesional normal appearing white matter in multiple sclerosis. *J Neurol* 2002; 249: 1382-90.

Truyen L, van Waesberghe JH, van Walderveen MA, van Oosten BW, Polman CH, Hommes OR, et al. Accumulation of hypointense lesions ("black holes") on T1 spin-echo MRI correlates with disease progression in multiple sclerosis. *Neurology* 1996; 47: 1469-76.

Tubridy N, Ader HJ, Barkhof F, Thompson AJ, Miller DH. Exploratory treatment trials in multiple sclerosis using MRI: sample size calculations for relapsing-remitting and secondary progressive subgroups using placebo controlled parallel groups. *J Neurol Neurosurg Psychiatry* 1998; 64: 50-5.

Urenjak J, Williams SR, Gadian DG, Noble M. Proton nuclear magnetic resonance spectroscopy unambiguously identifies different neural cell types. *J Neurosci* 1993; 13: 981-9.

van Waesberghe JH, Kamphorst W, De Groot CJ, van Walderveen MA, Castelijns JA, Ravid R, et al. Axonal loss in multiple sclerosis lesions: magnetic resonance imaging insights into substrates of disability. *Ann Neurol* 1999; 46: 747-54.

van Waesberghe JH, van Walderveen MA, Castelijns JA, Scheltens P, Lycklama a Nijeholt GJ, Polman CH, et al. Patterns of lesion development in multiple sclerosis: longitudinal observations with T1-weighted spin-echo and magnetization transfer MR. *AJNR Am J Neuroradiol* 1998; 19: 675-83.

van Walderveen MA, Barkhof F, Pouwels PJ, van Schijndel RA, Polman CH, Castelijns JA. Neuronal damage in T1-hypointense multiple sclerosis lesions demonstrated in vivo using proton magnetic resonance spectroscopy. *Ann Neurol* 1999; 46: 79-87.

van Walderveen MA, Kamphorst W, Scheltens P, van Waesberghe JH, Ravid R, Valk J, et al. Histopathologic correlate of hypointense lesions on T1-weighted spin-echo MRI in multiple sclerosis. *Neurology* 1998; 50: 1282-8.

van Walderveen MA, Lycklama ANGJ, Ader HJ, Jongen PJ, Polman CH, Castelijns JA, et al. Hypointense lesions on T1-weighted spin-echo magnetic resonance imaging: relation to clinical characteristics in subgroups of patients with multiple sclerosis. *Arch Neurol* 2001; 58: 76-81.

Vymazal J, Righini A, Brooks RA, Canesi M, Mariani C, Leonardi M, et al. T1 and T2 in the brain of healthy subjects, patients with Parkinson disease, and patients with multiple system atrophy: relation to iron content. *Radiology* 1999; 211: 489-95.

Weiner HL, Guttmann CR, Khoury SJ, Orav EJ, Hohol MJ, Kikinis R, et al. Serial magnetic resonance imaging in multiple sclerosis: correlation with attacks, disability, and disease stage. *J Neuroimmunol* 2000; 104: 164-73.

Werring DJ, Toosy AT, Clark CA, Parker GJ, Barker GJ, Miller DH, et al. Diffusion tensor imaging can detect and quantify corticospinal tract degeneration after stroke. *J Neurol Neurosurg Psychiatry* 2000; 69: 269-72.

Whitwell JL, Crum WR, Watt HC, Fox NC. Normalization of cerebral volumes by use of intracranial volume: implications for longitudinal quantitative MR imaging. *AJNR Am J Neuroradiol* 2001; 22: 1483-9.

Wilson M, Morgan PS, Lin X, Turner BP, Blumhardt LD. Quantitative diffusion weighted magnetic resonance imaging, cerebral atrophy, and disability in multiple sclerosis. *J Neurol Neurosurg Psychiatry* 2001; 70: 318-22.

Zivadinov R, Bakshi R. Role of MRI in multiple sclerosis II: brain and spinal cord atrophy. *Front Biosci* 2004; 9: 647-64.

Zivadinov R, Locatelli L, Stival B, Bratina A, Grop A, Nasuelli D, et al. Normalized regional brain atrophy measurements in multiple sclerosis. *Neuroradiology* 2003; 45: 793-8.

Zivadinov R, Rudick RA, De Masi R, Nasuelli D, Ukmar M, Pozzi-Mucelli RS, et al. Effects of IV methylprednisolone on brain atrophy in relapsing-remitting MS. *Neurology* 2001a; 57: 1239-47.

Zivadinov R, Sepcic J, Nasuelli D, De Masi R, Bragadin LM, Tommasi MA, et al. A longitudinal study of brain atrophy and cognitive disturbances in the early phase of relapsing-remitting multiple sclerosis. *J Neurol Neurosurg Psychiatry* 2001b; 70: 773-80.

Zivadinov and Zorzon. Is gadolinium enhancement predictive of the development of brain atrophy in multiple sclerosis? A review of the literature. *J Neuroimaging* 2002; 12, 302-309.

In: Brain and Spinal Cord Atrophy in Multiple Sclerosis
Editors: R. Zivadinov and R. Bakshi, pp. 113-136
ISBN 1-59454-160-4

Chapter VIII

Neurologic Disability and Central Nervous System Atrophy in Multiple Sclerosis

***Robert Zivadinov*[1-3*] *and Rohit Bakshi*[4]**
[1]Department of Neurology, SUNY–University at Buffalo School of Medicine and Biomedical Sciences, Buffalo, NY, USA.
[2]Buffalo Neuroimaging Analysis Center, Buffalo, NY, USA.
[3]The Jacobs Neurological Institute, Buffalo, NY, USA.
[4]Center for Neurological Imaging, Partners Multiple Sclerosis Center, Brigham & Women's Hospital, Harvard Medical School, Boston, MA, USA.

Introduction

The evaluation of brain atrophy seems to be of growing clinical relevance as a biomarker of the disease process of multiple sclerosis (MS) (Giovannoni et al., 1998; Losseff and Miller, 1998; Miller et al., 2002; Simon, 2000; Simon, 2001; Thompson, 1998; Zivadinov and Bakshi, 2004c). Several studies have examined the relationship between both disease course and duration in patients with MS and the rate of central nervous system (CNS) atrophy. Whether the rate of brain atrophy varies within the same individual or among subjects in the different stages of MS is still an open question. We do not yet know with certainty when this process begins, whether brain atrophy develops to the same degree in all disease subtypes, or whether the rate of brain atrophy is fairly constant in an individual over time.

Longitudinal studies have demonstrated that magnetic resonance imaging (MRI) represents a potentially powerful tool to monitor the rate of CNS atrophy as a surrogate marker of disease progression in MS (Chard et al., 2002; Fisher et al., 2000; Fisher et al., 2002; Fox et al., 2000; Hardmeier et al., 2003; Hohol et al., 1997; Ingle et al., 2002; Ingle et

* Correspondence to: Robert Zivadinov, MD, PhD, Department of Neurology, University at Buffalo, SUNY, The Jacobs Neurological Institute, 100 High Street, Buffalo, NY 14203, USA. Tel. 716 859 7031; Fax. 716 859 7874; E-mail: rzivadinov@thejni.org

al., 2003; Kalkers et al., 2002a; Losseff et al., 1996; Paolillo et al., 2002; Rovaris et al., 2003; Rudick et al., 2000; Rudick et al., 1999; Sailer et al., 2003; Sailer et al., 2001; Stevenson et al., 2000; Taylor et al., 2004; Zivadinov et al., 2001b; Zivadinov et al., 2001c; Zorzon et al., 2002). Several long-term longitudinal studies have shown that progression of brain atrophy is a fairly robust predictor of subsequent neurologic deterioration (Fisher et al., 2002; Ingle et al., 2003; Molyneux et al., 2000; Paolillo et al., 2002; Zivadinov et al., 2001b). The extent to which CNS atrophy leads to neurologic impairment and disability is probably influenced by the topography of the atrophic process, the underlying pathologic substrate of the damaged areas and the reserve capacity of relatively unaffected areas (Zivadinov and Bakshi, 2004c). When compared with conventional MRI lesion measurements, brain atrophy is a better predictor of neurologic deterioration such as physical disability, cognitive impairment, mood disorders, urodynamic and sexual dysfunction, and decreased quality of life (QOL). It is likely that once the level of CNS atrophy reaches a critical threshold, patients begin to suffer clinical impairment and disease progression (Zivadinov and Bakshi, 2004c).

In this review, we will focus on clinical aspects of CNS atrophy including the relationship between atrophy and disability, disease course, disease duration, QOL, and fatigue. These relationships will be gleaned from a variety of cross-sectional and longitudinal studies, both studies of untreated patients and those potentially contaminated by disease modifying treatments. We will not focus on the effect of treatment on CNS atrophy, because this is presented separately in the present collection of works (Rovaris and Filippi, 2004). Similarly, a discussion on relationship between neuropsychological impairment and CNS atrophy is presented separately (Benedict and Carone, 2004).

Relationship between CNS Atrophy and Neurologic Disability

Several cross-sectional (Bakshi et al., 2002; Bakshi et al., 2001b; Berg et al., 2000; Bermel et al., 2002; Bermel et al., 2003b; De Stefano et al., 2002a; De Stefano et al., 2002b; Filippi et al., 1998; Kalkers et al., 2001; Paolillo et al., 2000; Pelletier et al., 2003; Rudick et al., 2001; Sailer et al., 2003; Ukkonen et al., 2003; Wilson et al., 2001; Zivadinov et al., 2001a; Zivadinov et al., 2003a) and longitudinal studies (Fisher et al., 2000; Fisher et al., 2002; Ingle et al., 2003; Paolillo et al., 2002; Rudick et al., 2000; Zivadinov et al., 2001c) (Table 1; Fig 1) have shown that the development of CNS atrophy is a moderate but significant predictor of neurologic impairment. The salient themes that emerge from these studies are: 1) CNS atrophy shows a partial but significant relationship with physical disability including moderate predictive value towards the subsequent development of neurologic impairment. 2) The association between atrophy and disability is independent of the effect of MRI lesions 3) Atrophy shows better predictive value than conventional lesion measures in this regard. 4) The relationship between spinal cord atrophy and disability is particularly strong. These studies suggest that measurement of atrophy can help to resolve the "clinical-MRI paradox" that has historically limited the perception of the role of MRI as a disease biomarker (Barkhof, 1999). For example, Dastidar and colleagues (1999) measured the volume of intracranial CSF spaces in 28 patients with MS and found that measurement of atrophy was significantly associated with neurologic disability as assessed by the Expanded

Disability Status Scale (EDSS) score while T1-hypointense and T2-hyperintense lesion volumes were not. Loseff and colleagues (1996) showed that the rate of progression of brain atrophy over 18-months was significantly higher in patients who sustained deterioration in EDSS score while only trends were seen for a relationship between disability change and progression of T2-hyperintense lesions. Bermel et. al. (2003b) measured whole brain atrophy using brain parenchymal fraction (BPF) in 78 patients with MS. Stepwise regression compared the relative abilities of MRI variables to predict clinical data. By regression of age, BPF, 3rd ventricular width, whole brain T2-hyperintense lesion volume, and T1-hypointense lesion volume, BPF was the best predictor of disability score (R2=.204, *P*<.001).

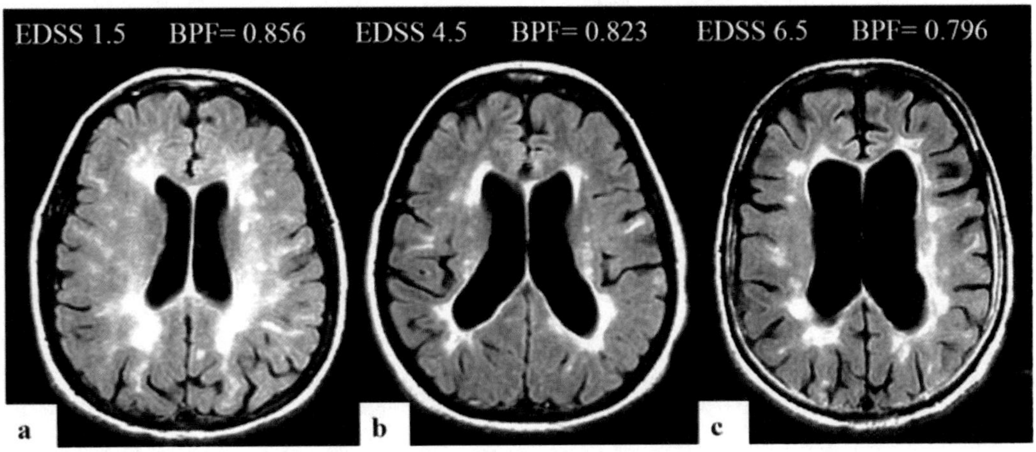

Fig 1. Adapted from Zivadinov and Bakshi (2004b). Progressive brain atrophy in a patient with multiple sclerosis over 9 years on representative axial fast fluid-attenuated inversion recovery images (**A–C**). A 32-year-old man with relapsing-remitting MS and 5-year disease duration showed mild physical disability, with an Expanded Disability Status Scale (EDSS) score of 1.5 (**A**). Brain parenchymal fraction (BPF), performed at the Buffalo Neuroimaging Analysis Center, was 0.856. Although receiving treatment with disease-modifying therapy for several years, the patient continued to have frequent relapses and disease progression. At 9 years, physical disability increased to a severe level, with an EDSS score of 6.5. Follow-up MRI was performed on a different scanner at year 4 (**B**) and year 9 (**C**), after the initial MRI. Note the marked enlargement of the cortical sulci, sylvian fissures, and lateral ventricles. BPF decreased by 6% at year 9 compared with baseline (annual rate of atrophy 0.66% per year).

Table 1. Estimated Annualized Brain Atrophy Progression Rate in Prospective Natural History Studies and Therapeutic Trials of Patients Treated with Placebo, According to Different Disease Course.

Reference/Year	Mean Age at Baseline (y)	Mean Disease Duration at Baseline	Number of Patients	Natural Course or Placebo-Treated Patients	Disease Course	Follow-up Time (mo)	EAPC of Regional Brain Atrophy (Method)	EAPC of Whole-Brain Atrophy (Method)
Brex et al., 2000	31.5	12 mo	16	NH	**CIS**	12	+15.1% (VE)	N.A.
Dalton et al., 2002	N.A.	12 mo	55	NH	**CIS**	12	+1.7% (VE)	N.A.
Comi et al., 2002	N.A	24 mo	99	P	CIS	24	N.A.	-0.84% (PBVC)
Redmond et al., 2000	33	46 mo	7	NH	**Early RR**	6	+29.8% (VE)	N.A.
Saindane et al., 2000	37	3.8 y	24	NH	**Early RR**	24	N.A.	-0.92% (BPV)
Ge et al., 2000a	34.4	4.2 y	13	P	**Early RR**	24	N.A.	-0.9% (BPV)
Zivadinov et al., 2001c	30.1	3.8 y	53	NH	**Early RR**	24	N.A.	-1.33% (BPV)
Leist et al., 2001	29.7	Early RR	16	NH	**Early RR**	16	+17.6% (VE) (16 mo)	N.A.
Kalkers et al., 2002a	35	4.2 y	42	NH	**Early RR**	24-48	+3.9% (VF)	-0.7% (BPF)
Simon et al., 1999	36.9	6.4 y	143	P	**RR**	24	+4.5% (3VW) + 5.5% (LVV) -4.9% (CCA)	-0.64% (WBW)
Rudick et al., 1999	36.4	6.2 y	72	P	**RR**	24	N.A.	-0.61% (BPF)
Luks et al., 2000	36	6 y	15	NH	**RR**	18	+20.2% (VE) (18 mo)	N.A.
Fox et al., 2000	36.7	5.6 y	6	NH	**RR**	12	+2.1% (VE)	-0.8% (BBSI)
Rovaris et al., 2001	34	8.3 y	114	P	**RR**	9	-0.7% (7SM) (9 mo)	N.A.
Zivadinov et al., 2001b	32.3	5.8 y	45	NH	**RR**	60	N.A.	-1.2% (BPV)
Jones et al., 2001	N.A.	N.A.	172	P	**RR**	24	N.A.	-0.68% (WBR)
Hardmeier et al., 2003	N.A.	7.6 y	128	NH	**RR**	76 days	N.A.	-1.06% (BPF)

Table 1. Continued

Reference/Year	Mean Age at Baseline (y)	Mean Disease Duration at Baseline	Number of Patients	Natural Course or Placebo-Treated Patients	Disease Course	Follow-up Time (mo)	EAPC of Regional Brain Atrophy (Method)	EAPC of Whole-Brain Atrophy (Method)
Redmond et al., 2000	44	138 mo	7	NH	**SP**	6	-0.8% (VE)	N.A.
Fox et al., 2000	43.7	19.3 y	6	NH	**SP**	12	+1% (VE)	-0.6% (BBSI)
Kalkers et al., 2002a	41.9	5.2 y	21	NH	**SP**	24-48	+3.9% (VF)	-0.8% (BPF)
Molyneux et al., 2000	39.6	13.1 y	46	P	**SP**	36	-0.85% (7SM)	N.A.
Filippi et al., 2000	44.2	12.3 y	54	P	**SP + PP**	12	-0.4% (4SM)	N.A.
Kidd et al., 1996	40.1	9 y	10	NH	**PP**	12	-2.34% (CA)	N.A.
Redmond et al., 2000	48	72 mo	5	NH	**PP**	6	-2.4% (VE)	N.A.
Fox et al., 2000	49.3	11.3 y	9	NH	PP	12	+2.9% (VE)	-0.9%
Stevenson et al., 2000	N.A	N.A	137	NH	**PP**	12	-1.3% (6SM) -3.73% (CA)	N.A.
Ingle et al., 2002	47	8 y	100	NH	**PP**	24	-1.35% (6SM) -1.9% (CA)	N.A.
Kalkers et al., 2002a	47.9	7.1 y	20	NH	**PP**	24-48	+2.4% (VF)	-0.5% (BPF)
Ingle et al., 2003	55.7	16.3 y	41	NH	**PP**	60	-0.74% (6SM) +7.7% (VE) -2.2% (CA)	N.A.
Leary et al., 2003	43	8 y	20	P	**PP**	24	+6% (VE) -0.94% (CA)	N.A.

3VW = third ventricle width, 4SM = 4-slice method, 6SM = 6-slice method, 7SM = 7-slice method, BBSI= brain boundary shift integral, BPF = brain parenchymal fraction, BPV = brain parenchymal volume, CA = cord cross-sectional area, CCA = corpus callosum area, CIS = clinically isolated syndrome, EAPC = estimated annualized percentage change, LVV = lateral ventricle width, N.A. = not available, NH = natural history patients, P = patients treated with placebo, PBVC = percentage brain volume change, PP = primary progressive, RR = relapsing-remitting, SP = secondary progressive, VE = ventricular enlargement, VF = ventricular fraction, WBR = whole brain ratio.

For some studies, the estimated annualized percentage changes have been calculated from raw data, when not available in the original reports. In studies performed by Leist et al. (2001), Luks et al. (2000), and Rovaris et al. (2001), it was not possible to obtain the estimated annualized percentage change. The reported values represent end-of-study changes.

Regarding the important question of predictive value of CNS atrophy towards long term disability, longitudinal studies have shown that the development of brain atrophy is a fairly reliable predictor of subsequent neurologic impairment accumulation in the long term (Table 1; Fig 1) (Fisher et al., 2000; Fisher et al., 2002; Ingle et al., 2003; Paolillo et al., 2002; Rudick et al., 2000; Zivadinov et al., 2001c). Results from these studies indicate that once brain atrophy occurs, the damage is irreversible. Fisher et al. (2002) found that the change in BPF from year 2 to the 8-year follow-up visit correlated with the change in EDSS score ($r = -0.31$; $P = .0005$) and change in the Multiple Sclerosis Functional Composite score ($r = -0.30$; $P = .001$) during the same period (Table 1). The relationship between BPF change and disability measured at subsequent time points indicated that patients with more atrophy during the first 2 years had greater disability at the 8-year follow-up visit. Furthermore, the change in BPF over the first 2 years was the best MRI predictor of the subsequent 8-year disability score after accounting for the 2 year change in T2-hyperintense lesions, T1-hypointense lesions, and Gd-enhancing lesions. Patients who developed the largest amount of brain atrophy were approximately 4 times more likely to develop an EDSS score of >6.0 at 8 years. Thus, it appears that CNS atrophy is emerging as a clinically relevant measure of disease progression in MS, supported by its relationship to physical disability.

Spinal cord atrophy in patients with MS has particularly good predictive value towards the development of physical disability. Cross-sectional studies showed that patients with MS have a lower spinal cord cross-sectional area than healthy controls (Kidd et al., 1993; Lycklama et al., 2003). Spinal cord atrophy may be focal or generalized (Tartaglino et al., 1995). Kidd et al. (1996) found that patients with MS and spinal cord atrophy had higher levels of disability, as measured by EDSS, than patients without atrophy ($P = .006$). No difference in cord cross-sectional area was found among patients with SPMS, PPMS, and benign MS. A longitudinal study of patients with primary progressive (PP) and secondary progressive (SP) MS showed a decrease in the mean of the cord cross-sectional area over 1 year; however, no correlation was observed with disability progression (Kidd et al., 1996). Another study demonstrated that the cord cross-sectional area of patients with PPMS and SPMS was significantly lower than patients with RRMS (Stevenson et al., 2000). Cord atrophy correlated strongly with disability ($r = -0.7$; $P < .0001$) and disease duration ($r = -0.52$; $P < .0001$); whereas T2 lesion load and T1 hypointense lesion load did not. Over 5 years, an association was seen between increased EDSS score and decreased cord area ($r = -0.31$; $P < 0.05$) (Ingle et al., 2003). The Nottingham group (Lin et al., 2003b; Turner et al., 2003) showed that both cerebral brain atrophy and spinal cord atrophy developing over 4 years closely paralleled the accumulation of progressive disability, regardless of whether the patients were receiving disease modifying therapy.

While MS is traditionally thought of as a white matter (WM) disease, a number of studies (Bakshi et al., 2001a; Bakshi et al., 2002; Bermel et al., 2003a; Chard et al., 2002; Cifelli et al., 2002; De Stefano et al., 2003; Fabiano et al., 2003; Ge et al., 2001; Quarantelli et al., 2003; Rovaris et al., 2002; Sharma et al., 2001) have called attention to gray matter (GM) involvement including the presence of lesions, atrophy, and diffuse damage. Using MRI analysis methods, the brain can be divided into GM, WM, and CSF compartments, each providing information on the topography of atrophy (Zivadinov and Bakshi, 2004c). Recent case-controlled studies have shown that atrophy affects both GM and WM compartments from the earliest stages of MS (Chard et al., 2002; De Stefano et al., 2003; Ge et al., 2001; Quarantelli et al., 2003). The results of the first GM vs. WM tissue segmentation study in patients with RRMS (Ge et al., 2001) suggested that the progression of brain atrophy was predominantly confined to the WM compartment. Conversely, recent reports in patients with RRMS have shown that atrophy disproportionately affects GM (Chard et al., 2002; De Stefano et al., 2003; Quarantelli et al., 2003). A significant amount of GM atrophy may also be present in patients with PPMS (De Stefano et al., 2003); however, the extent to which GM atrophy contributes to neurologic impairment is unclear. Several reports have failed to associate the loss of GM volume with accumulation of neurologic impairment (on EDSS) (Chard et al., 2002; Ge et al., 2001; Quarantelli et al., 2003). However, one study showed a significant relationship between neocortical GM volume loss and disability in patients with RRMS ($r = -0.27$ to -0.56; $P = .04$-.01) and PPMS ($r = -0.64$; $P < 0.0001$) (De Stefano et al., 2003). Additional cross-sectional and longitudinal studies are warranted to examine the predictive value of GM vs. WM atrophy on clinical impairment.

Relationship between CNS Atrophy and Urodynamic and Sexual Dysfunction, Fatigue, and Quality of Life

A retrospective study of 90 patients with MS did not show a relationship between urodynamic symptoms (impaired compliance or detrusor-external sphincter dyssynergia) and any MRI finding, including atrophy, Gd-enhancing lesions, and total number or size of lesions (103). In another study, autonomic dysfunction in 75 patients with MS (25 each with RRMS, SPMS, and PPMS) was related to spinal cord atrophy but not lesions (de Seze et al., 2001). Moreover, a recently published study showed that urodynamic abnormalities in 24 patients with PPMS were associated with increased lesion load and whole-brain atrophy (Ukkonen et al., 2004). Patients with hypotonicity of the bladder had a smaller brain volume than those with normal bladder function ($P = .02$).

Recently, we examined the relationship between sexual dysfunction and the severity and location of pathological lesions and atrophy, as shown on brain MRI in 62 patients with MS (46 with RRMS, 6 with SPMS, and 10 with PPMS) (Zorzon et al., 2003). When comparing patients with and without sexual dysfunction, no differences were observed in measures of whole-brain atrophy, frontal atrophy, or total brain, frontal, and pontine T1 and T2 lesion load. The only significant difference was found in pontine atrophy ($P = .026$). Another study showed that impaired QOL with respect to sexual functioning in patients with MS was associated with WM lesions in the inferior parietal lobe, pontine atrophy, and enlargement of the lateral ventricles (Janardhan and Bakshi, 2000). It has been suggested that pontine atrophy and lesions in the parietal lobe may be related to sexual dysfunction because they are related to a disruption in the circuits of the caudal brainstem which controls sexual behavior, and to the areas of the primary sensory cortex that are essential for sexual responses (Janardhan and Bakshi, 2000). These assumptions are corroborated by the results obtained in our study (Zorzon et al., 2003). Recently, we studied 31 patients with RRMS on whom we performed a urodynamic analysis: pudendal cortical evoked potentials, tibial cortical evoked potentials, and cranial and cervical spine MRI (Zivadinov et al., 2003b). The results confirmed that parenchymal pontine atrophy and destructive lesions in the pons were associated with sexual dysfunction, confirming the crucial role of the caudal brainstem in the regulation of sexual behavior.

Fatigue is a frequent complaint of patients with MS; however, little is known about its pathogenesis (Bakshi, 2003). The relationship between fatigue and the extent of brain abnormalities on MRI has been investigated in 45 patients reported to be seriously fatigued at least several times a week over the previous 3 months (van der Werf et al., 1998). Fatigue severity was not related to the total extent of brain abnormalities, or to MRI-based atrophy measures. In another study, Bakshi et al. (1999) assessed fatigue in 71 patients and identified MS-related and non–MS-related fatigue groups. Fatigue severity did not correlate with regional or global lesion load or atrophy, as assessed by conventional MRI sequences. No significant differences were noted in any MRI measures between the MS-related and non–MS-related fatigue groups or across MRI variables and fatigue scores in the entire cohort. This study suggests that disease topography or severity seen on MRI does not explain fatigue in patients with MS and that fatigue is likely due to mechanisms poorly characterized on conventional MRI. However, advanced MRI techniques measuring metabolic changes appear to show some correlations with MS-fatigue (Filippi et al., 2002; Tartaglia et al., 2004).

Several studies have examined the association between health-related QOL and CNS atrophy (Bakshi et al., 2001b; Janardhan and Bakshi, 2000; Miller et al., 2003; Rudick et al., 2001; Rudick et al., 2002). In a prospective cross-sectional study of 60 consecutive patients with MS, Janardhan and Bakshi (2000) investigated whether impaired QOL in patients with MS was related to any regional brain lesions or atrophy detected by conventional MRI. Assessment of QOL was quantified with the MSQOL-54 Instrument. Brain lesions and atrophy on MRI were found to be associated with impaired QOL with respect to sexual dysfunction, overall mental health, and limitations resulting from physical and emotional dysfunction. Data from the phase III study of patients with RRMS treated with IFNβ-1a (Jacobs et al., 1996) and reassessed approximately 8 years after study initiation (Miller et al., 2003) were used to investigate whether QOL was related to brain atrophy at baseline, at year 2, and after an average of 8.1 years from study initiation. The data collected during a clinic visit were available for 137 of the original 172 participants. Results of the correlation analysis suggested that the change in BPF from baseline to year 2 and from year 2 to the 8-year follow-up visit were related to a dynamic component of physical disability, as measured by the Sickness Impact Profile ($r = -0.28$, $P < .01$; and $r = -0.25$, $P < .01$, respectively). The associations between MRI abnormalities and QOL have been more robust for T1-hypointensities and widespread brain atrophy than for T2-hyperintense or Gd-enhancing lesions (Janardhan and Bakshi, 2000), reinforcing the link between destructive brain pathology and clinical impairment that has been evident from studies looking at disability assessments and MRI.

Relationship between CNS Atrophy and Disease Course/Duration

Recent reports have shown that patients exhibit significant brain (Brex et al., 2000; Dalton et al., 2002; Kalkers et al., 2002a; Leist et al., 2001; Redmond et al., 2000; Comi et al., 2002; Zivadinov et al., 2001a; Zivadinov et al., 2001c) and spinal cord atrophy (Brex et al., 2001) in the earliest stages of MS. However, it is not clear whether the rate of atrophy is constant throughout a patient's disease course. Some studies have shown higher rates of atrophy and axonal loss early in the disease course (Brex et al., 2000; Comi et al., 2002), while other reports have suggested that the rate of atrophy is greater in more advanced relapsing-remitting (RR) phases (Fox et al., 2000; Hardmeier et al., 2003; Zivadinov et al., 2001b). Still other reports have shown that CNS atrophy develops more rapidly in the later progressive stages of MS when clinical and MRI disease activity decreases but patients experience progression of disability (Coles et al., 1999; Losseff et al., 1996; Molyneux et al., 2000; Saindane et al., 2000). Therefore, it is likely that the rate of atrophy is heterogeneous in each stage of MS both within and among individuals (Miller et al., 2002; Simon, 2000; Simon, 2001; Zivadinov and Bakshi, 2004c).

Many of the longitudinal studies that monitored the rate of CNS atrophy progression were biased by a possible "treatment effect" of disease-modifying drugs during the observational period. As we review the published data in these natural history studies and therapeutic trials, we will try to determine the rate of CNS atrophy progression in different disease subtypes. For a discussion on the effect of treatment of CNS atrophy, the reader is referred to a separate piece in the present collection of works (Rovaris and Filippi, 2004).

Clinically Isolated Syndromes

In patients with clinically isolated syndromes (CIS) suggestive of MS, the brain MRI lesion load predicts the development of clinically definite MS (Brex and D, 2002; O'Riordan, 1998; Sailer, 1999). Three studies investigated whether the rate of brain atrophy from clinical onset predicts the development of clinically definite MS (Brex et al., 2000; Comi et al., 2002; Dalton et al., 2002). One natural history study evaluated 55 patients with CIS who had MRI done within 3 months of symptom onset and again after 1 year (Table 2) (Dalton et al., 2002). Significant ventricular enlargement (+0.5cm^3, +9.3% median change; P = .006) was seen in the 18 patients who developed clinically definite MS (i.e., who had a second clinical relapse). Moreover, 27 of 55 patients who met the McDonald MRI criteria for MS (McDonald et al., 2001) developed significant ventricular enlargement after 1 year (+0.3 cm^3, +5% median change; P = .005). In contrast, no change was seen in ventricular volume in the 15 patients with normal MRI at baseline (–0.2 cm^3, –4.7% median change). A recently concluded placebo-controlled study of interferon beta-1a (IFNβ-1a; Rebif®, Ares-Serono, Geneva, Switzerland) in patients with CIS (Comi et al., 2001) showed significant brain atrophy developing over 24 months in both the placebo group and treated patients (Comi et al, 2002). Brain volume decreased by 1.68% in the placebo group during the 24 months.

In a recently published cross-sectional study, 28 patients with CIS were followed for 14 years after the first onset of symptoms (Chard et al., 2003). The authors explored the association between changes in brain lesion load and subsequent development of brain atrophy. Disease-related atrophy was shown at the 14-year follow-up by lower normalized brain tissue volumes in the MS group vs. 29 healthy subjects (–3.6%; P = .0001). Change in lesion load during the first 5 years was more closely correlated to disease-related brain atrophy at 14 years than were later changes in lesion load; however, the correlation was only moderate (–0.53; P = .004). The study results suggested that development of brain atrophy in patients with MS was related to lesion activity in early RRMS, rather than in later progressive disease stages. An important limitation of this study was that the cohort was a relatively small subgroup of those originally recruited (Filippi, 1994). Moreover, the subgroup of patients had a relatively benign disease course, including only 3 patients with MS who developed SP MS after 14 years. Brain atrophy progression was not assessed prospectively; rather, cross-sectional evaluations of brain volumes in patients with MS and the control group were performed at the end of 14 years.

Table 2. Long-Term Longitudinal Correlations (≥5 Years) Between Development of Brain Atrophy and Accumulation of Subsequent Neurologic Impairment in Patients With Multiple Sclerosis.

Reference (Years)	Atrophy Measure vs. Neurologic Impairment	*r*	P
Zivadinov et al., 2001b (5 y)	BPAV vs EDSS	–0.38	.025
Ingle et al., 2003 (5 y)	CA vs EDSS	–0.31	.038
	VE vs MSFC	–0.31	<.05
Paolillo et al., 2002 (6 y)	SBV vs EDSS	–0.46	.001
Fisher et al., 2000; Fisher et al., 2002; Rudick et al., 2000 (8 y)	BPF vs EDSS	–0.31	.0005
	BPF vs MSFC	0.30	.001

BPAV = brain parenchymal absolute volume, BPF = brain parenchymal fraction, CA = cord cross-sectional area, EDSS = Expanded Disability Status Scale, MSFC = Multiple Sclerosis Functional Composite, SBV = supratentorial brain volume, VE = ventricular enlargement.

Recent evidence suggests that spinal cord atrophy begins early in the disease process. Brex et al (Brex et al., 2001) evaluated the development of cord atrophy over 1 year in 43 patients presenting with CIS and in 15 age-matched controls. The spinal cord area was significantly lower vs. controls in the 74% of patients with an abnormal brain MRI at baseline. However, spinal cord atrophy did not occur in patients with normal baseline brain MRI. At 1-year follow-up, no significant difference was seen in spinal cord area between members of the control group and patients with MS. This study suggests that spinal cord atrophy may occur in a subgroup of patients with CIS and a high risk for developing clinically definite MS. The lack of a detectable change in spinal cord area over 1 year of follow-up suggests that the spinal cord atrophy rate increases as the disease progresses.

These longitudinal studies suggest that CNS atrophy begins in patients with CIS even before their first clinical symptoms, especially in those at high risk for developing MS. The subgroup of patients with abnormal brain MRI who have met McDonald MRI criteria may develop brain atrophy over a 1-year period. The estimated annualized percentage change of brain atrophy varies across studies and methods but seems to be around 0.8% per year (Table 2). Additional studies are needed to establish the dynamics of CNS atrophy in patients with CIS.

Relapsing-Remitting Multiple Sclerosis

Several natural history studies have evaluated the rate of brain atrophy in early RRMS. In a recently published 2-year study, we monitored 53 patients with clinically definite RRMS, disease duration of 1 to 5 years, and an Expanded Disability Status Scale (EDSS) score of ≤5.0 at baseline (Zivadinov et al., 2001c). Over the 2 years, patients had a significant decrease of brain parenchymal volume (BPV) (–32.3 mL, –2.7%; $P < .0001$). The progression of brain atrophy was even higher in patients with cognitive dysfunction (–66 mL, 5.4%; $P = .0031$) and in patients with progressive physical disability (an increase in EDSS score of ≥1.0) during the follow-up period (–99 mL, 8%; $P = .005$). This longitudinal study of a homogeneous untreated patient group in the early phase of RRMS, suggests that whole-brain atrophy develops at a faster rate in patients with early RRMS than in those with CIS. Two other studies have investigated the progression of ventricular enlargement in patients with early RRMS over relatively shorter time periods (Table 2) (Leist et al., 2001; Redmond et al., 2000). The results from these studies indicate that significant ventricular enlargement may occur in early RRMS at an annualized rate of +17.6 to +29.8% (Table 2). Two other natural history studies monitored the progression of whole brain atrophy over 1-2 years. In one study, 42 patients with early RRMS were followed for 2 to 4 years (Table 2) (Kalkers et al., 2002a). Two different brain volume measurements were obtained in this study: the BPF, as a marker of global brain atrophy; and the ventricular fraction, as a marker of central brain atrophy. Over the study period, patients developed significant brain atrophy (BPF, –0.7%; ventricular fraction, +3.9%). A potential confounding factor was that 25% of patients received a disease modifying therapy during the study. However, the rate of brain atrophy did not differ significantly when the group receiving treatment was excluded from the analysis. In another study conducted over a period of 2 years, brain atrophy progression was detected in 24 patients with early RRMS (–1.84%; $P = .0003$) (Table 2) (Saindane et al., 2000). In a subgroup of 13 patients given a placebo (Ge et al., 2000a) who participated in the original study of glatiramer acetate (Copaxone®, Teva Pharmaceuticals, Montgomeryville, PA) of RRMS (Johnson et al., 1995), members of the placebo group developed a significant decrease in BPV over 2 years (–1.8% $P = .008$).

Several other natural history studies and therapeutic trials of patients treated with placebo monitored the brain atrophy progression rate in patients with RRMS over shorter (9 months) (Hardmeier et al., 2003; Rovaris et al., 2001; Zivadinov et al., 2004a) or longer time periods (1-5 years) (Fox et al., 2000; Inglese et al., 1999; Jones et al., 2001; Rudick et al., 1999; Simon et al., 1999; Zivadinov et al., 2001b) (Table 2). In a 2-year, placebo-controlled study of Avonex® (IFNβ-1a; Biogen, Inc., Cambridge, MA) of RRMS (Jacobs et al., 1996), the rate of brain atrophy progression was measured in 72 patients on placebo by yearly scans using the BPF (Table 2) (Rudick et al., 1999). The mean decrease in BPF in year 1 (–0.70%) was similar to year 2 (–0.52%). In a follow-up study, 134 patients originally included in this study were reassessed for brain atrophy after 8 years (Fisher et al., 2002). Many patients in the placebo arm received disease modifying therapy after the original study had concluded. The mean yearly reduction in BPF over 8 years was 0.38% in the whole group of patients, which is about half the rate seen during the 2 years of the original study. In a 9-month, placebo-controlled study of glatiramer acetate in RRMS, a mean reduction of central brain volume was observed in 114 patients on placebo (–0.7%; $P = .003$) (Table 2) (Rovaris et al., 2001). At 9 months, all patients on placebo who participated in the original study were converted to active treatment. In both treatment arms, significant progression of brain atrophy occurred over 18 months (–1.4%, $P = .0001$ in patients originally on placebo; –1.2%, $P = .0001$ in patients on glatiramer acetate from the beginning of the study). In a randomized, controlled trial of pulse intravenous methylprednisolone in 81 patients with RRMS, the rate of brain atrophy progression was monitored over 5 years (Table 2) (Zivadinov et al., 2001b). BPVs were measured at baseline and at the end of the study. Patients in the control arm showed significant changes in BPV after 5 years (5.9%; $P = .003$). Separate studies evaluated the rate of CNS atrophy progression in patients with RRMS (Gasperini et al., 2002; Ge et al., 2000b; Hohol et al., 1997; Lin et al., 2003a; Losseff et al., 1996; Paolillo et al., 2002; Sailer et al., 2001; Taylor et al., 2004; Turner et al., 2003; Wolinsky et al., 2001; Zorzon et al., 2002). Monitoring of the natural history of CNS atrophy progression in these studies was potentially biased by a "treatment effect," because most patients were on a disease modifying therapy during the study period. However, the estimated annual rate of CNS atrophy progression was only slightly lower than the rate found in natural history studies and therapeutic trials of patients treated with placebo (Table 2).

Longitudinal natural history studies and therapeutic trials of patients treated with placebo suggest that CNS atrophy is common in patients with RRMS from the earliest stages of the disease. The estimated annual rate of whole-brain atrophy varies across studies and methods but is slightly higher in patients with early stage RRMS (range, –0.7% to 1.33%) than in those with advanced stages of RRMS (range, –0.61% to 1.2%). A meta-analysis from currently available therapeutic trials of patients given placebo might be useful to establish the dynamics of CNS atrophy progression in patients with RRMS.

Secondary Progressive Multiple Sclerosis

The rate of brain atrophy progression in patients with SPMS has been investigated in 3 natural history studies (Fox et al., 2000; Kalkers et al., 2002a; Redmond et al., 2000) and 2 therapeutic trials of patients given placebo (Table 2). These studies reported slightly lower annual rates of whole-brain atrophy (range, –0.6% to –0.8%) and regional brain atrophy (range, –0.8% to +1% for ventricular enlargement) than that observed in patients with RRMS. A European trial of Betaseron® (IFNβ-1b, Berlex Laboratories, Montville, NJ) in patients with SPMS provided an opportunity to assess the rate of brain atrophy using serial MRI (Molyneux et al., 2000). Brain volume was estimated on 4 contiguous, 5-mm, brain-hemisphere slices using an algorithm with a high level of reproducibility and automation. By month 35, a significant, progressive reduction in brain volume was seen in the placebo group, with a mean reduction of 3.9%. A double-blind, placebo-controlled study assessed the efficacy of 2 doses of cladribine (0.7 mg/kg and 2.1 mg/kg) in patients with SPMS and PP MS. Over 12 months, significant progression of brain atrophy was observed in the placebo group (–0.4%) groups. This study confirmed that in a large cohort of patients with progressive MS, brain atrophy develops over a short period of time and that inflammation and new lesion formation play a marginal role in the development of brain atrophy in advanced stages of MS. Contributory clarification of this issue was also derived from human antileukocytic (CD52) monoclonal antibody (Campath-1H; alemtuzumab) studies (Coles et al., 1999; Paolillo et al., 1999). Paolillo et al. (1999) found that brain atrophy progressed in the SPMS population despite effective suppression of Gd+ lesion activity. In the same clinical sample, Coles et al. (1999) suggested that the dissociation between mechanisms underlying brain atrophy and Gd-enhancement activity could be explained by a delayed expression of sustained axonal damage during the acute inflammatory phase, preconditioned by the extent of previous inflammatory activity. T

Other longitudinal "treatment-effect–biased" studies have investigated the rate of brain atrophy progression in patients with SPMS (Hohol et al., 1997; Losseff et al., 1996; Sailer et al., 2001; Taylor et al., 2004; Zorzon et al., 2002). The results indicate that the annual rate of CNS atrophy is very similar to that found in previously reported natural history studies and therapeutic trials of patients treated with placebo (Table 2).

Primary Progressive Multiple Sclerosis

Natural history studies and therapeutic trials of patients treated with placebo showed significant progression of CNS atrophy in both the short and long term in patients with PPMS (Table 2). Of particular interest are studies derived from an MRI collaborative project involving 6 European centers (Ingle et al., 2002; Ingle et al., 2003; Stevenson et al., 2000). Of the 191 patients with progressive MS originally studied at baseline, 137 patients with PPMS were evaluated after a 1-year follow-up period (Stevenson et al., 2000). The authors found spinal cord atrophy (mean change of cord cross-sectional area: –3.7%; $P < .001$) and brain atrophy (mean change of central 6-slice atrophy: –1.3%; $P < .001$) over the 12-month period. A similar rate of central brain atrophy was seen after 2 years (a total of –2.7% from baseline) (Ingle et al., 2002). In contrast, a lower rate of spinal cord atrophy was seen at year 2 (a total of –3.8% from baseline). Only patients with spinal cord symptoms at baseline developed cord atrophy over 2 years. Of those who participated in a 2-year follow-up MRI study, 59 patients were asked to return for further clinical and MRI examination at year 5 (Ingle et al., 2003). Of the 41 patients included in the study, 15 participated in the phase II trial of Avonex during years 2 and 3; 9 of the included patients were on active treatment (Leary et al., 2003). Therefore, the CNS atrophy progression rate at 5 years should be interpreted with caution. After 5 years, significant deterioration was seen in all clinical and MRI measures ($P < .01$ and $P < .001$, respectively). An association was observed between an increase in disability and a decrease in the cord cross-sectional area. The rate of atrophy was lower in the last 3 years of follow-up compared with year 1 and year 2 evaluations (Table 2). A 2-year exploratory, randomized, controlled study of Avonex in patients with PPMS evaluated the progression of CNS atrophy in 20 patients given placebo and 30 given Avonex (30 μg and 60 μg). Patients given placebo had decreased a cord cross-sectional area (–1.88%) and increased ventricular volume (+12%) over 2 years. Other longitudinal studies have investigated the rate of CNS atrophy progression in patients with PPMS (Kalkers et al., 2002b; Kidd et al., 1996; Thorpe et al., 1996; Zorzon et al., 2002). A small, uncontrolled study of 16 patients with PPMS evaluated whether the neuroprotective agent riluzole could reduce the rate of spinal cord atrophy (Kalkers et al., 2002b). Patients were followed untreated for 1 year, then were given riluzole for 1 year. During the pretreatment phase, the cord cross-sectional area was reduced by 2%.

The results from natural history studies, therapeutic trials of patients treated with placebo, and other open-label and longitudinal studies suggest that patients with PPMS have a slightly higher annual rate of ventricular enlargement (range, –2.4 % to +7.7%) than patients with SPMS (Table 2), but this is lower than in patients with RRMS (range +2.1% to +29.8%). The loss of cord cross-sectional area develops at a faster rate than brain atrophy in patients with

PPMS (Table 2). The finding of modest inflammatory activity in the demyelinated lesions of patients with PPMS, despite the progression of brain atrophy (Fox et al., 2000; Ingle et al., 2002; Ingle et al., 2003; Kalkers et al., 2002a; Leary et al., 2003; Redmond et al., 2000; Stevenson et al., 2000), supports the concept that different pathological mechanisms underlie the development of brain atrophy in these patients. For further discussion on the relationship between MRI markers of lesions/inflammation and CNS atrophy, the reader is referred to a separate piece in the present collection of works (Meier and Guttmann, 2004).

The pathological processes responsible for the development of brain atrophy in patients with MS are uncertain; however, a combination of demyelination and axonal loss most likely plays a major role (Zivadinov and Bakshi, 2004c; Zivadinov and Zorzon, 2002). Reduced axonal diameter and tissue contraction caused by astrogliosis may also be contributing factors. It is not entirely clear, however, whether processes other than demyelination and axonal loss contribute to the progressive development of atrophy in the chronic-progressive stages of MS. Some authors hypothesize that mechanisms of neurotoxicity separate from inflammation might contribute to axonal loss. Some of these mechanisms are chronic demyelination (Brex et al., 2000; Trapp et al., 1999), loss of tropic support of axons (Kaplan et al., 1997), altered electrical conduction (Pfrieger and Barres, 1997), and iron deposition (Bakshi et al., 2002). For further discussion on the pathogenesis of CNS atrophy, the reader is referred to a separate piece in the present collection of works (Minagar et al., 2004).

The Rate of CNS Atrophy vs. Observational Period

Short-Term Studies (Less than 1 Year)

A few studies have monitored the development of brain atrophy over the short term (Hardmeier et al., 2003; Zivadanov et al., 2004a Redmond et al., 2000; Rovaris et al., 2001). Brain volume changes in the short term may be affected by factors other than tissue loss—mainly changes in hydration, steroid treatment, and edema caused by acute inflammation (Hoogervorst et al., 2002; Miller et al., 2002; Rao et al., 2002; Zivadinov and Bakshi, 2004c). Two studies have demonstrated that patients with MS develop significant brain atrophy within 6 to 12 months (Redmond et al., 2000; Rovaris et al., 2001). Recently, a group of very active patients with RRMS were monitored monthly for 3 months during a run-in phase preceding entry into a clinical trial (Clanet et al., 2002). The study determined that detectable brain volume loss can be shown in this short time period (Hardmeier et al., 2003). The authors reported a significant decrease in BPF from baseline scan to month 3 (–0.218%; $P < .001$). In another short-term study of a smaller sample, we did not observe significant brain atrophy progression in a group of patients with early RRMS at any time point over 3 months (Zivadinov et al., 2004c). Some differences in demographic (age and disease duration), clinical (EDSS and relapse rate) and MRI (number of Gd+ lesions at baseline) characteristics of patients with RRMS may help to explain the divergent findings in the 2 studies. Serial MRI studies aimed at investigating short-term brain volume changes in patients with MS are still needed to determine the usefulness of brain atrophy as an outcome measure in short-term exploratory treatment studies.

Mid-Term Studies (From 1 to 3 Years)

Although in the last few years a number of serial MRI studies have been performed to determine the time course of brain atrophy in patients with MS and various disease duration (Table 2), the dynamics of mid-term (≥1 to 3 years) CNS volume changes are still debatable. A growing body of evidence shows that significant CNS atrophy progression may occur over 3 years of follow-up, independent of disease duration and disease course (Table 2) (Brex et al., 2000; Coles et al., 1999; Comi et al., 2002; Dalton et al., 2002; Filippi et al., 2000; Fox et al., 2000; Gasperini et al., 2002; Ge et al., 2000a; Hohol et al., 1997; Inglese et al., 1999; Jones et al., 2001; Kidd et al., 1996; Leary et al., 2003; Leist et al., 2001; Losseff et al., 1996; Luks et al., 2000; Paolillo et al., 1999; Rovaris et al., 2001; Rudick et al., 1999; Sailer et al., 2001; Simon et al., 1999; Stevenson et al., 2000; Thorpe et al., 1996; Zivadinov et al., 2001c; Zorzon et al., 2002).

Long-Term Studies (3 or More Years)

A number of long-term studies have monitored the progression of CNS atrophy (≥3 years) (Table 2) (Chard et al., 2003; Fisher et al., 2000; Fisher et al., 2002; Ingle et al., 2003; Kalkers et al., 2002a; Lin et al., 2003b; Molyneux et al., 2000; Paolillo et al., 2002; Rudick et al., 2000; Taylor et al., 2004; Turner et al., 2003; Wolinsky et al., 2001; Zivadinov et al., 2001c). A study of 68 patients with RRMS treated over a 6-year period with IFNβ explored whether decreases in supratentorial brain atrophy and the corpus callosum area could predict long-term clinical outcome (Paolillo et al., 2002). Six MRI scans were performed monthly before treatment and another 13 during treatment with IFNβ; the last MRI scan was done 6 years after treatment ended. Of 67 patients, 55 had an MRI evaluation at 6 years. A median decrease of 1% was observed during the first year and 1.7% during the first 2 years; in the subsequent 4 years, the supratentorial brain volume decrease was 1.2%. A similar trend was also seen for changes in the corpus callosum area. From baseline scan to final scan, supratentorial brain atrophy decreased by 2.7%. The 6-year analysis showed a lower rate of brain atrophy progression in the subsequent 4 years of treatment when compared with the first 2 years.

Brain atrophy progression was studied over 8 years (Fisher et al., 2000; Fisher et al., 2002; Rudick et al., 2000) in the subgroup of patients with RRMS (n = 106) included in the phase III clinical trial of Avonex (Jacobs et al., 1996) who had analyzable MRI scans at all 4 time points (at baseline, at years 1 and 2 of the original study, and at 8 years). The progression of brain atrophy was significant between baseline and the 8-year follow-up period. The mean change in BPF over the 6 years from the end of the phase III trial to the 8-year follow-up visit was –2.0%. BPF was weakly correlated with age ($r = -0.18$; $P = .039$) and disease duration ($r = -0.29$; $P < .001$) at baseline; however, these correlations were not observed at the 8-year follow-up visit (Fisher et al., 2002).

A possible explanation for the lower rate of brain atrophy in the subsequent 4 to 6 years when compared with the first 2 years can be found in the studies of Paolillo et al. (2002) and Fisher et al. (2002). The results indicate that these lower rates may be related to the natural history of brain atrophy progression. It is probable that the rate of brain atrophy progression decreases over time in patients with MS, just as the frequency of Gd+ lesions decreases over time (Liu et al., 1999; Redmond et al., 2000). Another explanation may be that treatment with disease modifying therapy over 8 years exerted an immediate effect on inflammation but a delayed effect on atrophy. A number of other technical limitations could also have contributed to the slower rate of brain atrophy progression over time (i.e., scanner upgrades, pulse sequence parameters, and spatial resolution). Additional studies are needed to investigate the natural history of brain atrophy progression in clinical and open-label studies.

Conclusions

CNS atrophy is a powerful predictor of subsequent neurological disability in the long-term. The relationship between spinal cord atrophy and disability is stronger than the association between brain atrophy and disability. CNS atrophy correlates better with disability than do conventional lesion measures. Brain atrophy is associated with impaired QOL, as well as urodynamic and sexual dysfunction. It is likely that once the level of CNS atrophy reaches a critical threshold, patients begin to suffer clinical impairment and disease progression. Conversely, fatigue does not correlate with brain atrophy. Longitudinal natural history studies in patients with CIS, RR, SP and PPMS indicate that CNS atrophy is common and progressive. The annual rate of whole brain atrophy is slightly higher in early RRMS than in advanced stages of RRMS. Patients with PPMS have higher annual rates of brain atrophy than patients with SPMS, but definitively lower rates than patients with RRMS. The rate of spinal cord atrophy in patients with PPMS appears to be faster than the rate of brain atrophy. CNS atrophy appears to occur independent of disease duration and disease course. This is probably related to a higher rate of atrophy early in the disease course and the heterogeneity of the rate of atrophy among patients with MS. We conclude that measurement of atrophy of the CNS is emerging as a clinically relevant biomarker of the disease process. Measurement of atrophy can help to resolve the "clinical-MRI paradox" that has historically limited the perception of the role of MRI as a biomarker in MS.

Acknowledgments

We thank Eve Salczynski for technical support. This work was supported in part by a research grant to R. Bakshi from the National Institutes of Health (NIH-NINDS 1 K23 NS42379).

References

Bakshi R. Fatigue associated with multiple sclerosis: diagnosis, impact and management. *Mult Scler* 2003; 9: 219-27.

Bakshi R, Ariyaratana S, Benedict RH, Jacobs L. Fluid-attenuated inversion recovery magnetic resonance imaging detects cortical and juxtacortical multiple sclerosis lesions. *Arch Neurol* 2001a; 58: 742-8.

Bakshi R, Benedict RH, Bermel RA, Caruthers SD, Puli SR, Tjoa CW, et al. T2 hypointensity in the deep gray matter of patients with multiple sclerosis: a quantitative magnetic resonance imaging study. *Arch Neurol* 2002; 59: 62-8.

Bakshi R, Benedict RH, Bermel RA, Jacobs L. Regional brain atrophy is associated with physical disability in multiple sclerosis: semiquantitative magnetic resonance imaging and relationship to clinical findings. *J Neuroimaging* 2001b; 11: 129-36.

Bakshi R, Miletich RS, Henschel K, Shaikh ZA, Janardhan V, Wasay M, et al. Fatigue in multiple sclerosis: cross-sectional correlation with brain MRI findings in 71 patients. *Neurology* 1999; 53: 1151-3.

Barkhof F. MRI in multiple sclerosis: correlation with expanded disability status scale (EDSS). *Mult Scler* 1999; 5: 283-6.

Benedict RH, Carone DA. In: Zivadinov R, Bakshi R, eds. *Brain and Spinal Cord Atrophy in Multiple Sclerosis. Brain atrophy, cognitive dysfunction and emotional disturbances in multiple sclerosis* . New York: Nova Science Publisher 2004; (p139-168).

Berg D, Maurer M, Warmuth-Metz M, Rieckmann P, Becker G. The correlation between ventricular diameter measured by transcranial sonography and clinical disability and cognitive dysfunction in patients with multiple sclerosis. *Arch Neurol* 2000; 57: 1289-92.

Bermel RA, Bakshi R, Tjoa C, Puli SR, Jacobs L. Bicaudate ratio as a magnetic resonance imaging marker of brain atrophy in multiple sclerosis. *Arch Neurol* 2002; 59: 275-80.

Bermel RA, Innus MD, Tjoa CW, Bakshi R. Selective caudate atrophy in multiple sclerosis: a 3D MRI parcellation study. *Neuroreport* 2003a; 14: 335-9.

Bermel RA, Sharma J, Tjoa CW, Puli SR, Bakshi R. A semiautomated measure of whole-brain atrophy in multiple sclerosis. *J Neurol Sci* 2003b; 208: 57-65.

Brex P, D S. A Longitudinal Study of Abnormalities on MRI and Disability from Multiple Sclerosis. *New England Journal of Medicine* 2002; 346: 158-164.

Brex PA, Jenkins R, Fox NC, Crum WR, O'Riordan JI, Plant GT, et al. Detection of ventricular enlargement in patients at the earliest clinical stage of MS. *Neurology* 2000; 54: 1689-91.

Brex PA, Leary SM, O'Riordan JI, Miszkiel KA, Plant GT, Thompson AJ, et al. Measurement of spinal cord area in clinically isolated syndromes suggestive of multiple sclerosis. *J Neurol Neurosurg Psychiatry* 2001; 70: 544-7.

Chard DT, Brex PA, Ciccarelli O, Griffin CM, Parker GJ, Dalton C, et al. The longitudinal relation between brain lesion load and atrophy in multiple sclerosis: a 14 year follow up study. *J Neurol Neurosurg Psychiatry* 2003; 74: 1551-4.

Chard DT, Griffin CM, Parker GJ, Kapoor R, Thompson AJ, Miller DH. Brain atrophy in clinically early relapsing-remitting multiple sclerosis. *Brain* 2002; 125: 327-37.

Cifelli A, Arridge M, Jezzard P, Esiri MM, Palace J, Matthews PM. Thalamic neurodegeneration in multiple sclerosis. *Ann Neurol* 2002; 52: 650-3.

Clanet M, Radue EW, Kappos L, Hartung HP, Hohlfeld R, Sandberg-Wollheim M, et al. A randomized, double-blind, dose-comparison study of weekly interferon beta-1a in relapsing MS. *Neurology* 2002; 59: 1507-17.

Coles AJ, Wing MG, Molyneux P, Paolillo A, Davie CM, Hale G, et al. Monoclonal antibody treatment exposes three mechanisms underlying the clinical course of multiple sclerosis. *Ann Neurol* 1999; 46: 296-304.

Comi G, Filippi M, Barkhof F, Durelli L, Edan G, Fernandez O, et al. Effect of early interferon treatment on conversion to definite multiple sclerosis: a randomised study. *Lancet* 2001; 357: 1576-82.

Comi G, Inglese M, De Stefano N, Smith S, Barkhof F, Durelli L, et al. Brain volume changes in patients at presentation with suspected multiple sclerosis: results from the ETOMS study. *Multiple Sclerosis* 2002; 8: S10.

Dalton CM, Brex PA, Jenkins R, Fox NC, Miszkiel KA, Crum WR, et al. Progressive ventricular enlargement in patients with clinically isolated syndromes is associated with the early development of multiple sclerosis. *J Neurol Neurosurg Psychiatry* 2002; 73: 141-7.

Dastidar P, Heinonen T, Lehtimaki T, Ukkonen M, Peltola J, Erila T, et al. Volumes of brain atrophy and plaques correlated with neurological disability in secondary progressive multiple sclerosis. *J Neurol Sci* 1999; 165: 36-42.

de Seze J, Stojkovic T, Gauvrit JY, Devos D, Ayachi M, Cassim F, et al. Autonomic dysfunction in multiple sclerosis: cervical spinal cord atrophy correlates. *J Neurol* 2001; 248: 297-303.

De Stefano N, Iannucci G, Sormani MP, Guidi L, Bartolozzi ML, Comi G, et al. MR correlates of cerebral atrophy in patients with multiple sclerosis. *J Neurol* 2002a; 249: 1072-7.

De Stefano N, Matthews PM, Filippi M, Agosta F, De Luca M, Bartolozzi ML, et al. Evidence of early cortical atrophy in MS: relevance to white matter changes and disability. *Neurology* 2003; 60: 1157-62.

De Stefano N, Narayanan S, Francis SJ, Smith S, Mortilla M, Tartaglia MC, et al. Diffuse axonal and tissue injury in patients with multiple sclerosis with low cerebral lesion load and no disability. *Arch Neurol* 2002b; 59: 1565-71.

Fabiano AJ, Sharma J, Weinstock-Guttman B, Munschauer FE, 3rd, Benedict RH, Zivadinov R, et al. Thalamic involvement in multiple sclerosis: a diffusion-weighted magnetic resonance imaging study. *J Neuroimaging* 2003; 13: 307-14.

Filippi M. Quantitative brain MRI lesion load predicts the course of clinically isolated syndromes suggestive of multiple sclerosis. *Neurology* 1994; 44: 635-641.

Filippi M, Mastronardo G, Rocca MA, Pereira C, Comi G. Quantitative volumetric analysis of brain magnetic resonance imaging from patients with multiple sclerosis. *J Neurol Sci* 1998; 158: 148-53.

Filippi M, Rocca MA, Colombo B, Falini A, Codella M, Scotti G, et al. Functional magnetic resonance imaging correlates of fatigue in multiple sclerosis. *Neuroimage* 2002; 15: 559-67.

Filippi M, Rovaris M, Iannucci G, Mennea S, Sormani MP, Comi G. Whole brain volume changes in patients with progressive MS treated with cladribine. *Neurology* 2000; 55: 1714-8.

Fisher E, Rudick RA, Cutter G, Baier M, Miller D, Weinstock-Guttman B, et al. Relationship between brain atrophy and disability: an 8-year follow-up study of multiple sclerosis patients. *Mult Scler* 2000; 6: 373-7.

Fisher E, Rudick RA, Simon JH, Cutter G, Baier M, Lee JC, et al. Eight-year follow-up study of brain atrophy in patients with MS. *Neurology* 2002; 59: 1412-20.

Fox NC, Jenkins R, Leary SM, Stevenson VL, Losseff NA, Crum WR, et al. Progressive cerebral atrophy in MS: a serial study using registered, volumetric MRI. *Neurology* 2000; 54: 807-12.

Gasperini C, Paolillo A, Giugni E, Galgani S, Bagnato F, Mainero C, et al. MRI brain volume changes in relapsing-remitting multiple sclerosis patients treated with interferon beta-1a. *Mult Scler* 2002; 8: 119-23.

Ge Y, Grossman RI, Udupa JK, Babb JS, Nyul LG, Kolson DL. Brain atrophy in relapsing-remitting multiple sclerosis: fractional volumetric analysis of gray matter and white matter. *Radiology* 2001; 220: 606-10.

Ge Y, Grossman RI, Udupa JK, Fulton J, Constantinescu CS, Gonzales-Scarano F, et al. Glatiramer acetate (Copaxone) treatment in relapsing-remitting MS: quantitative MR assessment. *Neurology* 2000a; 54: 813-7.

Ge Y, Grossman RI, Udupa JK, Wei L, Mannon LJ, Polansky M, et al. Brain atrophy in relapsing-remitting multiple sclerosis and secondary progressive multiple sclerosis: longitudinal quantitative analysis. *Radiology* 2000b; 214: 665-70.

Giovannoni G, Green AJ, Thompson EJ. Are there any body fluid markers of brain atrophy in multiple sclerosis? *Mult Scler* 1998; 4: 138-42.

Hardmeier M, Wagenpfeil S, Freitag P, Fisher E, Rudick RA, Kooijmans-Coutinho M, et al. Atrophy is detectable within a 3-month period in untreated patients with active relapsing remitting multiple sclerosis. *Arch Neurol* 2003; 60: 1736-9.

Hohol MJ, Guttmann CR, Orav J, Mackin GA, Kikinis R, Khoury SJ, et al. Serial neuropsychological assessment and magnetic resonance imaging analysis in multiple sclerosis. *Arch Neurol* 1997; 54: 1018-25.

Hoogervorst EL, Polman CH, Barkhof F. Cerebral volume changes in multiple sclerosis patients treated with high-dose intravenous methylprednisolone. *Mult Scler* 2002; 8: 415-9.

Ingle GT, Stevenson VL, Miller DH, Leary SM, Rovaris M, Barkhof F, et al. Two-year follow-up study of primary and transitional progressive multiple sclerosis. *Mult Scler* 2002; 8: 108-14.

Ingle GT, Stevenson VL, Miller DH, Thompson AJ. Primary progressive multiple sclerosis: a 5-year clinical and MR study. *Brain* 2003; 126: 2528-36.

Inglese M, Rovaris M, Giacomotti L, Mastronardo G, Comi G, Filippi M. Quantitative brain volumetric analysis from patients with multiple sclerosis: a follow-up study. *J Neurol Sci* 1999; 171: 8-10.

Jacobs LD, Cookfair DL, Rudick RA, Herndon RM, Richert JR, Salazar AM, et al. Intramuscular interferon beta-1a for disease progression in relapsing multiple sclerosis. The Multiple Sclerosis Collaborative Research Group (MSCRG). *Ann Neurol* 1996; 39: 285-94.

Janardhan V, Bakshi R. Quality of life and its relationship to brain lesions and atrophy on magnetic resonance images in 60 patients with multiple sclerosis. *Arch Neurol* 2000; 57: 1485-91.

Johnson KP, Brooks BR, Cohen JA, Ford CC, Goldstein J, Lisak RP, et al. Copolymer 1 reduces relapse rate and improves disability in relapsing-remitting multiple sclerosis: results of a phase III multicenter, double-blind placebo-controlled trial. The Copolymer 1 Multiple Sclerosis Study Group. *Neurology* 1995; 45: 1268-76.

Jones CK, Riddehough A, Li DKB, Zhao G, Paty DW, Group PSGUMMR. MRI cerebral atrophy in relapsing-remitting MS: results from the PRISMS trial (abstract). *Neurology* 2001; 56: A379.

Kalkers NF, Ameziane N, Bot JC, Minneboo A, Polman CH, Barkhof F. Longitudinal brain volume measurement in multiple sclerosis: rate of brain atrophy is independent of the disease subtype. *Arch Neurol* 2002a; 59: 1572-6.

Kalkers NF, Barkhof F, Bergers E, van Schijndel R, Polman CH. The effect of the neuroprotective agent riluzole on MRI parameters in primary progressive multiple sclerosis: a pilot study. *Mult Scler* 2002b; 8: 532-3.

Kalkers NF, Hintzen RQ, van Waesberghe JH, Lazeron RH, van Schijndel RA, Ader HJ, et al. Magnetization transfer histogram parameters reflect all dimensions of MS pathology, including atrophy. *J Neurol Sci* 2001; 184: 155-62.

Kaplan MR, Meyer-Franke A, Lambert S, Bennett V, Duncan ID, Levinson SR, et al. Induction of sodium channel clustering by oligodendrocytes. *Nature* 1997; 386: 724-8.

Kidd D, Thorpe JW, Kendall BE, Barker GJ, Miller DH, McDonald WI, et al. MRI dynamics of brain and spinal cord in progressive multiple sclerosis. *J Neurol Neurosurg Psychiatry* 1996; 60: 15-9.

Kidd D, Thorpe JW, Thompson AJ, Kendall BE, Moseley IF, MacManus DG, et al. Spinal cord MRI using multi-array coils and fast spin echo. II. Findings in multiple sclerosis. *Neurology* 1993; 43: 2632-7.

Leary SM, Miller DH, Stevenson VL, Brex PA, Chard DT, Thompson AJ. Interferon beta-1a in primary progressive MS: an exploratory, randomized, controlled trial. *Neurology* 2003; 60: 44-51.

Leist TP, Gobbini MI, Frank JA, McFarland HF. Enhancing magnetic resonance imaging lesions and cerebral atrophy in patients with relapsing multiple sclerosis. *Arch Neurol* 2001; 58: 57-60.

Lin X, Blumhardt LD, Constantinescu CS. The relationship of brain and cervical cord volume to disability in clinical subtypes of multiple sclerosis: a three-dimensional MRI study. *Acta Neurol Scand* 2003a; 108: 401-6.

Lin X, Tench CR, Turner B, Blumhardt LD, Constantinescu CS. Spinal cord atrophy and disability in multiple sclerosis over four years: application of a reproducible automated technique in monitoring disease progression in a cohort of the interferon beta-1a (Rebif) treatment trial. *J Neurol Neurosurg Psychiatry* 2003b; 74: 1090-4.

Liu C, Edwards S, Gong Q, Roberts N, Blumhardt LD. Three dimensional MRI estimates of brain and spinal cord atrophy in multiple sclerosis. *J Neurol Neurosurg Psychiatry* 1999; 66: 323-30.

Losseff NA, Miller DH. Measures of brain and spinal cord atrophy in multiple sclerosis. *J Neurol Neurosurg Psychiatry* 1998; 64 Suppl 1: S102-5.

Losseff NA, Wang L, Lai HM, Yoo DS, Gawne-Cain ML, McDonald WI, et al. Progressive cerebral atrophy in multiple sclerosis. A serial MRI study. *Brain* 1996; 119 (Pt 6): 2009-19.

Luks TL, Goodkin DE, Nelson SJ, Majumdar S, Bacchetti P, Portnoy D, et al. A longitudinal study of ventricular volume in early relapsing-remitting multiple sclerosis. *Mult Scler* 2000; 6: 332-7.

Lycklama G, Thompson A, Filippi M, Miller D, Polman C, Fazekas F, et al. Spinal-cord MRI in multiple sclerosis. *Lancet Neurol* 2003; 2: 555-62.

McDonald WI, Compston A, Edan G, Goodkin D, Hartung HP, Lublin FD, et al. Recommended diagnostic criteria for multiple sclerosis: guidelines from the International Panel on the diagnosis of multiple sclerosis. *Ann Neurol* 2001; 50: 121-7.

Meier D, Guttmann C. In: Zivadinov R, Bakshi R, eds. *Brain and Spinal Cord Atrophy in Multiple Sclerosis. MRI measures of pathology and their relationship to central nervous system atrophy in multiple sclerosis.* New York: Nova Science Publisher 2004 (in press).

Miller DH, Barkhof F, Frank JA, Parker GJ, Thompson AJ. Measurement of atrophy in multiple sclerosis: pathological basis, methodological aspects and clinical relevance. *Brain* 2002; 125: 1676-95.

Miller DM, Rudick RA, Baier M, Cutter G, Doughtery DS, Weinstock-Guttman B, et al. Factors that predict health-related quality of life in patients with relapsing-remitting multiple sclerosis. *Mult Scler* 2003; 9: 1-5.

Molyneux PD, Kappos L, Polman C, Pozzilli C, Barkhof F, Filippi M, et al. The effect of interferon beta-1b treatment on MRI measures of cerebral atrophy in secondary progressive multiple sclerosis. European Study Group on Interferon beta-1b in secondary progressive multiple sclerosis. *Brain* 2000; 123: 2256-63.

O'Riordan J. The prognostic value of brain MRI in clinically isolated syndromes of the CNS: A 10-year follow-up. *Brain* 1998; 121: 495-503.

Paolillo A, Coles AJ, Molyneux PD, Gawne-Cain M, MacManus D, Barker GJ, et al. Quantitative MRI in patients with secondary progressive MS treated with monoclonal antibody Campath 1H. *Neurology* 1999; 53: 751-7.

Minagar A, Gonzalez Toledo E, Alexander JS. In: Zivadinov R, Bakshi R, eds. *Brain and Spinal Cord Atrophy in Multiple Sclerosis. Central nervous system atrophy in multiple sclerosis: mechanisms.* New York: Nova Science Publisher 2004 (in press).

Paolillo A, Pozzilli C, Gasperini C, Giugni E, Mainero C, Giuliani S, et al. Brain atrophy in relapsing-remitting multiple sclerosis: relationship with 'black holes', disease duration and clinical disability. *J Neurol Sci* 2000; 174: 85-91.

Paolillo A, Pozzilli C, Giugni E, Tomassini V, Gasperini C, Fiorelli M, et al. A 6-year clinical and MRI follow-up study of patients with relapsing-remitting multiple sclerosis treated with Interferon-beta. *Eur J Neurol* 2002; 9: 645-55.

Pelletier D, Nelson SJ, Oh J, Antel JP, Kita M, Zamvil SS, et al. MRI lesion volume heterogeneity in primary progressive MS in relation with axonal damage and brain atrophy. *J Neurol Neurosurg Psychiatry* 2003; 74: 950-2.

Pfrieger FW, Barres BA. Synaptic efficacy enhanced by glial cells in vitro. *Science* 1997; 277: 1684-7.

Quarantelli M, Ciarmiello A, Morra VB, Orefice G, Larobina M, Lanzillo R, et al. Brain tissue volume changes in relapsing-remitting multiple sclerosis: correlation with lesion load. *Neuroimage* 2003; 18: 360-6.

Rao AB, Richert N, Howard T, Lewis BK, Bash CN, McFarland HF, et al. Methylprednisolone effect on brain volume and enhancing lesions in MS before and during IFNbeta-1b. *Neurology* 2002; 59: 688-94.

Redmond IT, Barbosa S, Blumhardt LD, Roberts N. Short-term ventricular volume changes on serial MRI in multiple sclerosis. *Acta Neurol Scand* 2000; 102: 99-105.

Rovaris M, Agosta F, Sormani MP, Inglese M, Martinelli V, Comi G, et al. Conventional and magnetization transfer MRI predictors of clinical multiple sclerosis evolution: a medium-term follow-up study. *Brain* 2003; 126: 2323-32.

Rovaris M, Bozzali M, Iannucci G, Ghezzi A, Caputo D, Montanari E, et al. Assessment of normal-appearing white and gray matter in patients with primary progressive multiple sclerosis: a diffusion-tensor magnetic resonance imaging study. *Arch Neurol* 2002; 59: 1406-12.

Rovaris M, Comi G, Rocca MA, Wolinsky JS, Filippi M. Short-term brain volume change in relapsing-remitting multiple sclerosis: effect of glatiramer acetate and implications. *Brain* 2001; 124: 1803-12.

Rovaris, Filippi M. In: Zivadinov R, Bakshi R, eds. *Brain and Spinal Cord Atrophy in Multiple Sclerosis. Treatment effect on MRI measures of central nervous system atrophy in multiple sclerosis*. New York: Nova Science Publisher 2004 (in press).

Rudick RA, Cutter G, Baier M, Fisher E, Dougherty D, Weinstock-Guttman B, et al. Use of the Multiple Sclerosis Functional Composite to predict disability in relapsing MS. *Neurology* 2001; 56: 1324-30.

Rudick RA, Cutter G, Reingold S. The multiple sclerosis functional composite: a new clinical outcome measure for multiple sderosis trials. *Mult Scler* 2002; 8: 359-65.

Rudick RA, Fisher E, Lee JC, Duda JT, Simon J. Brain atrophy in relapsing multiple sclerosis: relationship to relapses, EDSS, and treatment with interferon beta-1a. *Mult Scler* 2000; 6: 365-72.

Rudick RA, Fisher E, Lee JC, Simon J, Jacobs L. Use of the brain parenchymal fraction to measure whole brain atrophy in relapsing-remitting MS. Multiple Sclerosis Collaborative Research Group. *Neurology* 1999; 53: 1698-704.

Sailer M. Quantitative MRI in patients with clinically isolated syndromes suggestive of demyelination. *Neurology* 1999; 52: 599-606.

Sailer M, Fischl B, Salat D, Tempelmann C, Schonfeld MA, Busa E, et al. Focal thinning of the cerebral cortex in multiple sclerosis. *Brain* 2003; 126: 1734-44.

Sailer M, Losseff NA, Wang L, Gawne-Cain ML, Thompson AJ, Miller DH. T1 lesion load and cerebral atrophy as a marker for clinical progression in patients with multiple sclerosis. A prospective 18 months follow-up study. *Eur J Neurol* 2001; 8: 37-42.

Saindane AM, Ge Y, Udupa JK, Babb JS, Mannon LJ, Grossman RI. The effect of gadolinium-enhancing lesions on whole brain atrophy in relapsing-remitting MS. *Neurology* 2000; 55: 61-5.

Sharma R, Narayana PA, Wolinsky JS. Grey matter abnormalities in multiple sclerosis: proton magnetic resonance spectroscopic imaging. *Mult Scler* 2001; 7: 221-6.

Simon JH. From enhancing lesions to brain atrophy in relapsing MS. *J Neuroimmunol* 1999; 98: 7-15.

Simon JH. Brain and spinal cord atrophy in multiple sclerosis. *Neuroimaging Clin N Am* 2000; 10: 753-70 ,ix.

Simon JH. Brain and spinal cord atrophy in multiple sclerosis: role as a surrogate measure of disease progression. *CNS Drugs* 2001; 15: 427-36.

Simon JH, Jacobs LD, Campion MK, Rudick RA, Cookfair DL, Herndon RM, et al. A longitudinal study of brain atrophy in relapsing multiple sclerosis. The Multiple Sclerosis Collaborative Research Group (MSCRG). *Neurology* 1999; 53: 139-48.

Stevenson VL, Miller DH, Leary SM, Rovaris M, Barkhof F, Brochet B, et al. One year follow up study of primary and transitional progressive multiple sclerosis. *J Neurol Neurosurg Psychiatry* 2000; 68: 713-8.

Tartaglia MC, Narayanan S, Francis SJ, Santos AC, De Stefano N, Lapierre Y, et al. The relationship between diffuse axonal damage and fatigue in multiple sclerosis. *Arch Neurol* 2004; 61: 201-7.

Tartaglino LM, Friedman DP, Flanders AE, Lublin FD, Knobler RL, Liem M. Multiple sclerosis in the spinal cord: MR appearance and correlation with clinical parameters. *Radiology* 1995; 195: 725-32.

Taylor I, Butzkueven H, Litewka L, MacGregor LR, Szoeke C, Cook M, et al. Serial MRI in multiple sclerosis: a prospective pilot study of lesion load, whole brain volume and thalamic atrophy. *J Clin Neurosci* 2004; 11: 153-8.

Thompson AJ. Identification of brain atrophy with MRI in MS. *Mult Scler* 1998; 4: 257-9.

Thorpe JW, Kidd D, Moseley IF, Kenndall BE, Thompson AJ, MacManus DG, et al. Serial gadolinium-enhanced MRI of the brain and spinal cord in early relapsing-remitting multiple sclerosis. *Neurology* 1996; 46: 373-8.

Trapp BD, Ransohoff R, Rudick R. Axonal pathology in multiple sclerosis: relationship to neurologic disability. *Curr Opin Neurol* 1999; 12: 295-302.

Turner B, Lin X, Calmon G, Roberts N, Blumhardt LD. Cerebral atrophy and disability in relapsing-remitting and secondary progressive multiple sclerosis over four years. *Mult Scler* 2003; 9: 21-7.

Ukkonen M, Dastidar P, Heinonen T, Laasonen E, Elovaara I. Volumetric quantitation by MRI in primary progressive multiple sclerosis: volumes of plaques and atrophy correlated with neurological disability. *Eur J Neurol* 2003; 10: 663-9.

Ukkonen M, Elovaara I, Dastidar P, Tammela TL. Urodynamic findings in primary progressive multiple sclerosis are associated with increased volumes of plaques and atrophy in the central nervous system. *Acta Neurol Scand* 2004; 109: 100-105.

van der Werf SP, Jongen PJ, Lycklama a Nijeholt GJ, Barkhof F, Hommes OR, Bleijenberg G. Fatigue in multiple sclerosis: interrelations between fatigue complaints, cerebral MRI abnormalities and neurological disability. *J Neurol Sci* 1998; 160: 164-70.

Wilson M, Morgan PS, Lin X, Turner BP, Blumhardt LD. Quantitative diffusion weighted magnetic resonance imaging, cerebral atrophy, and disability in multiple sclerosis. *J Neurol Neurosurg Psychiatry* 2001; 70: 318-22.

Wolinsky JS, Comi G, Filippi M, Ladkani D, Kadosh S, Shifroni G. Copaxone's effect on MRI-monitored disease in relapsing MS is reproducible and sustained. *Neurology* 2002; 59: 1284-6.

Wolinsky JS, Narayana PA, Johnson KP. United States open-label glatiramer acetate extension trial for relapsing multiple sclerosis: MRI and clinical correlates. Multiple Sclerosis Study Group and the MRI Analysis Center. *Mult Scler* 2001; 7: 33-41.

Zivadinov R, Bagnato F, Nasuelli D, Bastianello S, Bratina A, Locatelli L, Watts K, Finamore L, Grop A, Dwyer M, Catalan M, Clemenzi M, Millefiorini E, Bakshi R, Zorzon M. Short-term brain atrophy changes in relapsing-remitting multiple sclerosis. *J Neurol Sci* 2004; 223: 185-93.

Zivadinov R, Bakshi R. Central nervous system atrophy and clinical status in multiple sclerosis. *J Neuroimaging* 2004b; 9: 647-64.

Zivadinov R, Bakshi R. Role of MRI in multiple sclerosis II: brain and spinal cord atrophy. *Front Biosci* 2004c; 9: 647-64.

Zivadinov R, De Masi R, Nasuelli D, Bragadin LM, Ukmar M, Pozzi-Mucelli RS, et al. MRI techniques and cognitive impairment in the early phase of relapsing-remitting multiple sclerosis. *Neuroradiology* 2001a; 43: 272-8.

Zivadinov R, Locatelli L, Stival B, Bratina A, Grop A, Nasuelli D, et al. Normalized regional brain atrophy measurements in multiple sclerosis. *Neuroradiology* 2003a; 45: 793-8.

Zivadinov R, Rudick RA, De Masi R, Nasuelli D, Ukmar M, Pozzi-Mucelli RS, et al. Effects of IV methylprednisolone on brain atrophy in relapsing-remitting MS. *Neurology* 2001b; 57: 1239-47.

Zivadinov R, Sepcic J, Nasuelli D, De Masi R, Bragadin LM, Tommasi MA, et al. A longitudinal study of brain atrophy and cognitive disturbances in the early phase of relapsing-remitting multiple sclerosis. *J Neurol Neurosurg Psychiatry* 2001c; 70: 773-80.

Zivadinov R, Zorzon M. Is gadolinium enhancement predictive of the development of brain atrophy in multiple sclerosis? A review of the literature. *J Neuroimaging* 2002; 12: 302-9.

Zivadinov R, Zorzon M, Locatelli L, Stival B, Monti F, Nasuelli D, et al. Sexual dysfunction in multiple sclerosis: a MRI, neurophysiological and urodynamic study. *J Neurol Sci* 2003b; 210: 73-6.

Zorzon M, Zivadinov R, Locatelli L, Stival B, Nasuelli D, Bratina A, et al. Correlation of sexual dysfunction and brain magnetic resonance imaging in multiple sclerosis. *Mult Scler* 2003; 9: 108-10.

Zorzon M, Zivadinov R, Nasuelli D, Ukmar M, Bratina A, Tommasi MA, et al. Depressive symptoms and MRI changes in multiple sclerosis. *Eur J Neurol* 2002; 9: 491-6.

In: Brain and Spinal Cord Atrophy in Multiple Sclerosis
Editors: R. Zivadinov and R. Bakshi, pp. 137-166
ISBN 1-59454-160-4

Chapter IX

Brain Atrophy, Cognitive Dysfunction and Emotional Disturbances in Multiple Sclerosis

Ralph H. B. Benedict[1,2*] and Dominic A. Carone[1,2]
[1]Department of Neurology, SUNY–University at Buffalo School of Medicine and Biomedical Sciences, Buffalo, NY, USA; [2]The Jacobs Neurological Institute, Buffalo, NY, USA

Introduction

Multiple sclerosis (MS) is a degenerative, chronic inflammatory disease of the central nervous system that causes demyelination, sclerotic plaque formation and, eventually, cerebral atrophy. In addition to the well recognized motor and sensory defects of MS, cognitive and emotional sequelae have been recognized for over a century (Charcot, 1877). These more subtle neuropsychological (NP) impairments can be missed during routine neurological evaluation, yet are a significant source of caregiver distress (Knight et al., 1997), vocational disability (Rao et al., 1991b), social impairments, (Benedict et al., 2000; Rao et al., 1991b) and poor quality of life (Amato et al., 1995).

Since the early work of Young and colleagues (1981) demonstrating that magnetic resonance imaging (MRI) is sensitive and superior to computerized tomography in detecting MS lesions, MRI has become the "gold standard" for characterizing cerebral pathology in MS patients. Various conventional (e.g., T1, T2, and PD weighted imaging) and non-conventional (e.g., magnetization transfer imaging, diffusion weighted imaging) MRI techniques have been used to predict clinical phenomena such as cognitive, personality and affective disturbances. In addition to enhancing the understanding of NP impairment in MS, such research holds the promise of identifying imaging markers of specific cognitive and behavioral defects. In this chapter, we review what is known about NP syndromes in MS and propose cost-effective methods for objective evaluation. We then summarize research findings that have elucidated

* Corresponding author: Dr. Ralph H. B. Benedict, Neurology, D-6, Buffalo General Hospital, 100 High Street, Buffalo, NY 14203, USA, E-mail: benedict@buffalo.edu

the correlation between MRI and neuropsychological functions. We conclude with case examples, and suggestions for future work and clinical applications.

Neuropsychological Impairment in MS

Cognitive Dysfunction

Charcot (1877) is most often credited with the first description of cognitive impairment in MS. In 1877 he observed that some patients with disseminated sclerosis exhibited "enfeeblement of memory," "slow conceptual thoughts," and "blunted affective and intellectual life." For more than 100 years, most neurologists believed that cognitive impairment in MS was uncommon, only affecting a few severely impaired patients (McKhann, 1982). However, with recent advances in NP assessment, (Benedict et al., 2002b; Fischer et al., 1994; Peyser et al., 1990) we now know that rougly half of all patients are cognitively impaired, (Heaton et al., 1985; Rao et al., 1991a) and that a higher frequency may exist among clinic attendees (Medaer et al., 1984; Rao et al., 1984).

Little is known about the natural history of cognitive impairment. While a number of longitudinal studies have been published, variation in test-retest intervals and testing methods has limited conclusions (Bobholz and Rao, 2003). A major problem is that serial NP assessments can induce learning effects as patients become more accustomed to the testing milieu. Thus, in a recent clinical trial, the positive impact of interferon-beta-1a was demonstrated by a lack of across-exam learning in the placebo group, (Fischer et al., 2000) not the prevention of decline in test score as would be intuitively expected. Some of the better longitudinal studies have shown that MS patients with neuropsychological disorders early in the course of the illness are more likely to decline over three years, and that such decline is independent of decline in physical capacity (Kujala et al., 1997). In a 10-year longitudinal study, Amato et al. (2001) found that 20 of 37 patients who did not exhibit cognitive impairment at baseline were stable on follow-up evaluation. From these studies we can offer two conclusions. First, NP testing is more sensitive to cognitive impairment in cross-sectional than longitudinal research. Second, cognitive impairment, once established, seldom remits and is a risk factor for the development of dementia.

It is well known that the pattern of MS cognitive disorder varies significantly between patients, as would be expected in a disease where the localization of cerebral pathology is heterogeneous (Rao, 1986). Nevertheless, we know that defects on tests that emphasize processing speed, working memory, new learning and recent memory are most common (Benedict et al., 2002b; Bobholz and Rao, 2003; Rao, 1995). We now turn to a discussion of the specific domains of impairment in MS and a recommended battery for evaluation.

First, deficits in information processing speed, and in the capacity to temporarily store and simultaneously manipulate verbal or visuospatial information in working memory, are well documented in MS patients (Archibald and Fisk, 2000; Beatty et al., 1989; Camp et al., 1999; DeLuca et al., 1993; Demaree et al., 1999; Franklin et al., 1988; Kujala et al., 1994; Litvan et al., 1988; Rao et al., 1989d). Two NP tests commonly used to evaluate this domain are the Paced Auditory Serial Addition Test (PASAT; Gronwall, 1977) and the Symbol Digit Modalities Test (SDMT; Smith, 1982). The PASAT requires patients to monitor a series of audiotaped digits while adding each consecutive digit to the one preceding it. As such, the task emphasizes both rapid information processing and the allocation of attention to two concurrent tasks (i.e., working memory). The SDMT presents a series of nine symbols, each of which is paired with a single digit in a key at the top of an 8.5" x 11" sheet. The remainder of the page has a pseudo-randomized sequence of these symbols and patients respond by voicing the digit associated with each of these as quickly as possible. Visual scanning and working memory are involved. Both the PASAT and the SDMT were modified by Rao and colleagues (1991a) for use with MS patients, and these adapted versions were recommended for use by a recently convened consensus panel (Benedict et al., 2002b). The PASAT was also included in the MS Functional Composite (MSFC), a clinical outcome measure composed of quantitative measures of leg, arm/hand, and cognitive function (Cutter et al., 1999; Fischer et al., 1999; Rudick et al., 1996).

Deficits on tests requiring the recall of recently acquired information are often observed in MS patients (Beatty et al., 1996; DeLuca et al., 1994; DeLuca et al., 1998; Fischer, 1988; Grant et al., 1984; Rao et al., 1984). While memory deficits have been documented using a variety of standardized and experimental tasks, impairment on tasks emphasizing the free (or unaided) recall of recently presented information has been most often reported. Compared to normal controls, patients with MS recall less information on the first recall attempt, improve at a slower rate with repeated trials, but exhibit only slightly faster than normal rates of forgetting. Recognition memory is usually normal or at least not as affected as free recall, (Beatty, 1993) raising the argument that poor memory in MS is due to a deficit in retrieval rather than encoding or consolidation (Rao et al., 1989c). This contention was challenged by studies showing that delayed recall is preserved in patients when groups are equated on initial learning, (DeLuca et al., 1998) and work demonstrating that recall is also affected by the degree to which new associations are required during encoding (Thornton et al., 2002).

The second edition of the California Verbal Learning Test (CVLT-II) (Delis et al., 2000) and the Brief Visuospatial Memory Test – Revised (BVMT-R) (Benedict, 1997) are two tests that evaluate both learning and delayed recall capacities. The former is a measure of auditory/verbal learning and memory requiring oral recall of a 16-word list. In addition to learning efficiency over five successive trials, 25-min. delayed recall and recognition (yes/no and forced choice) are assessed. The CVLT-II has two alternate forms to control for learning effects and is sensitive to MS-associated cognitive impairment (Delis et al., 1987; Scarrabelotti and Carroll, 1998). The BVMT-R has an analogous format but requires visual/spatial learning and memory. Patients are asked to view and remember a matrix of six abstract designs, presented for 10 seconds, over 3 trials. As in the CVLT-II procedure, the learning assessment is followed by delayed recall and recognition (yes/no) tasks. The BVMT-R is sensitive to cerebral disease (Benedict et al., 1996; Benedict, 1997) and has been used with MS patients (Benedict et al., 2002a; Benedict et al., 2001). It offers six alternate forms, the equivalence of which is well established.

The term "executive functions" refers to a collection of related abilities comprising abstract reasoning, conceptual flexibility, and the planning and organization of behavior. Although less well studied than deficits in processing speed/working memory or learning/memory, deficits in executive functions occur with considerable frequency in MS (Beatty, 1995; Beatty and Monson, 1994; Beatty and Monson, 1996; Foong et al., 1999; Foong et al., 1997; Mendozzi et al., 1993). Moreover, impairments in executive functions can affect performance on tests of other cognitive abilities (Troyer et al., 1994). The familiar Wisconsin Card Sorting Test (WCST) has been widely studied in MS patients (Arnett et al.,

1994; Benedict et al., 2002a). A similar test, now called the Sorting Test from the Delis-Kaplan Executive Function System (D-KEFS Sorting Test), (Delis et al., 2001) places more emphasis on the verbal description of conceptual similarities and may be more useful in longitudinal cognitive studies of MS (Beatty and Monson, 1996) due to its equivalent alternate forms. Deficits in visual-spatial function are nearly as common as impairment in executive ability (Ryan et al., 1996; van den Burg et al., 1987; Vleugels et al., 2000). Benton's Judgment of Line Orientation Test (JLO) may be the best available measure of visual-spatial ability for cost effective MS assessment. The JLO, which requires patients to identify the angle defined by two stimulus lines from among those defined by a visual array of lines, often reveals deficits in MS patients (Benedict et al., 2002b; Rao et al., 1991a).

Performance on tests involving general intelligence and language is most often preserved in MS patients, (Beatty and Gange, 1977; Rao et al., 1991a) although some patients may present with deficient word retrieval (Beatty et al., 1989; Beatty et al., 1988) The Controlled Oral Word Association Test (COWAT; Benton, 1989) is one often used test that measures this capacity. Patients have one minute to generate as many words as possible beginning with each of three different stimulus letters, which are presented individually. Thus, the COWAT cannot be considered a "pure" language measure because performance is strongly affected by the efficiency and speed of lexical search. Two equivalent alternate forms of this test are available.

Recognizing that cognitive impairment is common in MS and that cognition is not routinely assessed in the clinical setting, we convened an international panel to generate consensus on an ideal, minimal record of cognitive dysfunction in MS. The panel was composed of neuropsychologists and psychologists from the United States, Canada, United Kingdom, and Australia. Our objectives were to: (a) propose a minimal battery for clinical monitoring and research, and (b) identify strategies for improving assessment MS patients in the future. A 90-minute NP battery (Table 1), the Minimal Assessment of Cognitive Function in MS (MACFIMS), emerged from this discussion. The MACFIMS is composed of seven NP tests, covering the aforementioned cognitive domains commonly impaired in MS. These tests are all commercially available, have acceptable reliability, and are well suited for serial assessments (Table 1).

Personality and Affective Disorders

In addition to cognitive impairments, patients with MS frequently experience personality, affect or emotional dysfunction. The three most common MS-associated problems in this domain are depressive disorder, pathological euphoria/eutonia, and pathological laughing and crying. In this section, we briefly describe each of these syndromes and offer recommended assessment techniques.

Primary or major depressive disorder refers to a constellation of symptoms that includes unusual and recurrent dysphoria, anhedonia, guilt rumination, feelings of worthlessness, apathy, and so-called neurovegetative symptoms such as reduced appetite and insomnia (A.P.A., 1994; Minden and Schiffer, 1990). Prevalence estimates place lifetime risk for major depressive disorder in MS at roughly 25-50% (Huber et al., 1993; Minden and Schiffer, 1990; Patten et al., 2000; Sadovnick et al., 1996). If minor depression is considered, lifetime prevalence estimates rise considerably (Feinstein and Feinstein, 2001). While the cause of depression in MS is unknown, multiple factors are associated with its presentation. Some observations support a relationship with stress (Gilchrist and Creed, 1994; LaRocca et al., 1993), as might be expected in a chronic illness with symptoms that are disabling and often unpredictable. On the other hand, depression is also associated with cerebral pathology (Bakshi et al., 2000; Zivadinov et al., 2001a; Zorzon et al., 2001; Zorzon et al., 2002). What is most important is that psychological coping responses and treatment of depression appear to have an impact on treatment adherence (Mohr et al., 1997) and neurological outcomes (Mohr et al., 2000; Mohr et al., 2002).

Table 1. Recommended Tests in for Clinical Monitoring and Neuropsychological Research in MS.

Test	Domain	Comment
North American Adult Reading Test	Estimated Premorbid Intelligence	Administration Time ~ 5 min.
Controlled Oral Word Association Test	Language	Administration Time ~ 5 min. Two alternate forms, letters C,F,L and P,R,W.
Judgment of Line Orientation Test	Spatial Processing	Administration Time ~ 5 min. The two published forms are actually the same test items administered in a different order. Odd/even item splits of the JLO have been evaluated but the full length test may be more valid.
California Verbal Learning Test - II	Learning and Recent Memory	Administration Time ~ 20 min. There are two equivalent alternate forms and many indices regarding the quality of learning, confabulation, and response bias tendencies.
Brief Visuospatial Memory Test - Revised	Learning and Recent Memory	Administration Time ~ 10 min. There are six equivalent alternate forms and other indices to assess drawing ability and recognition bias.
Paced Auditory Serial Addition Test	Processing Speed/Working Memory	Administration Time ~ 5 min. Rao's 3.0 and 2.0 ISI versions suggested.
Symbol Digit Modalities Test	Processing Speed/Working Memory	Administration Time ~ 5 min. Rao's oral administration recommended.
D-KEFS Sorting Test	Executive Function	Administration Time ~ 10 min. Two administration formats and two forms. To conserve time, recommended that only the "free sort" condition be administered.
Beck Depression Inventory – Fast Screen	Depression	Administration Time ~ 5 min. Brief screening version of the larger Beck scale emphasizing mood and self-appraisal.
NEO Personality Inventory – FFI	Personality	Administration Time ~ 15 min. Short form of the larger scale than includes patient self-report and informant report forms.
Neuropsychiatric Inventory	Psychiatric and Behavior Disorders	Administration Time ~ 20 min. Structured interview based entirely on informant report.

Like cognitive impairment, MS-associated changes in personality and behavior were known in Charcot's time. In his scholarly review of this topic, Finger (1998) noted that Charcot observed that some MS patients exhibit a peculiar "cheerful indifference without cause." In the MS literature, the terms euphoria and eutonia have been used to describe these patients. A proclivity for "cheerful complacency which is out of context to the patient's total situation" (Surridge, 1969) may be the core feature. A few recent studies attempted to measure euphoric personality and behavior change using modern psychometric instruments. Our group (Benedict et al., 2001) compared cognitively-impaired MS patients and controls on the NEO Personality Inventory (NEO-PI; Costa and McCrae, 1992). Patients had higher degrees of neuroticism, and lower degrees of extraversion, agreeableness and conscientiousness. Regression models demonstrated that decrements in agreeableness and conscientiousness were associated with cognitive impairment. We also found that MS patients overestimated their capacity for empathy and conscientiousness, thus demonstrating poor insight. Three tests of executive function were correlated with these presumed personality changes. Thus, frontal lobe dysfunction may be related to poor insight and personality change in MS. Another sample (Diaz-Olavarrieta et al., 1999) was assessed with the Neuropsychiatric Inventory (NPI) (Cummings et al., 1994). Neuropsychiatric disturbances were far more common in MS (95%) than controls (16%). While depression was most common, euphoria and disinhibition were also observed. Finally, we studied 75 consecutive, unselected MS patients using the NPI (Fishman et al., 2004). Factor analysis identified a cluster of symptoms—labeled euphoria/disinhibition—similar to the euphoria/eutonia described by Charcot (1877) and others (Brown and Davis, 1922; Cottrell and Wilson, 1926). A euphoria/disinhibition factor score was elevated in 9% of patients and associated with secondary-progressive (SP) course, low agreeableness on the NEO-PI, impaired cognition, and high caregiver distress.

Rather than an acute mood disorder or personality disposition, pathological laughter-crying (PLC) refers to an involuntary dissociation between the expression of affect (eg crying and laughter) and subjectively reported mood. PLC was reported in MS by O.R. Langworthy and colleagues (1941) and has since been studied primarily by Feinstein and colleagues (Feinstein et al., 1997; Feinstein et al., 1999; Ron and Feinstein, 1992). The lifetime prevalence of PLC in MS is estimated at 10% (Feinstein et al., 1997). Most patients with PLC have chronic MS and SP course (Langworthy et al., 1941; Surridge, 1969). Like patients with pathological euphoria syndrome, PLC patients tend to show impairment on executive function tasks (Feinstein et al., 1999).

In the clinical setting, it is important that clinicians routinely evaluate for depression because of its very high prevalence in MS. In addition, methods are now available for the assessment of personality and neuropsychiatric symptoms. Such evaluation is most valuable when informants (e.g., spouse or partner) are also available for interview. In our center, we have complemented the MACFIMS with some other available tests when concerns are raised about disturbance of affect, mood or personality (Table 1).

MRI Correlates of Neuropsychological Impairment

Conventional Measures of Lesion Burden

As MS is a demyelinating disease causing white-matter cerebral lesions, brain/behavior research in MS has emphasized the quantitative assessment of lesion burden. Lesions shown as hyperintense on conventional T2-weighted MRI have been useful in diagnosing MS (Fazekas et al., 1999) and have afforded longitudinal monitoring of cerebral disease during clinical trials (Miller et al., 1996). The advent of fluid attenuated inversion recovery (FLAIR) imaging increased the sensitivity of T2-weighted lesion measures, particularly for lesions bordering CSF or gray matter (Bakshi et al., 2001). T1-weighted MRI has been used to detect hypointense areas in the brain thought to represent more chronic necrosis or axonopathy. T1 lesion load or so-called "black holes" appear to correlate better with some clinical outcomes than T2 lesion load measurements (Truyen et al., 1996). In this section, we briefly review correlation between lesion burden and neuropsychological dysfunction in MS patients.

In 1987, Huber and colleagues (1987) reported that neither the number nor distribution of MRI lesion was associated with dementia in MS, and in the following year, Franklin and colleagues (1988) reported a significant but modest correlation between MRI lesion ratings and cognitive functioning ($r = 0.35$). Rao et al. (1989b) improved upon these studies by employing quantitative (not qualitative) MRI measures and found that total T2 lesion area predicted performance in several domains of cognitive function. There were 34 measures considered. Partial correlations, accounting for the effects of age and education, ranged from not significant to -0.54 (conceptual reasoning). These authors also found that 83% of patients with total lesion area >30 cm^2 had some degree of cognitive impairment while only 22% of patients with a burden of <30 cm^2 were defective. Similar results were reported by Swirsky-Sacchetti et al. (1992). Grading patients as impaired or normal on NP testing, Patti et al (1995) found that demented and non-demented groups of MS patients differed significantly in total T2 confluent lesion area.

Arnett et al. (1994) divided 43 patients into three groups based on the extent of T2 lesion burden in the frontal lobe. While the groups were comparable on measures of intelligence, the high frontal burden group was more impaired on the WCST (e.g., more perseverative responses) than the non-frontal MS group. Significant correlations between executive function tests and frontal lobe lesion burden were also reported by Foong et al. (1997) although when these authors divided patients into frontal and non-frontal groups, there were no significant differences on executive function tasks. Thus, there is an association between frontal lobe lesion burden and executive function testing, but the regional specificity of this finding is suspect.

Using a crude clinician rating, Reischies and colleagues (1988) reported that total lesion load discriminated between patients with and without depression, euphoria and lability of affect. Reports on the location of lesions in psychiatric disorders has been inconsistent, with some investigators finding frontal lobe lesions associated with psychiatric disturbance, and others reporting correlations with pathology in temporal and parietal areas. Bakshi et al. (2000) evaluated 19 depressed and 29 non-depressed MS patients. After correcting for EDSS, depression was correlated with superior frontal and superior parietal TI lesions ($P < 0.01$), but not T2 hyperintense lesions. In contrast, lesions in the left suprainsular region were associated with elevations on scales reflecting mood and somatic complaints (Pujol et al., 2000). Temporal lobe pathology was also implicated by Berg et al. (2000) who found that depressed MS patients identified by psychiatric interviews had significantly larger temporal lesion burden than their non-depressed counterparts, especially on the right side. Support for the hypothesis that abnormalities in temporal-limbic cortex mediate depression in MS is also found in studies of functional brain imaging (Sabatini et al., 1996). It should be noted that some research (Millefiorini et al., 1992) with relapsing-remitting (RR) MS patients has shown that depression is not associated with brain lesions, suggesting that depression in this group may also be related to psychological-reactive states and stress coping responses (Mohr et al., 1999).

Little is known about the relationship between the euphoric state or PLC and lesion burden in MS patients. Ron and Logsdail (1989) found that euphoria in MS is associated with higher total MRI lesion load. In an effort to highlight the potential significance of frontal lobe lesion, Arnett's group (1994) reported a case study of a patient who showed increasing frontal lesion burden correlated with worsening performance on executive function tasks. This same patient exhibited increasing degrees of disinhibition, euphoria and indifference. The euphoric state is probably closely tied to dementia in MS, an assertion to which we will return below.

Non-Conventional MRI Techniques

Although T2-weighted imaging is sensitive to MS lesions, it does not provide information on the pathological substrate of MS lesions, which can range from edema and inflammation to axonal loss (McDonald et al., 1992; Trapp et al., 1999). This section focuses on newer MRI techniques with higher pathological specificity, including magnetization transfer imaging, magnetic resonance spectroscopy (MRS), and diffusion weighted imaging (DWI).

Magnetization transfer imaging (MTI), introduced in 1989, (Wolff and Balaban, 1989) has been a promising technique because it can test for pathological changes in normal appearing white matter. In brief, the magnetization transfer ratio (MTR) refers to signal intensity that is an indirect measure of the ability of myelin and other cell membranes to exchange energy with surrounding water molecules. Thus, MTR indicates the integrity or destruction of myelin and other cell membranes. Lower MTR indicates greater white matter pathology such as astrocytic hyperplasia and axonal damage (Grossman, 1994). Cognitive dysfunction is correlated with low MTR (Rovaris et al., 1998; van Buchem et al., 1998; Zivadinov et al., 2001a) and it accounts for more variance than lesion burden in regression models (Filippi et al., 2000). These studies have shown that it is possible to identify pathological processes within brain lesions and normal appearing white matter that are associated with cognitive impairment in MS.

NAA is an abundant amino acid in the brain that is a marker of axonal and neuronal integrity, making MRS a potentially sensitive measure of subtle white matter abnormalities (Arnold et al., 1998). MRS studies have revealed diminished *N*-acetyl aspartate/creatine ratio (NAA/Cr) in both acute and chronic MS lesions (Arnold et al., 1992; Arnold et al., 1998). Foong et al. (1999) found significantly reduced NAA/Cr ratios in the normal appearing white matter and frontal lesions of 25 MS patients. These authors did not find significant MRS/executive function correlations in group analyses,, but patients (n=5) with severely reduced N-acetyl aspartate (NAA)/Cr ratios performed worse than other patients (n=20) on a spatial working memory task.

Bakshi's group (Fabiano et al., 2003) has shown that DWI can assess tissue damage with greater sensitivity than conventional MRI in MS. The objective was to assess thalamic gray matter damage. Apparent diffusion coefficients were correlated with measures of atrophy and FLAIR lesion burden, and were higher in SP than RR MS patients. It is likely that atrophy of deep gray matter structures such as the thalamus contributes to neuropsychological impairment in MS, although to date this hypothesis has not been tested.

Brain Atrophy and NP Dysfunction

In this section we examine the correlation between brain MRI indices of brain atrophy and neuropsychological dysfunction in MS. We concern ourselves with two general groups of imaging measures: (1) linear measures of ventricle or corpus callosum size, and (2) quantitative measures of whole brain atrophy. There is intense interest in the potential measurement of regional cortical atrophy, but research in this domain is nascent.

While this chapter is focused on MRI, it seems fitting to begin our discussion with some early, seminal work that utilized computed tomography (CT). In 1985, Rao and colleagues (Rao et al., 1985) examined three linear measures, the length of the distance between the most lateral portion of each of the frontal horns of the lateral ventricles (bifrontal span), the width of the lateral ventricles in the region of the caudate (bicaudate span), and the maximum width of the third ventricle. All CT measures were significantly correlated with measures of cognitive function, and as can be seen in Table 2, some of the correlations were large. This study was followed the next near by Rabins et al's (1986) oft cited study which demonstrated an association between central atrophy and both depression and pathological euphoria. Atrophy was measured by a ratio of the width of the lateral ventricles at their widest point over the width of the brain at the same level. Mean depression scores were similar in MS and spinal cord injury patients, but MS patients with cerebral lesions were more depressed than those with only cord lesions ($P = 0.05$). Patients judged to be euphoric by clinical interview were more likely to have cerebral lesions and enlarged ventricles ($P = 0.04$).

These early studies were followed by the first comprehensive study investigating correlations between cerebral disease and neuropsychological impairment using semi-automated, quantified MRI techniques (Rao et al., 1989b). Fifty-three patients were studied to yield measures of total lesion area (TLA), ventricle-brain ratio, and corpus callosum size. Corpus callosum size was hypothesized to be an important predictor because pathology in this structure should cause slowed processing speed and deficient interhemispheric transfer (Pelletier et al., 1993; Rao et al., 1989a). Regression analyses indicated that TLA and corpus callosum size were both robust predictors of performance on a wide range of cognitive tests while ventricle-brain ratio was a predictor of each variable. Corpus callosum size or area was found to be a significant predictor of neuropsychological dysfunction in some subsequent studies, (Huber et al., 1992; Tsolaki et al., 1994) but linear ventricle measures were seldom employed in neuropsychological research until more recently (see below).

Table 2. Summary of Non-Longitudinal Correlational Studies on MS, CT/MRI Atrophy Measures, and Neuropsychological Measures*

Authors	Imaging Measures	Correlation with Neuropsychological Measures*		Controlled for
Rao et al., 1985	3VW	WMS-LM (-0.41) ± 7/24 DESIGN B (-0.37) ± WMS-ASSOC (-0.34) + WAIS-R SIM (-0.33) + FVRT-LISTAR (-0.32) + WMS-INF (-0.29) + 7/24-A RECALL (-0.28) + WAIS-R COMP (-0.26) + WAIS-R-LISTAD (-0.26) +	WMS-MQ (-0.37) ± WMS-VR (-0.35) ± FVRT-LISTB (-0.34) + WMS-DIGIT (-0.32) + 7/24 A (-0.32) + FVRT-LISTATR (-0.28) + WAIS-R VIQ (-0.27) +	Age
	Bicaudate Span	WMS-MQ (-0.32) + WMS-DIGIT (-0.29) + 7/24 DESIGN A (-0.29) +	FVRT-LISTB (-0.30) + WMS-VR (-0.29) + WMS-ASSOC (-0.26) +	Age
	Bifrontal Span	WMS-DIGIT (-0.26) +	WMS-INF (-0.25) +	Age
Rao et al., 1989	SCC	BCT ERRORS (-0.48) ± JLO (0.47) ± WAIS-R ARITH (0.39) ± WAIS-R VIQ (0.37) +	MEMSCAN (-0.48) ± PASAT (0.40) ± COWAT (0.39) +	Age, Education
Huber et al., 1992	SCC	TPT (0.57) ± TACTILE RH (0.48) ±	TMT B (0.55) ±	No variables
Tsolaki et al., 1994	3VW	WORD LIST (NR) +		No variables
Hohol et al. 1997	Brain/ ICV	SRT-LTS (0.32) + 10/36 (0.53) § PASAT (0.56) §	SRT-Del (0.35) + SDMT (0.63) §	Age, gender,, education
Camp et al. 1999	Linear estimate of CV	VESPAR (-0.40) ± BRB (-.32) +	Cog. Impairment Index (-0.35)	±No variables
van Buchem et al., 1998	Linear estimate of CV	VISSPFOR (0.67) § MAP (0.58) § DIGSPBACK (0.54) § PASAT (0.47) ± VISPUR (0.37) +	REYCOPY (0..61) ± REYIMEMREC (0.56)± VISSPBACK (0.52) § WORDSPAN (0.41) ±	No variables

Table 2. Continued*

Authors	Imaging Measures	Correlation with Neuropsychological Measures*		Controlled for
Zivadinov et al., 2001b	BPV	Overall cognitive impairment (.89) ±		No variables
Zorzon et al. 2001	Right temporal BV	HDRS (0.29) ±		No variables
	Total temporal BV	HDRS (0.26) ±		
	Right hemisphere BV	HDRS (0.25) ±		
Benedict et al., 2002	3VW	PASAT (0.22) ±		None
	SFA right	CVLT Trials 1-5 (0.52) ± PASAT (0.44) ±	BVMT Trials 1-3 (0.45) ±	TLA
	SFA left	BCT (0.39) ±		
Bermel et al., 2002	BCR	SDMT (-0.42) +		Age
Christodolou et al., 2003	CA	SDMT (-.70) ±	Overall NPP (-0.64) ±	Age, education
		10/36 SRT Total (-0.52) ±	10/36 SRT DR (-0.50) ±	
		PASAT (-0.48) ±	TOH (-0.47) ±	
		COWAC (-0.44) ±	SRT Delayed Recall (-0.38) +	
Benedict et al., 2004	3VW	SDMT (-0.71) §	PASAT (-0.57) ±	Age, Premorbid IQ
		BVMT-R DR (-0.47) §	CVLT-II LEARNING (-0.45)	
		CVLT-II DR (-0.45) §		
	3VW	SDMT (-0.71) §	PASAT (-0.57) §	Age, Premorbid IQ
		BVMT-R DR (-0.47) ±	CVLT-II DR (-0.45) ±	
		CVLT-II LEARNING (-0.44) +	Depression	

Note: Only correlation significant less than or equal to .05 are reported.

* Only the Rao et al., 1985 study includes CT measures. The remaining studies include MRI measures.

**Values are Spearman's correlation coefficients

\+ Correlations with p values between 0.01 and 0.05

±Correlations with p value between 0.001 and 0.01

§ Correlation with p <.001

NR = Correlation coefficient not reported

MRI Measure Abbreviations: 3VW = Third Ventricle Width; BCR = Bicaudate ratio; BPF = Brain Parenchymal Fraction; BV = Brain volume; CCA = Corpus callosum atrophy; CA = Cerebral Atrophy; CV = Cerebral Volume; SCC = Size of corpus callosum; SFA = Superior frontal atrophy; TLA = Total T2 Lesion Area

Neuropsychological Measures and Abbreviations: 7/24 DESIGN A = 7/24 Test (Design A); 7/24 AR = 7/24 Test (Design A Total Recall); 7/24 DESIGN B = 7/24 Test (Design B); 10/36 SRT = 10/36 Spatial Recall Test; 10/36 SRT DR = 10/36 Spatial Recall Test Delayed Recall; BCT = Booklet Category Test; BCT ERRORS = BCT Total Errors; BVMT-R DR = Brief Visuospatial Memory Test-Revised, Delayed Recall; CAT FLUENCY = Category Fluency; Cog. Impairment Index = Cognitive Impairment Index; BRB = Brief Repeatable Battery; COWAC = Controlled Oral Word Association Categories; COWAT = Controlled Oral Word Association Test; CVLT-II DR= California Verbal Learning Test – Second Edition, Delayed Recall; CVLT-II LEARNING = California Verbal Learning Test – Second Edition, Learning; DIGSPBACK = Digit Span Backwards Task; FVRT-LISTAD = Free Verbal Recall Test List A Delayed; FVRT-LISTAR = Free Verbal Recall Test List A Recall; FVRT-LISTATR = Free Verbal Recall Test List A Total Recall; FVRT-LISTB = Free Verbal Recall Test List B; HDRS = Hamilton Depression Rating Scale; JLO = Judgment of Line Orientation; MAP = Road Map Test; MEMSCAN = Sternberg Memory Scanning Test, Scan rate (msec per digit); NPP = Neuropsychological performance; PASAT = Paced Auditory Serial Addition Test; PHON FLUENCY = Phonetic Verbal Fluency; REYCOPY = Rey-Osterrieth Complex Figure Test (Copy); REYIMMEMREC= Rey-Osterrieth Complex Figure Test (Copy) with immediate recall of complex design; SDMT = Symbol Digit Modalities Test; SRT = Selective Reminding Test; TACTILE RH = Tactile Forms Right Hand; TMT B Trail Making Test part B; TOH = Tower of Hanoi; TPT = Tactual Performance Test; VISPUR = Visual Pursuits Test of the Employee Aptitude Survey; VISSPBACK = Visual Memory Span Backward Test; VISSPFOR = Visual Memory Span Forward Test; VESPAR = Verbal and Spatial Reasoning Test; WAIS-R ARITH = Wechsler Adult Intelligence Scale-Revised Arithmetic subtest; WAIS-R COMP = Wechsler Adult Intelligence Scale-Revised Comprehension subtest; WAIS-R SIM = Wechsler Adult Intelligence Scale-Revised Similarities subtest; WAIS-R VIQ = Wechsler Adult Intelligence Scale-Revised Verbal IQ; WMS-ASSOC = Wechsler Memory Associate Learning subtest; WMS-DIGIT = Wechsler Memory scale Digit Span subtest; WMS-INF = Wechsler Memory Scale Information subtest; WMS-LM = Wechsler Memory Scale Logical Memory subtest; WMS-MQ = Wechsler Memory Scale Memory Quotient; WMS-VR = Wechsler Memory Scale Visual Reproduction subtest; WORDSPAN = Word Span Test

Thus far, we have been discussing regional measures of brain atrophy. But over the past five years there has been increasing interest in measures of whole-brain atrophy that involve fully- or semi-automated measures of parenchymal volume, or a ratio of brain volume to cranial space or some other measure that accounts for CSF volume. Rudick et al. (1999) found that a reproducible measure of whole brain atrophy worsened in MS patients over two years, independent of clinical disease activity. Brain Parenchymal Fraction (BPF) was defined as the ratio of brain parenchymal volume over the total volume within the brain surface contour. Earlier, Hohol et al. (1997) had shown that a similar measure of brain to intracranial volume ratio was correlated with Brief Repeatable Neuropsychological Battery measures of nonverbal memory, processing speed and attention. This was not replicated by Rovaris et al. (2002) who found no correlation between their measure of brain volume and cognitive performance.

A related measure of whole brain atrophy involves the segmentation of the MRI signal into gray matter, white matter, and CSF. It may be that one of these three indices is a more robust predictor of neuropsychological outcomes. Along these lines, Edwards et al. (2001) reported that a general cognitive index derived from neuropsychological testing was significantly correlated with corpus callosum and white matter volume loss but not gray matter volume. They proposed that subcortical axonal loss is most important in predicting cognitive function in MS.

While cognitive dysfunction is correlated with measures of lesion burden and atrophy, it is unclear which of these conventional dimensions is most predictive. We would like to close this discussion of the cross-sectional atrophy research with more detailed presentations of three studies completed or published during the past year that address this question (Benedict et al., 2004; Bermel et al., 2002; Christodoulou et al., 2003). They share in common (1) a hierarchical regression approach that accounted for multiple atrophy and lesion MRI predictors, (2) the finding that the SDMT is a parsimonious NP outcome, and (3) the conclusion that linear measures of atrophy account for more variance in cognitive function than measures of lesion burden.

Bermel and colleagues (2002) set out to determine whether bicaudate ratio (BCR), the minimum intercaudate distance divided by brain width along the same line, is comparable to other MRI markers in predicting cognitive impairment. Sixty patients with MS and 50 age- and sex-matched control subjects were evaluated. In addition to BCR, regression models accounted for T1 and FLAIR lesion burden, and whole brain atrophy. The SDMT was selected as the primary neuropsychological outcome due to its suspected sensitivity to MS-associated cognitive disorder. BCR was higher in patients than controls and regression modeling selected BCR but not lesion volume in the final model. The authors concluded that BCR is abnormal in MS and more closely correlated with cognitive dysfunction than other magnetic resonance imaging markers.

Christodoulou and others (2003) examined a similar question but with different MRI predictors and a wider range of NP outcomes. Thirty-seven MS patients meeting liberal entrance criteria for cognitive impairment ($z<-.5$) were studied. T2 lesion burden was measured, as was central atrophy, assessed as the percent of central CSF/intracranial volume. In addition, left and right posterior periventricular regions were examined with MRS looking for abnormalities in NAA/Cr and NAA/Cho. NP tests included components of the Brief Repeatable Battery of NP Tests in MS, (Rao, 1991a) which included the SDMT. Partial correlations controlling for age and education were calculated, followed by regression analysis. Among these MRI measures, central atrophy accounted for the most variance in all cognitive tests, and the correlation between SDMT and CSF-parenchyma fraction was very high, at $r = -.70$.

In a similar vein, we (Benedict et al., 2004) studied 37 MS patients and 27 healthy volunteers, group matched on age, education, race and gender. The median Expanded Disability Status Scale (EDSS) was 2.5 (range = 0-7.5). Thirty patients had RR and the remainder SP course. MRI predictors were T1 hypointense lesion volume (T1LV), FLAIR lesion volume (FLV), BCR determined using the method of Bermel et al. (2002) third ventricle width (TVW), and BPF. To obtain TVW, a line ROI was drawn through the long axis of the ventricle, parallel to the inter-hemispheric fissure in the slice where the third ventricle was most visible (Fig 1). Width was measured by drawing a second line perpendicular to the first at its midpoint and recording its length. BPF was based on a semi-automated technique (Bermel et al., 2003), defined as the ratio of brain parenchymal volume to the total brain volume within the surface contour. Neuropsychological testing was based on the MACFIMS position paper (Benedict et al., 2002b) and included the PASAT, SDMT, CVLT-II, BVMT-R, COWAT, BNT, JLO, and WCST. Regression analysis was limited to neuropsychological variables that discriminated patients and controls ($P <0.01$). Covariates, entered and retained in block 1 included age and North American Adult Reading Test (NAART) in the first model, and age, NAART and depression scale in the second. The MRI measures (T1LV, FLV, BCR, TVW, BPF) were then entered in block 2. After controlling for age and premorbid intelligence, TVW accounted for significant variance in the processing speed and memory tests (CVLT-II Learning, CVLT-II Delayed Recall, BVMT-R Delayed

Recall, PASAT, SDMT). Similar results were obtained when depression was added to the covariates. When the models were repeated with TVW removed, BPF accounted for most variance. The partial r effect between TVW and SDMT, controlling for age, education and depression, was quite large (r = -0.71) as in the Christodoulou (2003) study.

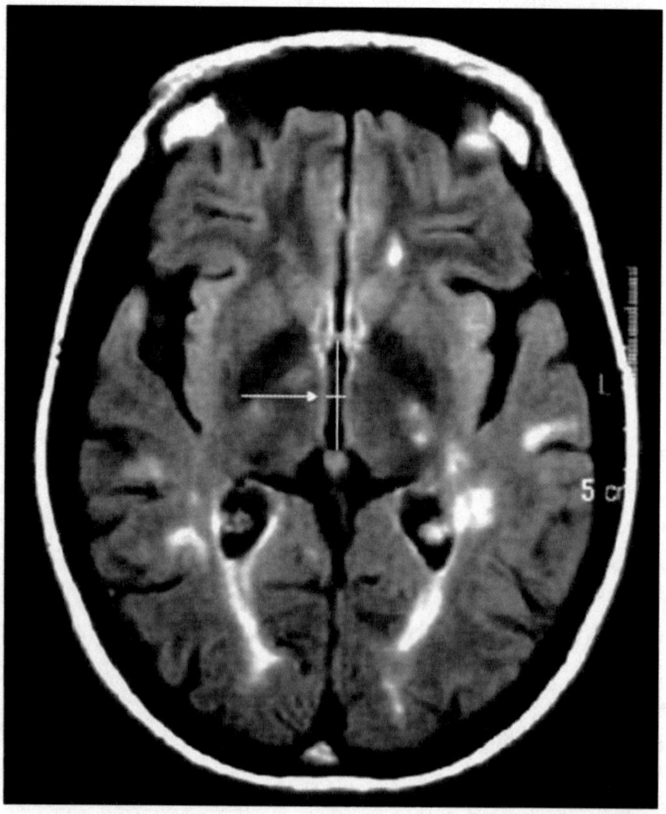

Fig 1. Calculation of third ventricle width (TVW) (Benedict et al., 2004). A line region of interest (ROI) is drawn through the long axis of the third ventricle, parallel to the interhemispheric fissure in the FLAIR axial slice where the third ventricle was most visible. The width was measured by drawing a second line ROI perpendicular to the first at its midpoint (arrow).

Altogether, these studies accounted for multiple MRI predictors including T1 lesion volume, FLAIR or T2 lesion volume, MRS, BPF, and various measures of central atrophy. In all three studies, measures of central atrophy accounted for most predictive variance in NP testing and the SDMT was the NP measure most strongly correlated with MRI. The studies were rigorous methodologically in that they controlled for multiple co-variates, including age, education and, in one case, depression. As was noted by Christodoulou, the SDMT, despite its brevity and ease of administration, has been shown to be sensitive to other neurological disorders.

Quantified studies of cortical atrophy and cognition in MS are yet to appear in the literature, as it has proven quite difficult to measure atrophy exclusively in the cortex in a reliable and semi-automated fashion. We (Benedict et al., 2002a) conducted a preliminary study of sulcal widening using an ordinal rating scale shown in previous studies to have good reliability (Bakshi et al., 1999). Cortical atrophy was rated in six lobar regions in each hemisphere as follows: superior frontal, inferior frontal, temporal, superior parietal, inferior parietal, occipital. The degree of atrophy was graded as 0 mild to 3 severe. Regression models were developed to predict cognitive functioning based first on general measures of lesion burden (FLAIR lesion volume) and central atrophy (TVW), followed by the ordinal rankings. Four of five memory and executive function tests were predicted by superior frontal atrophy after accounting for the general measures. That this region was selected by the regression analysis is not surprising, considering the importance of the superior frontal cortex for a wide range of cognitive tasks in functional imaging studies, (Braver et al., 1997; Grasby et al., 1994; Sarazin et al., 1998) and evidence for prominent hypometabolism in the superior versus inferior frontal cortex of MS patients (Bakshi et al., 1998).

While only modest correlations were recently reported between whole brain volumes and clinician ratings of depression and anxiety (Zorzon et al., 2001), Bakshi et al. (2000) found that depression was associated with ordinal ratings of frontal atrophy and enlargement of the lateral and third ventricles. Other literature has suggested an association between general atrophy measures and other neuropsychiatric states, such as euphoria, behavioral disinhibition, social aggression, and apathy (Hotopf et al., 1994; Rabins, 1990; Rabins et al., 1986). It may be that as patients become more vulnerable cognitively, they also become more inclined to develop affect or personality syndromes.

A promising, innovative method for measuring atrophy in multiple brain regions has been proposed by Feinstein and colleagues in their recent study of depression (Feinstein et al., 2004). Automated segmentation was used to divide the MRI signal into gray matter, white matter, and CSF. A semi-automatic method was then used to parcel the brain into 13 regions of interest per hemisphere (inter rater reliability varied across regions from an ICC of .93 to .97). Gray, white and CSF volumes in each region were as expressed a proportion of the entire regional volume. Compared with euthymic patients, depressed MS patients had less gray matter volume ($p=.01$) and more csf volume in the left anterior temporal lobe ($p=.005$).

Finally, the few longitudinal studies of atrophy and cognitive dysfunction (Table 3) should be discussed. In Hohol's study (1997), changes in cognitive function at one-year follow-up were correlated with increasing whole brain atrophy. Pelletier et al. (2001) investigated corpus callosum atrophy and cognitive dysfunction in RR patients over a 5-year period. Experimental tasks thought to involve interhemispheric transfer of motor, auditory, and sensory information were the primary neuropsychological outcomes. The authors found significant correlation between corpus callosum atrophy and performance. While correlations between change scores were not examined, the authors noted that the significant relationship between atrophy and impairment persisted after five years, suggesting that atrophy and cognitive impairment follow a progressive and parallel course.

Piras and collegues (2003) showed that cognitive dysfunction was correlated with atrophy and lesion burden at baseline and after 8.5 years, although there was no association between indices of progression in cognition and MRI pathology. In contrast, such an association was reported by Zivadinov et al. (2001b) who studied 53 RR MS patients over two years. BPVs were obtained and the relationship between cognitive impairment and MRI was assessed. Overall, 14 patients (26.4%) were judged to be cognitively impaired at baseline and 28 (52.8%) follow up. Five (9.4%) of patients were considered cognitively improved, 33 (62.3%) stable, and 15 (28.3%) worsened over 2 years. T2 and T1 volume changes in improved, stable, and worsened patients did not differ significantly whereas BPV decline was greater in those cognitively worsened. Thus, even in the early stages of RRMS, cognitive deterioration relies more on the development of brain atrophy than on lesion burden.

Case Examples

One of the advantages of linear measurement of atrophy is that indices are easily derived in the clinical setting. We now describe three cases wherein the imaging was performed on the same scanner, and the aforementioned methods were used to calculate TVW (Benedict et al., 2004) and BCR (Bermel et al., 2002). Axial T1-weighted (TR/TE: 400/10) and FLAIR) images (TR/TE/TI: 8000/120/2200) were obtained on a Philips Gyroscan ACS-NT 1.5-T scanner. Analysis was performed on a Unix workstation (Sun Microsystems) using Java Image software by a trained technician, blind to clinical data. TVW and BCR were measured from FLAIR images (Figs 2, 4 and 6). BCR was calculated as the ratio of the inter-caudate distance to the brain width along the same line. TVW was measured by drawing a line through the long axis of the ventricle, parallel to the inter-hemispheric fissure in the slice where the third ventricle was most visible, and measuring width by drawing a second line perpendicular to the first. BPF was obtained based a semi-automated technique developed by Bakshi's group (Bermel et al., 2003). In our normal sample, we obtained the following mean values: TVW = 1.65 (SD = 0.33), BCR = 0.08 (SD = 0.01), BPF = 0.90 (SD = 0.05).

The patients described also underwent a standard neuropsychological examination based largely on the MACFIMS (Benedict et al., 2002b). Also employed were assessments of personality, (Benedict et al., 2001), mood (Benedict et al., 2003), and behavior (Fishman et al., 2004), as suggested by our published work in these areas. From a sample of 40 normal controls, matched to our MS sample on demographic variables, we obtained z scores (Figs. 3, 5, and 7) on all cognitive measures.

Case HJ, a 23 year-old woman, was diagnosed with MS just three years prior to assessment. She has RR disease. Her EDSS is 2.5. She has 12 years of education and is employed full time. Her MRI atrophy indices are TVW = 3.0, BCR = 0.05, and BPF = 0.87 (Fig 2). While outside of the normal range, these indices are modest in comparison to patients with more advanced disease (see below). It can also be seen that she is cognitively intact. Neuropsychological testing reveals no z scores below -1.0 (Fig 3). Her primary complaint is fatigue. She has only minimal complaints of depression and her Neuropsychiatric Inventory index is normal. At the time of this writing, this patient is functioning well from a vocational and social perspective.

Case LD is a 43 year-old single woman, with a 17-year history of MS. Her EDSS is 6.5. Well known to our clinic, LD has long been regarded as an example of patients with mostly physical, and not mental, disability. Although she is disabled vocationally, she volunteers 20-30 hours per week in a technical position, and is a part-time student. Her MRI atrophy indices are TVW = 5.1, BCR = 0.15, and BPF = 0.81 (Fig 4). Depression scales are normal. Her spouse reports a modest elevation of 12 on the Neuropsychiatric Inventory, with the strongest weightings found on the depression and anxiety scales. This patient has no psychosocial defects and she describes healthy family relationships. While she does not consider herself to be cognitively disabled, we note that she is cognitively impaired (Fig 5), not employed, and that she has struggled in the academic setting.

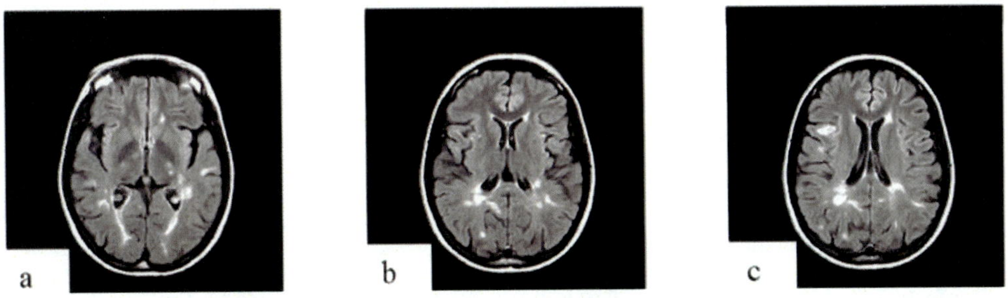

Fig. 2. Patient HJ with little cognitive impairment. FLAIR images taken at the level of third ventricle (**2a**), inferior lateral ventricle and caudate nucleus (**2b**), and dorsal aspect of lateral ventricle (**2c**).

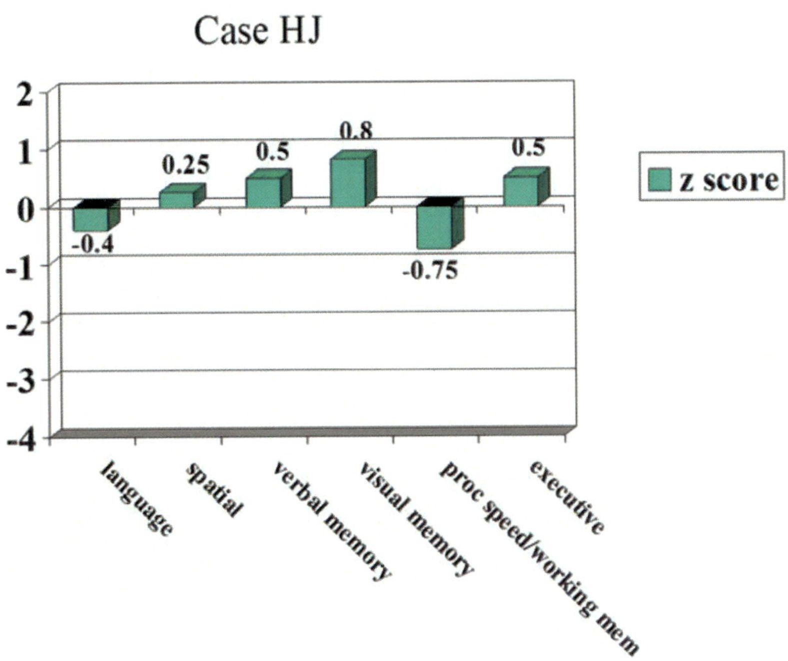

Fig 3 shows z scores in cognitive domains assessed with the MACFIMS battery.

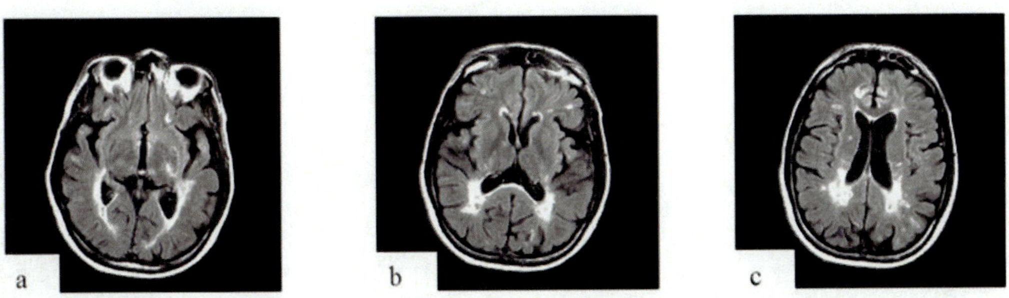

Fig 4. Patient LD with moderate cognitive impairment. FLAIR images taken at the level of third ventricle (**4a**), inferior lateral ventricle and caudate nucleus (**4b**), and dorsal aspect of lateral ventricle (**4c**).

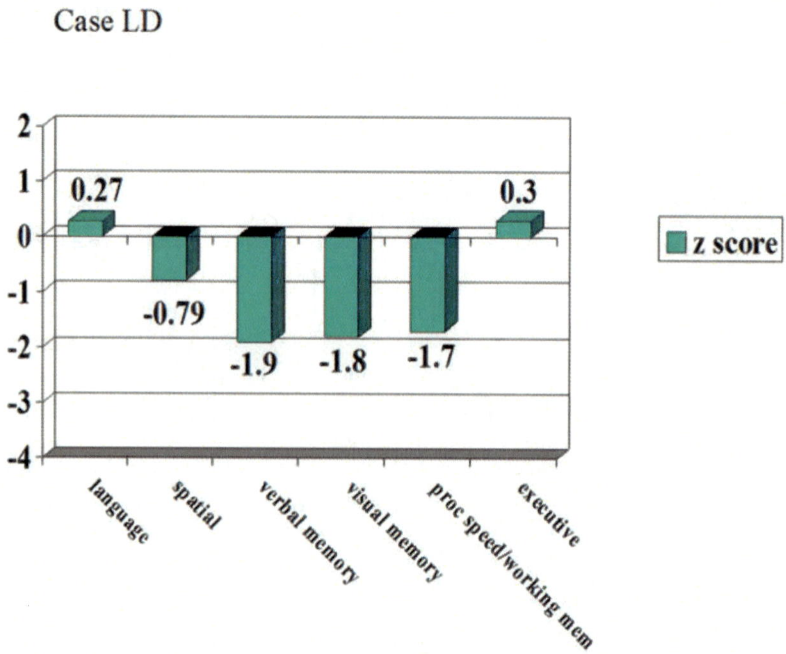

Fig 5 shows z scores in cognitive domains assessed with the MACFIMS battery.

Case BK is a 26 year-old female MS patient who has already entered into a progressive course of the disease, despite her youth. She was diagnosed just seven years ago. Her EDSS is 4.0. Her MRI atrophy indices are all markedly abnormal (TVW = 6.4, BCR = 0.12, and BPF = 0.79) (Fig 6). What are the effects of this pathology? First, she is totally disabled from vocational function and unlike LD, she does not volunteer nor is she active in the community. Objective cognitive testing reveals a severe defect in processing speed and working memory (Fig 7). She is also more moderately impaired on tests of memory. She is only mildly depressed on the BDI-FS. However, her spouse reports frequent episodes of emotional dyscontrol. Indeed, on the Neuropsychiatric Inventory, her general severity index is markedly elevated at 44, and there are severe problems in depression, agitation/aggression, irritability and disinhibition. Fortunately, this patient has responded well to antidepressant and mood stabilizing therapies.

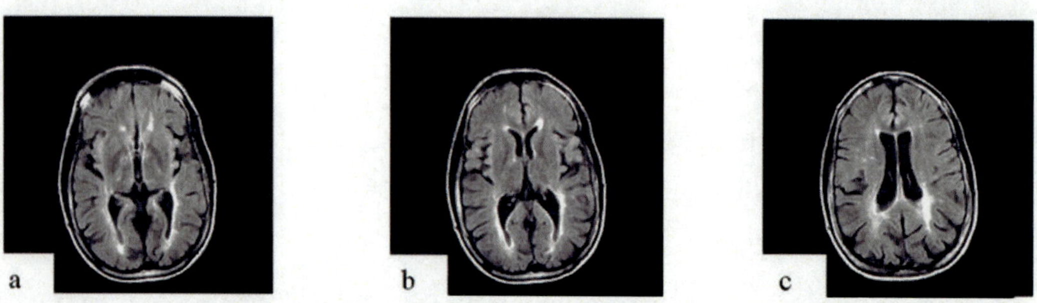

Fig 6. Patient BK with MS-associated dementia with early personality/behavior disorder. FLAIR images taken at the level of third ventricle (**6a**), inferior lateral ventricle and caudate nucleus (**6b**), and dorsal aspect of lateral ventricle (**6c**).

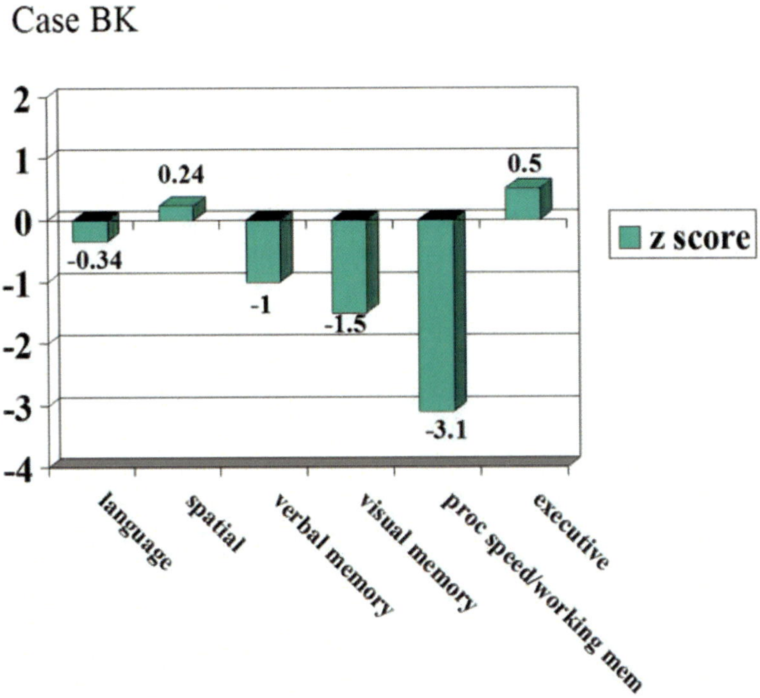

Fig 7 shows z scores in cognitive domains assessed with the MACFIMS battery.

Conclusions and Future Directions

The research reviewed in this chapter strongly supports the notion that a wide range of MRI measures of cerebral disease in MS are correlated with standardized measures of neuropsychological dysfunction. While there are far more published studies of cognitive function than emotional disorders, the existing data indicate that MRI predicts cognitive dysfunction, depression, euphoria/eutonia, and PLC. Some of the effects reported in this literature have been large, approaching r= 0.7 in the more recent studies. These large effects have been obtained in studies using ventricle size as opposed to lesion burden.

Correlations between neuropsychological dysfunction and measures of whole brain atrophy, such as the familiar BPF, have been disappointing. The reason is unclear. These measures attempt to account for pathology throughout the brain. Because they are semi- or fully-automated, they are very reliable and useful for monitoring the progression of atrophy over time. However, they are general measures. Low BPF may reflect central atrophy in one patient and cortical atrophy in another. In contrast, third ventricle width reflects only central atrophy and perhaps more specific pathological changes that are relevant for processing speed (as measured by SDMT). We also encourage researchers to pursue the distinction between white and gray matter volumes (Edwards et al., 2001). Of the more recently developed, non-conventional, MRI technologies, analysis of microscopic pathological changes within the normal appearing white matter have shown considerable promise. In one recent study, low MTR accounted for more variance in predicting cognitive dysfunction than did lesion burden in regression models (Filippi et al., 2000). In sum, we can now account for roughly half of the variance in MS associated cognitive dysfunction using structural MRI. In the near future, we will see continuing efforts to build optimal statistical models that better predict neuropsychological phenomena using various combinations of the reviewed techniques.

A related but different question concerns the regional specificity of these MRI findings. The case examples presented above highlight the clinical utility of these correlative studies. Ventricular enlargement that is readily apparent on visual inspection of axial images would seem to predict a much higher risk of neuropsychological dysfunction. One would hope that we would some day develop the technology and expertise to identify MRI features that are specific for regional neurobehavioral syndromes. Clinically, it can be difficult to disentangle premorbid personality states from neurogenic personality syndromes. We know that ventricle enlargement (Rabins et al., 1986) and cognitive dysfunction (Benedict et al., 2001) are risk factors for euphoria/eutonia. Future research will hopefully explore the predictive validity of regional cortical atrophy that has heretofore been difficult to measure in a reliable way. Our rating scale estimates of dorsal-frontal cortical atrophy predicted executive dysfunction in MS, (Benedict et al., 2002a) but these measures are of questionable reliability and utility across multiple research centers. A semi-automatic brain region extraction technique (Feinstein et al., 2004) shows considerable promise in this regard. At the time of this writing, we are attempting to use this same methodology to predict euphoria/eutonia as can be measured with the NPI (Fishman et al., 2004).

There are a number of methodological points that bear mentioning. First, most of the studies cited in this chapter included patients with various types of MS, disease duration, clinical course, and disability severity. Unfortunately, these subjects were most often analyzed as a single group and compared to controls. While we know that cognitive impairment is more common in chronic or SP course and longer disease duration, we do not know whether the brain/behavior correlations described here hold equally well for these subtypes. To better understand the relationship between neuropsychological impairment and MRI abnormalities, future studies should compare relatively homogenous groups of MS patients. Second, there is clearly a need for more longitudinal studies regarding neuropsychological impairment and MS. The few published longitudinal studies involved short test-retest intervals (i.e., 2 to 4 years duration). In conducting these studies, future researchers will need to bear in mind that practice effects are common, and that alternate form tests with good reliability should be used when possible. Neuropsychological testing appears to be more sensitive to cognitive impairment in cross-sectional as opposed to longitudinal studies. Third, correlative research in this area should control for variables that could enhance or mitigate the relationship between cognitive function and MRI. As can be seen from Tables 2 and 3, there are many studies that have not controlled for covariates such as age, education, and depression. Studies controlling for these covariates have often yielded larger effects. At a minimum, age, education or estimated premorbid intelligence, and depression should be accounted for in future studies.

Table 3. Summary of Longitudinal Correlational Studies on MS, MRI Atrophy Measures, and Neuropsychological Measures

Authors	Time	MRI Measures	Correlation with Neuropsychological Measures*		Controlled for
Hohol et al., 1997	1 year	BICVR	% PASAT (0.83) +[RRMS]	% SRT TOTDEL (0.77) +[CPMS]	Not stated
			% SDMT (0.75) +[RRMS]	% 10/36 SRT (0.69) +[CPMS]	
			% SRT LTS (0.38) +	% SDMT (0.31) +	
Pelletier et al., 2001	5 years	CCA	DICHOTIC (-0.42) +	SENSORY TRN (-0.40) +	No variables
			MOTOR TRN (-.037) +		
Zivadinov et al., 2001b	1 year	Decreased BPV	CHANGED COG PERF (0.31) +		No variables
	2 years	MAC in BPV §	Cognitive impairment (0.51)		

*Values are Spearman's correlation coefficients
+ Correlations with p values between 0.01 and 0.05
±Correlations with p value between 0.001 and 0.01
§ Correlation with p <.001
% Represents percent change in the test
[CPMS] Correlation only found for chronic progressive MS patients
[RRMS] Correlation only found for relapsing remitting MS patients
MRI Measure Abbreviations: BICVR = Brain-Intracranial Cavity Volume Ratio; BPF = Brain parenchymal fraction; CCA = Corpus callosum atrophy; MAC = Mean absolute change
Neuropsychological Measure Abbreviations: 10/36 SRT = 10/36 Spatial Recall Test; CHANGED COG PERF = Changed cognitive performance; CORSI = Corsi span; DICHOTIC = Dichotic Listening Test; MOTOR TRN = Motor Transfer Test; MSFC = Multiple Sclerosis Functional Composite; PASAT = Paced Serial Auditory Addition Task; RAVENS = Raven's progressive coloured matrices; SDMT = Symbol Digit Modalities Test; SENSORY TRN = Sensory Transfer Test; SRT LTS = Selective Reminding Test Long Term Storage; SRT TOT DEL = Selective Reminding Test Total Delay

Finally, another important methodological issue is that more large-scale, multicenter studies using common testing methodology are needed. It is very difficult to compare studies employing different neuropsychological tests that vary in their psychometric properties and sensitivity to MS-associated cognitive impairment. Consensus panel neuropsychological batteries have been offered (Benedict et al., 2002b; Peyser et al., 1990; Rao, 1991a) but not consistently employed. The suggested battery proposed here represents a beginning point for future consensus on a minimal neuropsychological record for MS clinical care and research.

In conclusion, measures of cerebral atrophy account for much of the neuropsychological phenomenology observed in MS patients. Compared to lesion burden, atrophy is a more significant predictor of cognitive and emotional disorder in MS and, in turn, presumably a more important predictor of vocational and social disability. Brain atrophy in MS should thus be viewed as a clinically relevant phenomenon. Future work will shed more light on more specific brain/behaviour relationships and hopefully lead to reliable MRI predictors of specific cognitive and affective syndromes in MS patients.

References

A.P.A. *Diagnostic and Statistical Manual of Mental Disorders*. Washington, D.C.: American Psychiatric Association, 1994.

Amato MP, Ponziani G, Pracucci G, Bracco L, Siracusa G, Amaducci L. Cognitive impairment in early-onset multiple sclerosis. Pattern, predictors, and impact on everyday life in a 4-year follow-up. *Arch Neurol* 1995; 52: 168-72.

Amato MP, Ponziani G, Siracusa G, Sorbi S. Cognitive dysfunction in early-onset multiple sclerosis: a reappraisal after 10 years. *Arch Neurol* 2001; 58: 1602-6.

Archibald CJ, Fisk JD. Information processing efficiency in patients with multiple sclerosis. *J Clin Exp Neuropsychol* 2000; 22: 686-701.

Arnett PA, Rao SM, Bernardin L, Grafman J, Yetkin FZ, Lobeck L. Relationship between frontal lobe lesions and Wisconsin Card Sorting Test performance in patients with multiple sclerosis. *Neurology* 1994; 44: 420-5.

Arnold DL, Matthews PM, Francis GS, O'Connor J, Antel JP. Proton magnetic resonance spectroscopic imaging for metabolic characterization of demyelinating plaques. *Ann Neurol* 1992; 31: 235-41.

Arnold DL, Wolinsky JS, Matthews PM, Falini A. The use of magnetic resonance spectroscopy in the evaluation of the natural history of multiple sclerosis. *J Neurol Neurosurg Psychiatry* 1998; 64 Suppl 1: S94-101.

Bakshi R, Ariyaratana S, Benedict RH, Jacobs L. Fluid-attenuated inversion recovery magnetic resonance imaging detects cortical and juxtacortical multiple sclerosis lesions. *Arch Neurol* 2001; 58: 742-8.

Bakshi R, Czarnecki D, Shaikh ZA, Priore RL, Janardhan V, Kaliszky Z, Kinkel PR. Brain MRI lesions and atrophy are related to depression in multiple sclerosis. *NeuroReport* 2000; 11:1153-1158.

Bakshi R, Miletich RS, Henschel K, Shaikh ZA, Janardhan V, Wasay M, et al. Fatigue in multiple sclerosis: cross-sectional correlation with brain MRI findings in 71 patients. *Neurology* 1999; 53: 1151-3.

Bakshi R, Miletich RS, Kinkel PR, Emmet ML, Kinkel WR. High-resolution fluorodeoxyglucose positron emission tomography shows both global and regional cerebral hypometabolism in multiple sclerosis. *J Neuroimaging* 1998; 8: 228-34.

Beatty PA, Gange JJ. Neuropsychological aspects of multiple sclerosis. *J Nerv Ment Dis* 1977; 164: 42-50.

Beatty WW. Memory and "frontal lobe" dysfunction in multiple sclerosis. *J Neurol Sci* 1993; 115 Suppl: S38-41.

Beatty WW. Verbal abstraction deficit in multiple sclerosis. *Neuropsychol* 1995; 9: 198-205.

Beatty WW, Goodkin DE, Monson N, Beatty PA. Cognitive disturbances in patients with relapsing remitting multiple sclerosis. *Arch Neurol* 1989; 46: 1113-9.

Beatty WW, Goodkin DE, Monson N, Beatty PA, Hertsgaard D. Anterograde and retrograde amnesia in patients with chronic progressive multiple sclerosis. *Arch Neurol* 1988; 45: 611-9.

Beatty WW, Monson N. Picture and motor sequencing in multiple sclerosis. *J Clin Exp Neuropsychol* 1994; 16: 165-72.

Beatty WW, Monson N. Problem solving by patients with multiple sclerosis: comparison of performance on the Wisconsin and California Card Sorting Tests. *J Int Neuropsychol Soc* 1996; 2: 134-40.

Beatty WW, Wilbanks SL, Blanco CR, Hames KA, Tivis R, Paul RH. Memory disturbance in multiple sclerosis: reconsideration of patterns of performance on the selective reminding test. *J Clin Exp Neuropsychol* 1996; 18: 56-62.

Benedict RH, Bakshi R, Simon JH, Priore R, Miller C, Munschauer F. Frontal cortex atrophy predicts cognitive impairment in multiple sclerosis. *J Neuropsychiatry Clin Neurosci* 2002a; 14: 44-51.

Benedict RH, Fischer JS, Archibald CJ, Arnett PA, Beatty WW, Bobholz J, et al. Minimal neuropsychological assessment of MS patients: a consensus approach. *Clin Neuropsychol* 2002b; 16: 381-97.

Benedict RH, Fishman I, McClellan MM, Bakshi R, Weinstock-Guttman B. Validity of the Beck Depression Inventory-Fast Screen in multiple sclerosis. *Mult Scler* 2003; 9: 393-6.

Benedict RH, Priore RL, Miller C, Munschauer F, Jacobs L. Personality disorder in multiple sclerosis correlates with cognitive impairment. *J Neuropsychiatry Clin Neurosci* 2001; 13: 70-6.

Benedict RH, Schretlen D, Groninger L, Dobraski M, Shpritz B. Revision of the Brief Visuospatial Memory Test:Studies of normal performance, reliability, and validity. *Psychol Assessment* 1996; 8: 145-153.

Benedict RH, Shapiro A, Priore R, Miller C, Munschauer F, Jacobs L. Neuropsychological counseling improves social behavior in cognitively-impaired multiple sclerosis patients. *Mult Scler* 2000; 6: 391-6.

Benedict RH, Weinstock-Guttman B, Fishman I, Sharma J, Tjoa CW, Bakshi R. Prediction of neuropsychological impairment in multiple sclerosis: comparison of conventional magnetic resonance imaging measures of atrophy and lesion burden. *Arch Neurol* 2004; 61: 226-30.

Benedict RHB. *Brief Visuospatial Memory Test - Revised: Professional Manual.* Odessa, FL: Psychological Assessment Resources, Inc., 1997.

Benton AL. *Multilingual Aphasis Examination.* Iowa City, IA: AJA Associates, 1989.

Berg D, Supprian T, Thomae J, Warmuth-Metz M, Horowski A, Zeiler B, et al. Lesion pattern in patients with multiple sclerosis and depression. *Mult Scler* 2000; 6: 156-62.

Bermel RA, Bakshi R, Tjoa C, Puli SR, Jacobs L. Bicaudate ratio as a magnetic resonance imaging marker of brain atrophy in multiple sclerosis. *Arch Neurol* 2002; 59: 275-80.

Bermel RA, Sharma J, Tjoa CW, Puli SR, Bakshi R. A semiautomated measure of whole-brain atrophy in multiple sclerosis. *J Neurol Sci* 2003; 208: 57-65.

Bobholz JA, Rao SM. Cognitive dysfunction in multiple sclerosis: a review of recent developments. *Curr Opin Neurol* 2003; 16: 283-8.

Braver TS, Cohen JD, Nystrom LE, Jonides J, Smith EE, Noll DC. A parametric study of prefrontal cortex involvement in human working memory. *Neuroimage* 1997; 5: 49-62.

Brown S, Davis TK. The mental symptoms of multiple sclerosis. *Arch Neurol Psychiatry* 1922; 7: 629-634.

Camp SJ, Stevenson VL, Thompson AJ, Miller DH, Borras C, Auriacombe S, et al. Cognitive function in primary progressive and transitional progressive multiple sclerosis: a controlled study with MRI correlates. *Brain* 1999; 122: 1341-8.

Charcot JM. *Lectures on the Diseases of the Nervous System.* London, England: New Sydenham Society, 1877.

Christodoulou C, Krupp LB, Liang Z, Huang W, Melville P, Roque C, et al. Cognitive performance and MR markers of cerebral injury in cognitively impaired MS patients. *Neurology* 2003; 60: 1793-8.

Costa PT, McCrae RR. *NEO PI-R Professional Manual.* Odessa, FL: Psychological Assessment Resources, Inc., 1992.

Cottrell SS, Wilson SAK. The affective symptomatology of disseminated sclerosis. *J Neurol Psychopathol* 1926: 1-30.

Cummings JL, Mega M, Gray K, Rosenberg-Thompson S, Carusi DA, Gornbein J. The Neuropsychiatric Inventory: comprehensive assessment of psychopathology in dementia. *Neurology* 1994; 44: 2308-14.

Cutter GR, Baier ML, Rudick RA, Cookfair DL, Fischer JS, Petkau J, et al. Development of a multiple sclerosis functional composite as a clinical trial outcome measure. *Brain* 1999; 122: 871-82.

Delis DC, Kaplan E, Kramer JH. *Delis-Kaplan Executive Function System.* San Antonio, TX: Psychological Corporation, 2001.

Delis DC, Kramer JH, Kaplan E, Ober BA. *California Verbal Learning Test: Adult Version.* San Antonio, TX: Psychological Corporation, 1987.

Delis DC, Kramer JH, Kaplan E, Ober BA. *California Verbal Learning Test Manual: Second Edition, Adult Version.* San Antonio, TX: Psychological Corporation, 2000.

DeLuca J, Barbieri-Berger S, Johnson SK. The nature of memory impairments in multiple sclerosis: acquisition versus retrieval. *J Clin Exp Neuropsychol* 1994; 16: 183-9.

DeLuca J, Gaudino EA, Diamond BJ, Christodoulou C, Engel RA. Acquisition and storage deficits in multiple sclerosis. *J Clin Exp Neuropsychol* 1998; 20: 376-90.

DeLuca J, Johnson SK, Natelson BH. Information processing efficiency in chronic fatigue syndrome and multiple sclerosis. *Arch Neurol* 1993; 50: 301-4.

Demaree HA, DeLuca J, Gaudino EA, Diamond BJ. Speed of information processing as a key deficit in multiple sclerosis: implications for rehabilitation. *J Neurol Neurosurg Psychiatry* 1999; 67: 661-3.

Diaz-Olavarrieta C, Cummings JL, Velazquez J, Garcia de la Cadena C. Neuropsychiatric manifestations of multiple sclerosis. *J Neuropsychiatry Clin Neurosci* 1999; 11: 51-7.

Edwards SG, Liu C, Blumhardt LD. Cognitive correlates of supratentorial atrophy on MRI in multiple sclerosis. *Acta Neurol Scand* 2001; 104: 214-23.

Fabiano AJ, Sharma J, Weinstock-Guttman B, Munschauer FE, 3rd, Benedict RH, Zivadinov R, et al. Thalamic involvement in multiple sclerosis: a diffusion-weighted magnetic resonance imaging study. *J Neuroimaging* 2003; 13: 307-14.

Fazekas F, Barkhof F, Filippi M, Grossman RI, Li DK, McDonald WI, et al. The contribution of magnetic resonance imaging to the diagnosis of multiple sclerosis. *Neurology* 1999; 53: 448-56.

Feinstein A, Feinstein K. Depression associated with multiple sclerosis. Looking beyond diagnosis to symptom expression. *J Affect Disord* 2001; 66: 193-8.

Feinstein A, Feinstein K, Gray T, O'Connor P. Prevalence and neurobehavioral correlates of pathological laughing and crying in multiple sclerosis. *Arch Neurol* 1997; 54: 1116-21.

Feinstein A, O'Connor P, Gray T, Feinstein K. Pathological laughing and crying in multiple sclerosis: a preliminary report suggesting a role for the prefrontal cortex. *Mult Scler* 1999; 5: 69-73.

Feinstein A, Roy P, Lobaugh N, Feinstein K, O C, P., Black S. The relationship between multiple sclerosis and major depression: A MRI brain segmentation study. *Neurology* 2004; 62; 586-90..

Filippi M, Tortorella C, Rovaris M, Bozzali M, Possa F, Sormani MP, et al. Changes in the normal appearing brain tissue and cognitive impairment in multiple sclerosis. *J Neurol Neurosurg Psychiatry* 2000; 68: 157-61.

Finger S. A happy state of mind: a history of mild elation, denial of disability, optimism, and laughing in multiple sclerosis. *Arch Neurol* 1998; 55: 241-50.

Fischer J. Using the Wechsler Memory Scale--Revised to detect and characterize memory deficits in multiple sclerosis. *Clin Neuropsychol* 1988; 2: 149-172.

Fischer J, Foley KW, Aikens JE, Ericson GD, Rao SM, Shindell S. What do we really know about cognitive dysfunction, affective disorders, and stress in multiple sclerosis? A practitioner's guide. *J Neurol Rehab* 1994; 8: 151-164.

Fischer JS, Priore RL, Jacobs LD, Cookfair DL, Rudick RA, Herndon RM, et al. Neuropsychological effects of interferon beta-1a in relapsing multiple sclerosis. Multiple Sclerosis Collaborative Research Group. *Ann Neurol* 2000; 48: 885-92.

Fischer JS, Rudick RA, Cutter GR, Reingold SC. The Multiple Sclerosis Functional Composite Measure (MSFC): an integrated approach to MS clinical outcome assessment. National MS Society Clinical Outcomes Assessment Task Force. *Mult Scler* 1999; 5: 244-50.

Fishman I, Benedict RH, Bakshi R, Priore R, Weinstock-Guttman B. Construct validity and frequency of euphoria slcerotica in multiple sclerosis. *J Neuropsychiatry Clin Neurosci* 2004; (in press).

Foong J, Rozewicz L, Davie CA, Thompson AJ, Miller DH, Ron MA. Correlates of executive function in multiple sclerosis: the use of magnetic resonance spectroscopy as an index of focal pathology. *J Neuropsychiatry Clin Neurosci* 1999; 11: 45-50.

Foong J, Rozewicz L, Quaghebeur G, Davie CA, Kartsounis LD, Thompson AJ, et al. Executive function in multiple sclerosis. The role of frontal lobe pathology. *Brain* 1997; 120: 15-26.

Franklin GM, Heaton RK, Nelson LM, Filley CM, Seibert C. Correlation of neuropsychological and MRI findings in chronic/progressive multiple sclerosis. *Neurology* 1988; 38: 1826-9.

Gilchrist AC, Creed FH. Depression, cognitive impairment and social stress in multiple sclerosis. *J Psychosom Res* 1994; 38: 193-201.

Grant I, McDonald WI, Trimble MR, Smith E, Reed R. Deficient learning and memory in early and middle phases of multiple sclerosis. *J Neurol Neurosurg Psychiatry* 1984; 47: 250-5.

Grasby PM, Frith CD, Friston KJ, Simpson J, Fletcher PC, Frackowiak RS, et al. A graded task approach to the functional mapping of brain areas implicated in auditory-verbal memory. *Brain* 1994; 117: 1271-82.

Gronwall DM. Paced auditory serial-addition task: a measure of recovery from concussion. *Percept Mot Skills* 1977; 44: 367-73.

Grossman RI. Magnetization transfer in multiple sclerosis. *Ann Neurol* 1994; 36 Suppl: S97-9.

Heaton RK, Nelson LM, Thompson DS, Burks JS, Franklin GM. Neuropsychological findings in relapsing-remitting and chronic-progressive multiple sclerosis. *J Consult Clin Psychol* 1985; 53: 103-10.

Hohol MJ, Guttmann CR, Orav J, Mackin GA, Kikinis R, Khoury SJ, et al. Serial neuropsychological assessment and magnetic resonance imaging analysis in multiple sclerosis. *Arch Neurol* 1997; 54: 1018-25.

Hotopf MH, Pollock S, Lishman WA. An unusual presentation of multiple sclerosis. *Psychol Med* 1994; 24: 525-8.

Huber SJ, Bornstein RA, Rammohan KW, Christy JA, Chakeres DW, McGhee RB. Magnetic resonance imaging correlates of neuropsychological impairment in multiple sclerosis. *J Neuropsychiatry Clin Neurosci* 1992; 4: 152-8.

Huber SJ, Paulson GW, Shuttleworth EC, Chakeres D, Clapp LE, Pakalnis A, et al. Magnetic resonance imaging correlates of dementia in multiple sclerosis. *Arch Neurol* 1987; 44: 732-6.

Huber SJ, Rammohan K, Bornstein RA, Christy JA. Depressive symptoms are not influenced by severity of multiple sclerosis. *J Neuropsychiatr Neuropsychol Behav Neurol* 1993; 6: 177-180.

Knight RG, Devereux RC, Godfrey HP. Psychosocial consequences of caring for a spouse with multiple sclerosis. *J Clin Exp Neuropsychol* 1997; 19: 7-19.

Kujala P, Portin R, Revonsuo A, Ruutiainen J. Automatic and controlled information processing in multiple sclerosis. *Brain* 1994; 117 (Pt 5): 1115-26.

Kujala P, Portin R, Ruutiainen J. The progress of cognitive decline in multiple sclerosis. A controlled 3-year follow-up. *Brain* 1997; 120 (Pt 2): 289-97.

Langworthy OR, Kolb L, Androp S. Disturbances of behavior i patients with disseminated sclerosis. *Am J Psychiatry* 1941; 98: 243-249.

LaRocca NG, Kalb RC, Foley F, McGann CM. Psychosocial, affective, and behavioral consequences of multiple sclerosis: Treatment of the whole patient. *Neurorehab* 1993; 3: 30-38.

Litvan I, Grafman J, Vendrell P, Martinez JM. Slowed information processing in multiple sclerosis. *Arch Neurol* 1988; 45: 281-5.

McDonald WI, Miller DH, Barnes D. The pathological evolution of multiple sclerosis. *Neuropathol Appl Neurobiol* 1992; 18: 319-34.

McKhann GM. Multiple sclerosis. *Annu Rev Neu*rosci 1982; 5: 219-39.

Medaer R, De Smedt L, Swerts M, Geutjens J. Use of rating scales to reflect cognitive and mental functioning in multiple sclerosis. *Acta Neurol Scand Suppl* 1984; 101: 65-7.

Mendozzi L, Pugnetti L, Saccani M, Motta A. Frontal lobe dysfunction in multiple sclerosis as assessed by means of Lurian tasks: effect of age at onset. *J Neurol Sci* 1993; 115 Suppl: S42-50.

Millefiorini E, Padovani A, Pozzilli C, Loriedo C, Bastianello S, Buttinelli C, et al. Depression in the early phase of MS: influence of functional disability, cognitive impairment and brain abnormalities. *Acta Neurol Scand* 1992; 86: 354-8.

Miller DH, Albert PS, Barkhof F, Francis G, Frank JA, Hodgkinson S, et al. Guidelines for the use of magnetic resonance techniques in monitoring the treatment of multiple sclerosis. US National MS Society Task Force. *Ann Neurol* 1996; 39: 6-16.

Minden SL, Schiffer RB. Affective disorders in multiple sclerosis. Review and recommendations for clinical research. *Arch Neurol* 1990; 47: 98-104.

Mohr DC, Dick LP, Russo D, Pinn J, Boudewyn AC, Likosky W, et al. The psychosocial impact of multiple sclerosis: exploring the patient's perspective. *Health Psychol* 1999; 18: 376-82.

Mohr DC, Goodkin DE, Bacchetti P, Boudewyn AC, Huang L, Marrietta P, et al. Psychological stress and the subsequent appearance of new brain MRI lesions in MS. *Neurology* 2000; 55: 55-61.

Mohr DC, Goodkin DE, Likosky W, Gatto N, Baumann KA, Rudick RA. Treatment of depression improves adherence to interferon beta-1b therapy for multiple sclerosis. *Arch Neurol* 1997; 54: 531-3.

Mohr DC, Goodkin DE, Nelson S, Cox D, Weiner M. Moderating effects of coping on the relationship between stress and the development of new brain lesions in multiple sclerosis. *Psychosom Med* 2002; 64: 803-9.

Patten SB, Metz LM, Reimer MA. Biopsychosocial correlates of lifetime major depression in a multiple sclerosis population. *Mult Scler* 2000; 6: 115-20.

Patti F, Di Stefano M, De Pascalis D, Ciancio MR, De Bernardis E, Nicoletti F, et al. May there exist specific MRI findings predictive of dementia in multiple sclerosis patients? *Funct Neurol* 1995; 10: 83-90.

Pelletier J, Habib M, Lyon-Caen O, Salamon G, Poncet M, Khalil R. Functional and magnetic resonance imaging correlates of callosal involvement in multiple sclerosis. *Arch Neurol* 1993; 50: 1077-82.

Pelletier J, Suchet L, Witjas T, Habib M, Guttmann CR, Salamon G, et al. A longitudinal study of callosal atrophy and interhemispheric dysfunction in relapsing-remitting multiple sclerosis. *Arch Neurol* 2001; 58: 105-11.

Peyser JM, Rao SM, LaRocca NG, Kaplan E. Guidelines for neuropsychological research in multiple sclerosis. *Arch Neurol* 1990; 47: 94-7.

Piras MR, Magnano I, Canu ED, Paulus KS, Satta WM, Soddu A, et al. Longitudinal study of cognitive dysfunction in multiple sclerosis: neuropsychological, neuroradiological, and neurophysiological findings. *J Neurol Neurosurg* Psychiatry. 2003; 74: 878-85.

Pujol J, Bello J, Deus J, Cardoner N, Marti-Vilalta JL, Capdevila A. Beck Depression Inventory factors related to demyelinating lesions of the left arcuate fasciculus region. *Psychiatry Res* 2000; 99: 151-9.

Rabins PV. Euphoria in Multiple Sclerosis. In: Ral SM, editor. *Neurobehavioral Aspects of MS*. New York City, NY: Oxford University Press, 1990: 180-185.

Rabins PV, Brooks BR, O'Donnell P, Pearlson GD, Moberg P, Jubelt B, et al. Structural brain correlates of emotional disorder in multiple sclerosis. *Brain* 1986; 109 (Pt 4): 585-97.

Rao SM. Neuropsychology of multiple sclerosis: a critical review. *J Clin Exp Neuropsychol* 1986; 8: 503-42.

Rao SM. *A Manual for the Brief, Repeatable Battery of Neuropsychological Tests in Multiple Sclerosis*, 1991a.

Rao SM. *Neuropsychological Screening Battery for Multiple Sclerosis*, 1991b.

Rao SM. Neuropsychology of multiple sclerosis. *Curr Opin Neurol* 1995; 8: 216-20.

Rao SM, Bernardin L, Leo GJ, Ellington L, Ryan SB, Burg LS. Cerebral disconnection in multiple sclerosis. Relationship to atrophy of the corpus callosum. *Arch Neurol* 1989a; 46: 918-20.

Rao SM, Glatt S, Hammeke TA, McQuillen MP, Khatri BO, Rhodes AM, et al. Chronic progressive multiple sclerosis. Relationship between cerebral ventricular size and neuropsychological impairment. *Arch Neurol* 1985; 42: 678-82.

Rao SM, Hammeke TA, McQuillen MP, Khatri BO, Lloyd D. Memory disturbance in chronic progressive multiple sclerosis. *Arch Neurol* 1984; 41: 625-31.

Rao SM, Leo GJ, Bernardin L, Unverzagt F. Cognitive dysfunction in multiple sclerosis. I. Frequency, patterns, and prediction. *Neurology* 1991a; 41: 685-91.

Rao SM, Leo GJ, Ellington L, Nauertz T, Bernardin L, Unverzagt F. Cognitive dysfunction in multiple sclerosis. II. Impact on employment and social functioning. *Neurology* 1991b; 41: 692-6.

Rao SM, Leo GJ, Haughton VM, St Aubin-Faubert P, Bernardin L. Correlation of magnetic resonance imaging with neuropsychological testing in multiple sclerosis. *Neurology* 1989b; 39: 161-6.

Rao SM, Leo GJ, St Aubin-Faubert P. On the nature of memory disturbance in multiple sclerosis. *J Clin Exp Neuropsychol* 1989c; 11: 699-712.

Rao SM, St Aubin-Faubert P, Leo GJ. Information processing speed in patients with multiple sclerosis. *J Clin Exp Neuropsychol* 1989d; 11: 471-7.

Reischies FM, Baum K, Brau H, Hedde JP, Schwindt G. Cerebral magnetic resonance imaging findings in multiple sclerosis. Relation to disturbance of affect, drive, and cognition. *Arch Neurol* 1988; 45: 1114-6.

Ron MA, Feinstein A. Multiple sclerosis and the mind. *J Neurol Neurosurg Psychiatry* 1992; 55: 1-3.

Ron MA, Logsdail SJ. Psychiatric morbidity in multiple sclerosis: a clinical and MRI study. *Psychol Med* 1989; 19: 887-95.

Rovaris M, Filippi M, Falautano M, Minicucci L, Rocca MA, Martinelli V, et al. Relation between MR abnormalities and patterns of cognitive impairment in multiple sclerosis. *Neurology* 1998; 50: 1601-8.

Rovaris M, Iannucci G, Falautano M, Possa F, Martinelli V, Comi G, et al. Cognitive dysfunction in patients with mildly disabling relapsing-remitting multiple sclerosis: an exploratory study with diffusion tensor MR imaging. *J Neurol Sci* 2002; 195: 103-9.

Rudick R, Antel J, Confavreux C, Cutter G, Ellison G, Fischer J, et al. Clinical outcomes assessment in multiple sclerosis. *Ann Neurol* 1996; 40: 469-79.

Rudick RA, Fisher E, Lee JC, Simon J, Jacobs L. Use of the brain parenchymal fraction to measure whole brain atrophy in relapsing-remitting MS. Multiple Sclerosis Collaborative Research Group. *Neurology* 1999; 53: 1698-704.

Ryan L, Clark CM, Klonoff H, Li DK, Paty DW. Patterns of cognitive impairment in relapsing-remitting multiple sclerosis and their relationship to neuropathology on magnetic resonance images. *Neuropsychology* 1996; 10: 176-193.

Sabatini U, Pozzilli C, Pantano P, Koudriavtseva T, Padovani A, Millefiorini E, et al. Involvement of the limbic system in multiple sclerosis patients with depressive disorders. *Biol Psychiatry* 1996; 39: 970-5.

Sadovnick AD, Remick RA, Allen J, Swartz E, Yee IM, Eisen K, et al. Depression and multiple sclerosis. *Neurology* 1996; 46: 628-32.

Sarazin M, Pillon B, Giannakopoulos P, Rancurel G, Samson Y, Dubois B. Clinicometabolic dissociation of cognitive functions and social behavior in frontal lobe lesions. *Neurology* 1998; 51: 142-8.

Scarrabelotti M, Carroll M. Awareness of remembering achieved through automatic and conscious processes in multiple sclerosis. *Brain Cogn* 1998; 38: 183-201.

Smith A. *Symbol digit modalities test: Manual.* Los Angeles, CA: Western Psychological Services, 1982.

Surridge D. An investigation into some psychiatric aspects of multiple sclerosis. *Br J Psychiatry* 1969; 115: 749-64.

Swirsky-Sacchetti T, Mitchell DR, Seward J, Gonzales C, Lublin F, Knobler R, et al. Neuropsychological and structural brain lesions in multiple sclerosis: a regional analysis. *Neurology* 1992; 42: 1291-5.

Thornton AE, Raz N, Tucke KA. Memory in multiple sclerosis: contextual encoding deficits. *J Int Neuropsychol Soc* 2002; 8: 395-409.

Trapp BD, Ransohoff R, Rudick R. Axonal pathology in multiple sclerosis: relationship to neurologic disability. *Curr Opin Neurol* 1999; 12: 295-302.

Troyer AK, Graves RE, Cullum CM. Executive functioning as a mediator of the relationship between age and episodic memory in healthy aging. *Aging Neuropsychol Cogn* 1994; 1: 45-53.

Truyen L, van Waesberghe JH, van Walderveen MA, van Oosten BW, Polman CH, Hommes OR, et al. Accumulation of hypointense lesions ("black holes") on T1 spin-echo MRI correlates with disease progression in multiple sclerosis. *Neurology* 1996; 47: 1469-76.

Tsolaki M, Drevelegas A, Karachristianou S, Kapinas K, Divanoglou D, Routsonis K. Correlation of dementia, neuropsychological and MRI findings in multiple sclerosis. *Dementia* 1994; 5: 48-52.

van Buchem MA, Grossman RI, Armstrong C, Polansky M, Miki Y, Heyning FH, et al. Correlation of volumetric magnetization transfer imaging with clinical data in MS. *Neurology* 1998; 50: 1609-17.

van den Burg W, van Zomeren AH, Minderhoud JM, Prange AJ, Meijer NS. Cognitive impairment in patients with multiple sclerosis and mild physical disability. *Arch Neurol* 1987; 44: 494-501.

Vleugels L, Lafosse C, van Nunen A, Nachtergaele S, Ketelaer P, Charlier M, et al. Visuoperceptual impairment in multiple sclerosis patients diagnosed with neuropsychological tasks. *Mult Scler* 2000; 6: 241-54.

Wolff SD, Balaban RS. Magnetization transfer contrast (MTC) and tissue water proton relaxation in vivo. *Magn Reson Med* 1989; 10: 135-44.

Young IR, Hall AS, Pallis CA, Legg NJ, Bydder GM, Steiner RE. Nuclear magnetic resonance imaging of the brain in multiple sclerosis. *Lancet* 1981; 2: 1063-6.

Zivadinov R, De Masi R, Nasuelli D, Bragadin LM, Ukmar M, Pozzi-Mucelli RS, et al. MRI techniques and cognitive impairment in the early phase of relapsing-remitting multiple sclerosis. *Neuroradiology* 2001a; 43: 272-8.

Zivadinov R, Sepcic J, Nasuelli D, De Masi R, Bragadin LM, Tommasi MA, et al. A longitudinal study of brain atrophy and cognitive disturbances in the early phase of relapsing-remitting multiple sclerosis. *J Neurol Neurosurg Psychiatry* 2001b; 70: 773-80.

Zorzon M, de Masi R, Nasuelli D, Ukmar M, Mucelli RP, Cazzato G, et al. Depression and anxiety in multiple sclerosis. A clinical and MRI study in 95 subjects. *J Neurol* 2001; 248: 416-21.

Zorzon M, Zivadinov R, Nasuelli D, Ukmar M, Bratina A, Tommasi MA, et al. Depressive symptoms and MRI changes in multiple sclerosis. *Eur J Neurol* 2002; 9: 491-6.

In: Brain and Spinal Cord Atrophy in Multiple Sclerosis
Editors: R. Zivadinov and R. Bakshi, pp. 167-174
ISBN 1-59454-160-4

Chapter X

Relationship Between Central Nervous System Atrophy and Genetic-Immunological Markers in Multiple Sclerosis

Marino Zorzon[1*] and Robert Zivadinov[2-4]
[1] Department of Clinical Medicine and Neurology, University of Trieste, Trieste, Italy
[2] Department of Neurology, SUNY–University at Buffalo School of Medicine and Biomedical Sciences, Buffalo, NY, USA.
[3] Buffalo Neuroimaging Analysis Center, Buffalo, NY, USA.
[4] The Jacobs Neurological Institute, Buffalo, NY, USA.

Introduction

Cerebral volume loss and hypointense lesions on T1-weighted magnetic resonance imaging (MRI) are widely accepted as markers of axonal loss in patients with multiple sclerosis (MS). Evidence is mounting that these MRI measures correlate better with the progression of disability, than conventional MRI measures, such as the white matter lesion load (LL) on T2-weighted MRI and the presence of Gadolinium (Gd) enhancing lesions on T1-weighted MRI.

Genetic factors contribute to determining susceptibility to MS, and, recently, a hypothesis has been proposed which states that several genes, including human leukocyte antigen (HLA) class II, Apo E, IL-1ra and IL-1β, may exert a disease modifying effect, influencing the prognosis of patients with MS.

Understanding how genes affect disease expressivity could prove to be very useful, as this could assist in predicting the clinical course of the disease and provide information that

* Corresponding Author: Marino Zorzon, MD, Department of Clinical Medicine and Neurology, University of Trieste, Cattinara Hospital. Strada di Fiume 447, 34149 Trieste, Italy,.Phone: +390403994321; Fax: +39040910861; e-mail: m.zorzon@fmc.units.it

would affect the timing, intensity and duration of therapy. It could be hypothesized that expression of different genes may influence the heterogeneity and severity of MS pathological processes measured by the accumulation of disease activity on conventional and non-conventional long-term MRI measures. The diversity of disease expression in MS may reflect major differences in the underlying pathogenetic mechanisms.

In this perspective, study of the correlation between putative disease modifying genes, immunologic markers and MRI measures that have been shown to reflect axonal degeneration may be important.

Genetic Markers

Human Leukocyte Antigen

An association with the HLA-DPB1*501 allele has been recently reported in patients with opticospinal MS, a selective and severe form of MS common in Asians (Yamasaki et al., 1999). In HLA-DPB1*501-positive patients with opticospinal MS, the frequency of spinal cord atrophy was significantly higher than in patients showing disseminated lesions in the central nervous system (CNS), including the cerebrum, cerebellum and brainstem.

The relationship between HLA genotypes and disease severity as measured by brain MRI quantitative markers of demyelinating and destructive pathology in patients with MS was the objective of a case-control study that included 100 MS cases and 122 age-, sex-, ethnicity-, and residence- matched controls (Zivadinov et al., 2003). HLA-DQB1*02,-DQB1*03,-DRB1*15, and –DRB1*03 alleles were associated with MS. Clinical (i.e., Expanded Disability Status Scale [EDSS]) and MRI (i.e., T2-and T1-LL and brain parenchymal fraction [BPF]) measures of disease severity did not significantly differ according to the carriers' status of these HLA alleles. A trend towards higher T1-LL and more severe brain atrophy, considered to be MRI expressions of destructive pathology in MS, was not confirmed in carriers of DRB1*15 and DQB1*02 alleles after multiple comparison correction. Hence, the hypothesis raised by the authors—that these alleles may increase susceptibility to axonal loss and subsequently cause the accumulation of black holes and progression of brain atrophy—remains unconfirmed. Multiple regression analysis was used to establish whether any HLA allele and/or haplotype was able to predict MRI outcomes. With respect to MRI markers of axonal damage, B7 and DRB1*12 alleles were associated with T1-LL, whereas BPF was predicted only by the presence of the DRB1*12 allele. The authors suggested that some other HLA alleles may predict the destructive pathological processes visible on MRI, although the relatively small sample size prevented a definitive conclusion about genotype/phenotype correlation.

Apo E

Two studies investigated the extent of axonal damage and brain atrophy in patients with MS in relation to their Apo E genotypes. The rationale of these studies was the hypothesis that in MS patients carrying an Apo E ε4 allele, the course of the disease may be more severe, the progression of disability more rapid and the T1-hypointense LL higher. The disease-modifying effect of the Apo E genotype in MS may be related to more extensive tissue destruction and/or less efficient neuronal maintenance and repair in carriers of Apo E ε4. Preliminary results of these studies, presented in an abstract form, were conflicting (DeStefano et al., 2004; Pelletier et al., 2003). DeStefano et al., (2004) examined 27 relapsing-remitting (RR) MS patients with short disease duration (median = 1 year) and mild disability (median EDSS = 1.5). To evaluate cerebral volumes and axonal integrity, combined proton MRI and magnetic resonance spectroscopy (MRS) examinations were conducted. Twenty patients with the Apo E ε3/ ε3 genotype and seven patients with the ε4 allele were identified. Automated measurements of normalized brain volumes (NBV) showed a significant decrease in MS patients carrying the ε4 allele compared with normal controls and MS patients without the ε4 allele. Both patient groups showed a similar significant reduction in central brain N-Acetyl-aspartate (NAA) levels compared with normal controls. In the authors' opinion, the significant brain volume loss found only in early RRMS patients with the Apo E ε4 genotype suggests that the ε4 allele can be associated with more severe tissue destruction and that this effect may be measurable even in early disease stages.

A larger study examined 88 MS patients with either RR, secondary progressive (SP) or primary progressive (PP) MS with long-echo proton MRS to measure levels of NAA in a large brain region of interest centered at the corpus callosum. Volumetric high resolution images were also obtained to evaluate brain atrophy. Both non- Apo E ε4 (n=66) and Apo E ε4 (n=22) MS patient groups showed a significant decrease of NAA and more brain atrophy compared with controls, but no differences were found between Apo E ε4 and non- Apo E ε4 groups. The study failed to demonstrate more axonal injury or brain atrophy in carriers of Apo E ε4 versus non- Apo E ε4 patients and, therefore, the authors concluded that the effect, if any, of Apo E genotype on NAA and brain atrophy was modest.

Recently, Enzinger et al. (2004) studied longitudinally the impact of the Apo E genotype on evolution of focal black holes and of global brain volume changes. Ninety-nine MS patients underwent ApoE genotyping, clinical examination, and magnetic resonance imaging at baseline and after 2.7 years. In Apo E ε4 patients, the annual reduction in brain volume was fivefold higher than in those without ApoE ε4 ($p = 0.0001$). The results of this study showed that accelerated brain tissue loss and a higher proportion of lesions evolving into black holes were related to the presence of Apo E ε4.

Matrix Metalloproteinase-9

Matrix metalloproteinase-9 (MMP-9), a neutral zinc-dependent protease, may be implicated in MS pathophysiology. In fact, MMP-9 levels are higher in the tissue and serum of MS patients compared with healthy controls, and patients with RRMS, even during the remitting phases show a tendency to produce more MMP-9 at rest than controls. Changes in serum levels of MMP-9 have been correlated with clinical and MRI evidence of disease activity in MS patients. An increase in MMP-9 activity has been associated with the formation of new MS lesions, suggesting that serum levels of MMP-9 and tissue inhibitors of MMP type 1 may be surrogate markers of disease activity in RRMS, since high MMP-9 levels correlate with disease activity, as evidenced by the appearance of new enhanced MRI lesion.

A recent study evaluated the relationship between polymorphism (PM) in the microsatellite of the promoter region of MMP-9 and both the clinical and MRI characteristics of 95 patients with either the RR form (n=67), the SP form (n=15), or the PP form (n=13) of MS (Fiotti et al., 2004,). When patients were divided according to the number of Cytosine-Adenosine (CA) repeats in the MMP-9 promoter region, in carriers of ≤21 CA repeats and ≥22 CA repeats alleles no differences between clinical data and MRI measures (T2-, T1-LL and BPF) were found with the exception of age at disease onset, which was significantly lower in carriers of the longer microsatellite. Multiple regression models were used to verify whether the genotype having at least one allele with ≥22 CA repeats was associated with any of the clinical or MRI characteristics. After taking into account potential confounding variables such as age, disease duration, years of lifetime actual disease-modifying treatment and lifetime days of steroid use, the only variable that independently predicted the presence of this genotype in the MMP-9 promoter region was younger age at disease onset, whereas no relationship existed between any measure of LL or brain atrophy and MMP-9 PM. The conclusion was that no main clinical or MRI long-term measures of disease severity were associated with MMP-9 PM, although the results must be considered with caution due to the limited power of the study.

Immunological Markers

Cytokines and Adhesion Molecules

Although MRI is very useful for monitoring the course of MS and has the potential to identify atrophy and different types of lesions, it lacks specificity and correlates poorly with clinical outcomes. Therefore, the possibility of recognizing inflammatory or degenerative aspects of MS by means of cerebrospinal fluid (CSF) or serum analysis may provide useful information. Various cytokines and products of inflammation, demyelination and axonal loss have been analyzed in the serum, CSF and urine of MS patients, but none of them showed a relationship with disease activity so strong as to allow monitoring of disease progression.

Adhesion molecules expressed on vascular endothelial cells regulate the migration of activated autoreactive T-cells across the blood-brain-barrier and have an important role in the pathogenesis of MS.

To determine the levels of adhesion molecules in blood and CSF samples of patients with different subtypes of MS, the expressions of very late activation antigen 4 (VLA-4), lymphocyte function associated antigen 1 (LFA-1), vascular cell adhesion molecule 1 (VCAM-1) and intercellular adhesion molecule 1 (ICAM-1) were determined immunocytochemically, and levels of soluble VCAM-1, ICAM-1 and E-selectin were obtained by means of the enzyme immunoassay technique. To correlate the adhesion molecules' expressions with MRI markers of disease severity, T2- and T1-LL and brain atrophy were measured by means of a semiautomated MRI segmentation technique in 20 patients with SPMS (Elovaara et al., 2000). No significant correlations were found between MRI abnormalities and the expressions of adhesion molecules.

Soluble adhesion molecule levels were measured in 13 of 20 patients with SPMS and the levels were correlated with corresponding MRI measurements. A correlation was found only between the volumes of the T2-LL and the levels of s ICAM-1 in serum. These results confirmed the negative findings of most of the previous studies aimed at establishing an association between biological markers, including adhesion molecules, and MS-related MRI or EDSS changes.

The relationship between serum inflammatory markers and clinical and MRI markers of disease progression was investigated in 29 MS patients, 13 with a RR and 16 with a SP course, by Giovannoni and co-workers (Giovannoni et al., 2001). The aim of the study was to assess whether a series of pro-inflammatory immunological markers, when measured serially over an 18-month period, correlate with disease progression or putative MRI markers of axonal loss. Serial serum levels of s VCAM-1, s ICAM-1, nitric oxide (NO) metabolites nitrate and nitrite (NOx), C-reactive protein (CRP), neopterin and tumor necrosis alpha (TNFα) were measured. In addition, ex-vivo-stimulated whole blood TNFα production was quantitated as an inflammatory marker. MRI variables included the number and volume of Gd-enhancing lesions and the change in the T2-LL, T1-LL and brain volume between baseline and exit studies. Patients who developed significant brain atrophy during the study had lower mean serum CRP levels than those who did not; however, the mean levels of both groups were within the normal range. Overall, this study failed to show any link between several inflammatory markers and disease progression and putative MRI markers of axonal loss in patients with RRMS. In fact, no correlations were found between the mean levels of the inflammatory marker measures and the MRI parameters studied. The authors argued that the relatively small sample size (29 patients), a follow-up period that was too short (18 months), and immunological marker examinations that were too infrequent (monthly or every 3 months) may account for the negative results.

Antiganglioside Antibodies

A role for serum antiganglioside antibodies in the pathogenesis of disease progression in MS has been suggested because, in a cross-sectional study, increased circulating antiganglioside antibodies were reported in patients with PP and SPMS. The authors proposed that the elevated levels of these antibodies could be involved in the process of axonal damage which occurs in MS (Sadatipour et al., 1998).

These findings could not be confirmed in a longitudinal study conducted with the purpose of establishing whether antiganglioside antibodies were associated with progressive disease (Giovannoni et al., 2000). Circulating levels of IgG and IgM antibodies against gangliosides GM1, GM3, GD1a, GT1b, and GQ1b, as well as sulphatide, were measured in 29 patients with RR or SPMS who also underwent serial brain MRI and clinical examinations over an 18-month follow-up. There were no differences in circulating antiganglioside antibody levels between patients who progressed clinically or developed significant brain atrophy and those who did not during the 18 months of follow-up. Furthermore, no differences were noted between patients with RR and those with SP course, with frequent (two or more) or infrequent (none or one) relapses and with high or low Gd-enhancing MRI activity between the baseline and month 18 absorbance values.

Nitric Oxide

NO production has been implicated in immune-mediated cellular cytotoxicity and inflammatory processes that are of importance in the pathogenesis of MS. Furthermore, recent studies have suggested that NO may contribute to myelin and oligodendrocyte damage. In the above cited study of Giovannoni and co-workers (Giovannoni et al., 2001), however, no positive correlation was found between the mean serum level of NOx, a surrogate marker of NO production, and the immune response in vivo, and clinical and MRI markers of disease activity. On the contrary, mean levels of NOx were significantly higher in patients with RRMS than in patients with SP disease course, and in patients who had either a single relapse or no relapse during the 18-month follow-up compared with patients with multiple relapses. These data suggest that, in the short-term, increased serum NO metabolites may be associated with a better clinical outcome in the form of a non-progressive clinical course and fewer clinical relapses.

Serum and CSF NO metabolite levels and their relationship with MRI markers of axonal loss have been analyzed in MS patients either with RR or SP or PP course (Peltola et al., 2001; Yuceyar et al., 2001). MS patients exhibited significantly increased serum and CSF levels of nitrite and nitrate compared with controls in both RR and SP MS (Yuceyar et al., 2001), whereas in patients with PPMS the levels of NOx in CSF were fourfold higher than in controls, but the concentrations in serum were similar (Peltola et al., 2001). No significant correlation was found between NO metabolite levels and Gd-enhancing MRI or development of cortical atrophy on MRI in both RR and SPMS patients (Yuceyar et al., 2001). The concentration of NOx in the serum and CSF of patients with PPMS correlated with MRI decreased volumetric measurements of the brain and spinal cord (Peltola et al., 2001). A cytokine-mediated toxicity against oligodendrocytes in which NO may be involved has been advocated as an explanation for the mechanism of NO production in PPMS.

Neurofilaments

It has been suggested that intrathecal levels of axonal cytoskeletal proteins may be reliable markers of axonal damage. Neurofilaments are important axonal cytoskeletal proteins that are closely linked to axonal diameter and myelination. CSF levels of neurofilament light subunit (NfL) may be a marker of axonal damage in MS and elevated intrathecal production of antibodies to NfL has been reported in patients with SP and PPMS.

In a recent study, levels of heavy neurofilaments (NfH) and NfL and antibodies to neurofilaments (anti-NfL and anti-NfH) as well as total IgG were measured in 51 patients with MS (21 RR, 20 SP and 10 PP) in an attempt to correlate markers of axonal damage in the CSF and serum of patients with different subtypes of MS with measures of disease progression on MRI (Eikelenboom et al., 2003). For the total group of patients, significant correlations were found between the anti-NfL index and the parenchymal fraction (PF, defined as whole brain parenchyma/intracranial volume), T2-LL, ventricular fraction (VF, defined as ventricular volume/whole brain parenchyma), and T1-LL. For the anti-NfH index, a correlation was found with PF. No correlation was found between the IgG index and the MRI measures. Analyzing the subgroups separately, the correlations were mainly found in the RR subgroup: the anti-NfL index correlated with the PF, VF and T1-LL, whereas in the SP and PP subgroups, no correlation was found between the CSF proteins or antibodies and MRI measures. The strongest correlation was for the PF, one of the two atrophy measures used in this study. This would indicate that the anti-NfL index is more closely related to atrophy measures than to LL measures. The findings of this study suggest that intrathecal production of anti-NfL antibodies may serve as a marker of tissue damage, particularly axonal loss, in MS.

Beta-2 Microglobulin

Beta-2 microglobulin (β2-MG) and neopterin correlate with disease activity in several autoimmune disorders and are currently used as pharmacodynamic markers of interferon beta treatment in MS. However, both these molecules are unstable and rapidly eliminated by the kidneys, and, therefore, the serum, unlike CSF and urine, is not an ideal body fluid for measuring the concentration of these molecules to monitor disease activity in MS. In fact, urinary excretion of neopterin is higher during a clinical relapse, but blood levels of this molecule do not correlate with clinical and MRI measurements (Bagnato et al., 2004,).

To establish whether β2-MG is a marker of disease activity/progression, spontaneous fluctuations of β2-MG were analyzed in 30 free-treatment patients with RRMS who were clinically assessed and imaged monthly over a 3-month period (Bagnato et al., 2004,). The results of this study failed to demonstrate the validity of β2-MG as a surrogate marker of either inflammatory activity or axonal degeneration in patients with MS.

Conclusions

In conclusion, studies that investigated the relationship between CNS atrophy and genetic markers are few, whereas more studies have been performed trying to correlate CNS atrophy and immunological markers. The results of two studies suggested that some HLA alleles may predict more severe axonal damage in MS patients, but the size of the sample studied was small and did not permit firm conclusions (Yamasaki et al., 1999; Zivadinov et al., 2003). The influence of the Apo E ε4 genotype on disease severity remains doubtful (DeStefano et al., 2004; Pelletier et al., 2003) and larger studies are needed to establish its role in the causation of axonal damage (Enzinger et al., 2004). MMP-9 PM may be associated with an increased risk of MS, but whether it can influence the clinical expression of MS has yet to be demonstrated (Fiotti et al., 2004, in press). Most studies failed to show a correlation between serum and CSF immunological markers of inflammation and axonal damage and MRI measures of atrophy (Bagnato et al., 2004,); Elovaara et al., 2000; Giovannoni et al., 2001; Giovannoni et al., 2000; Yuceyar et al., 2001). Only a small study on patients with PPMS reported a correlation between plasma and CSF NOx concentrations and brain and spinal cord atrophy (Peltola et al., 2001). Finally, the finding that intrathecal production of antibodies against axonal cytoskeletal proteins correlates with CNS atrophy (Eikelenboom et al., 2003) must be reproduced by further studies.

References

Bagnato F, Zivadinov R, Cecchinelli D, Tancredi A, Grop A, Pieralini A, et al. ß2-microglobulin serum level is not a marker of disease activity in multiple sclerosis. *Eur J Neurol* 2004; 11: 455-60.

DeStefano N, Bartolozzi ML, Nacmias B, Zipoli V, Mortilla M, Guidi L, Siracusa G, Sorbi, S, Frederico A, Amato MP. Influence of apolipoprotein E epsilon4 genotype on brain tissue integrity in relapsing-remitting multiple sclerosis. *Arch Neurol* 2004;61: 536-40.

Eikelenboom MJ, Petzold A, Lazeron RH, Silber E, Sharief M, Thompson EJ, et al. Multiple sclerosis: Neurofilament light chain antibodies are correlated to cerebral atrophy. *Neurology* 2003; 60: 219-23.

Elovaara I, Ukkonen M, Leppakynnas M, Lehtimaki T, Luomala M, Peltola J, et al. Adhesion molecules in multiple sclerosis: relation to subtypes of disease and methylprednisolone therapy. *Arch Neurol* 2000; 57: 546-51.

Enzinger C, Ropele S, Smith S, Strasser-Fuchs S, Poltrum B, Schmidt H, et al. Accelerated evolution of brain atrophy and "black holes" in MS patients with APOE-epsilon 4. *Ann Neurol.* 2004; 55:563-9.

Fiotti N, Zivadinov R, Altamura N, Nasuelli D, Bratina A, Tommasi MA, et al. MMP-9 microsatellite polymorphism and multiple sclerosis. *Journal of Neuroimmunology* 2004; 52: 147-53.

Giovannoni G, Miller DH, Losseff NA, Sailer M, Lewellyn-Smith N, Thompson AJ, et al. Serum inflammatory markers and clinical/MRI markers of disease progression in multiple sclerosis. *J Neurol* 2001; 248: 487-95.

Giovannoni G, Morris PR, Keir G. Circulating antiganglioside antibodies are not associated with the development of progressive disease or cerebral atrophy in patients with multiple sclerosis. *Ann Neurol* 2000; 47: 684-5.

Pelletier D, Brassat D, Joonmi O, Swerdlin AR, Hauser SL, Oksenberg JR, et al. Magnetic resonance spectroscopy and brain atrophy measurements in relation with apoE genotypes of patients with multiple sclerosis. *Neurology* 2003; 60: A269.

Peltola J, Ukkonen M, Moilanen E, Elovaara I. Increased nitric oxide products in CSF in primary progressive MS may reflect brain atrophy. *Neurology* 2001; 57: 895-6.

Sadatipour BT, Greer JM, Pender MP. Increased circulating antiganglioside antibodies in primary and secondary progressive multiple sclerosis. *Ann Neurol* 1998; 44: 980-3.

Yamasaki K, Horiuchi I, Minohara M, Kawano Y, Ohyagi Y, Yamada T, et al. HLA-DPB1*0501-associated opticospinal multiple sclerosis: clinical, neuroimaging and immunogenetic studies. *Brain* 1999; 122: 1689-96.

Yuceyar N, Taskiran D, Sagduyu A. Serum and cerebrospinal fluid nitrite and nitrate levels in relapsing-remitting and secondary progressive multiple sclerosis patients. *Clin Neurol Neurosurg* 2001; 103: 206-11.

Zivadinov R, Uxa L, Zacchi T, Nasuelli D, Ukmar M, Furlan C, et al. HLA genotypes and disease severity assessed by magnetic resonance imaging findings in patients with multiple sclerosis. *J Neurol* 2003; 250: 1099-106.

In: Brain and Spinal Cord Atrophy in Multiple Sclerosis
Editors: R. Zivadinov and R. Bakshi, pp. 175-190
ISBN 1-59454-160-4

Chapter XI

Treatment Effects on MRI Measures of Central Nervous System Atrophy in Multiple Sclerosis

Marco Rovaris [*] ***and Massimo Filippi***
Neuroimaging Research Unit, Department of Neurology, Scientific Institute and University Ospedale San Raffaele, Milan, Italy

Introduction

Magnetic resonance imaging (MRI) is widely used to follow in vivo the evolution of multiple sclerosis (MS) pathology, mainly because of its sensitivity to the assessment of disease activity and accumulated burden, which is significantly greater than that achieved only on clinical grounds. For this reason, the number and volume of MRI-visible lesions have been used as paraclinical outcomes in phase II and III MS trials (Rovaris and Filippi, 1999), where it has been shown that several drugs exert a dramatic treatment effect on these MRI-derived parameters but without a commensurate clinical benefit, thus suggesting that other aspects of MS pathology warrant investigation.

In the last few years, there has been considerable interest in measuring brain and cord tissue volume decrease (atrophy) as a marker reflecting the more disabling aspects of MS pathology (Miller et al., 2002; Zivadinov and Bakshi, 2004). The assessment of atrophy in MS is, however, not without problems (Filippi and Grossman, 2002). First, the pathological basis of MS-related atrophy is still unclear and its measurements are also likely to be biased by fluctuations of tissue water content related to important aspects of MS pathology or therapy, such as the edema associated with active lesions or the administration of steroids. Secondly, it is conceivable that MRI-detectable brain volume decrease is an end-stage phenomenon preceded by other events (e.g., progressive myelin loss, inefficient

[*] Corresponding author: Marco Rovaris, Neuroimaging Research Unit, Department of Neurology, Scientific Institute Ospedale San Raffaele, via Olgettina 60, 20132 Milan, Italy. Phone: +39-02-26433054; Fax: +39-02-26433031; E-mail: rovaris.marco@hsr.it

remyelination, sublethal axonal injury, etc). Thirdly, atrophy is less sensitive to disease changes than other MRI-derived outcomes. On average, brain volume decreases by about 1% yearly in patients with different MS phenotypes (Ge et al., 2000; Inglese et al., 1999; Kalkers et al., 2002a; Rudick et al., 2000; Simon et al., 1999), despite evidence of highly variable disease activity and characteristics. Finally, the optimal methodology for MRI-based assessment of brain atrophy and the robustness of this approach are still debated (Miller et al., 2002; Zivadinov and Bakshi, 2004). Available studies widely differ in terms of types of measures (absolute vs. normalized, linear vs. three-dimensional, whole-brain vs. regional), acquisition schemes of source MRI data (two- vs. three-dimension, T2- vs. T1-weighted sequences) and methods of image postprocessing (semi- vs. fully-automated). This can lead to different accuracy in measurement, even though the assessment of brain atrophy seems to be, on the average, a "solid" approach, with limited intra-observer and inter-scanner variability (Fisher et al., 2000; Losseff et al., 1996a; Rovaris et al., 2000).

This chapter reviews the results from trials which assessed the efficacy of disease-modifying MS treatments in the prevention of brain atrophy. Preliminary results from studies of cord atrophy are also reported to provide a comprehensive picture of all the currently available data.

Treatment Effect on Brain Atrophy in Relapsing-Remitting MS

Evidence-based disease-modifying therapies for relapsing-remitting (RR) MS include recombinant interferon beta (IFNβ) 1a and 1b (Betaferon®, Avonex® and Rebif®), given at different dosages (IFNßMSSG, 1995; Jacobs et al., 1996; Paty and Li, 1993; PRISMS, 1998), and glatiramer acetate (GA; Copaxone®) (Johnson et al., 1995; Johnson et al., 1998). All the IFNβ formulations are known to significantly reduce the frequency of clinical relapses (IFNßMSSG, 1995; Jacobs et al., 1996; PRISMS, 1998), the extent of MRI-measured disease activity (IFNßMSSG, 1995; Li and Paty, 1999; Paty and Li, 1993; Simon et al., 1998), and the accumulation of T2-visible lesions (IFNßMSSG, 1995; Li and Paty, 1999; Paty and Li, 1993; Simon et al., 1998). IFNβ also has a partial effect on limiting the progression of MS disability. GA, which is the acetate salt of a mixture of synthetic polypeptides, appears to act via the production of specific T-suppressor cells that cross react with myelin basic protein in the central nervous system (CNS) (Neuhaus et al., 2001). GA significantly reduces the occurrence of relapses (Johnson et al., 1995; Johnson et al., 1998), as well as the activity and accumulated burden of disease, as measured by serial MRI scans of the brain (Comi et al., 2001b).

Interferon-Beta

Five studies (Gasperini et al., 2002; Kalkers et al., 2002a; Rudick et al., 1999; Jones et al., 2001; Comi et al., 2002) have investigated the effects of different dosages of IFNβ-1a on MRI measures of brain atrophy. In a post-hoc study, (Rudick et al., 1999) assessed brain volume from yearly MRI scans of patients participating into a double-blind, placebo-controlled trial originally designed to assess the effects of 30 mcg IFNβ-1a (Avonex®), given once a week, on clinical RRMS activity (Jacobs et al., 1996). The atrophy study cohort consisted of less than 60% of the original randomized population. A normalized measure of atrophy was obtained by calculating the brain parenchymal fraction (BPF), i.e., the ratio of brain parenchymal tissue volume to the total volume contained within the brain surface contour. Tissue segmentation was performed using an automated analysis method, which had to be modified to analyze dual echo T2-weighted images from the IFNβ-1a study, since the program was originally developed for the postprocessing of fluid-attenuated inversion recovery images (Fisher et al., 2000). In this study, the average BPF at baseline was significantly lower in MS patients than in a group of healthy controls. Over the study period, placebo patients showed an average 1.2% decrease of BPF values, with a similar pace during the first and the second year of observation. The percentage reductions in BPF were similar during the first year in the placebo and the IFNβ-1a group, whereas, in the second year, the percentage reduction in BPF was lower in the treated group (mean values [standard deviation] were -0.233 [0.74] % vs. –0.521 [0.80] % for treated and placebo patients; $P = 0.03$). BPF change over the whole study period was 18% less in the IFNβ-1a than in the placebo group, but this difference was not statistically significant. Corticosteroid use did not account for the observed differences between the treatment groups.

Gasperini et al. (2002) measured brain volume changes in 52 RRMS patients participating in a baseline-versus-treatment study, who, after a six-month observation period, were assigned to receive thrice weekly either 11 or 33 mcg IFNβ-1a (Rebif®) for 24 months. A measure of cerebral volume was obtained on MRI scans at study entry, at the end of the observation period and at the end of the treatment period. A semi-automated segmentation of brain tissue from T1-weighted images and subsequent volume quantification was used to measure the absolute parenchymal volume from four contiguous slices, with the most caudal one positioned at the level of the velum interpositum. This represents a measure of atrophy in brain regions which are most affected by MS pathology, with a high reproducibility and sensitivity to MS-related changes (Losseff et al., 1996a). Over the six months of pre-treatment observation, no significant changes in brain volume were found, whereas a mean 2.2% decrease in brain volume was observed at month 24 compared to the last pre-treatment scan ($P < 0.001$). A recent, open-label, six-year follow-up study of the same patient cohort (Paolillo et al., 2002) reported that brain atrophy continued to progress during the subsequent treatment period, when all patients were switched to receive either 99 mcg IFNβ-1a or 875 mcg IFNβ-1b weekly in three divided doses. Over the study period, brain volume decrease was significantly correlated with a worsening of disability. In another longitudinal study comparing the dynamics of brain atrophy in MS patients with different disease phenotypes, (Kalkers et al., 2002a) did not find any significant difference in the annualized decrease of total and central brain volume in patients who did and did not receive treatment with IFNβ-1a during the study period. However, this study was uncontrolled, at least partially unblinded, the duration of treatment was not similar for all patients and the treatment regimen was not specified.

A large-scale, double-blind, placebo-controlled, randomized trial (PRISMS Study) (Li and Paty, 1999; PRISMS, 1998) has demonstrated that two different doses of IFNβ-1a (Rebif®) (i.e., 22 and 44 mcg given subcutaneously three times a week) are both effective in reducing clinical and MRI-monitored RRMS activity. The complete results of brain atrophy analysis from this trial have not been fully published yet. However, data from 519 patients scanned at baseline, year 1 and year 2 were presented as an abstract (Jones et al., 2001) and did not show any evidence of treatment efficacy for either dose in the prevention of brain volume decreases, despite the strong effect on clinical and MRI outcomes.

Two studies (Comi et al., 2001a; Jacobs et al., 2000) have shown that, in patients at presentation with clinically isolated syndromes (CIS) suggestive of RRMS at its onset, IFNβ-1a (Avonex® or Rebif®) is effective in delaying the occurrence of a second relapse and in reducing MRI-measured disease activity. In a post-hoc analysis of the ETOMS (Early Treatment Of MS) trial (Comi et al., 2001a), treatment effects on brain volume changes over the two-year study period were also analyzed (Comi et al., 2002). MRI data for brain volume measurements at baseline, month 12 and month 24 were available from 131, 111 and 112 patients randomized to the treated arm (weekly 22 mcg of IFNβ-1a, Rebif®), and 132, 98 and 99 patients randomized to placebo. Normalized brain parenchymal volume (NBV) at baseline and percentage brain volume change (PBVC) over the study period were measured using a fully-automated normalized technique with whole brain coverage, the Structural Image Evaluation of Normalized Atrophy (SIENA) software (Smith et al., 2001). Mean NBV at study entry was similar for placebo and treated patients. Placebo patients experienced a mean PBVC of –0.83% during the first year, -0.67% during the second year and -1.68% during the entire study period. The corresponding values for treated patients were -0.62%, -0.61% and -1.18%, respectively. Within-each group, PBVC was significant at all time-points and for both study arms. A significant treatment effect was detected for month 24 vs. baseline PBVC ($P = 0.003$).

Glatiramer Acetate

The pivotal phase III, double-blind, placebo-controlled US GA trial (Johnson et al., 1995; Johnson et al., 1998) did not formally address the issue of treatment efficacy in preventing brain atrophy. However, in a pilot study of 27 patients enrolled at one site (University of Pennsylvania, Philadelphia), (Ge et al., 2000) measured brain volume changes on yearly MRI scans using a fully-automated technique. Surprisingly, no significant treatment effect on clinical (relapse rate) or MRI (number of contrast-enhancing and active T2-hyperintense lesions) measures of MS activity was observed in this subcohort of patients, whereas the rate of brain volume decrease was found to be significantly higher in placebo than in treated patients (-1.8% vs. –0.6% per year, respectively, p=0.0078). A recent, cross-sectional analysis of data from the extended, open-label follow-up of the US trial (Wolinsky et al., 2001) investigated the consequences of long-term GA treatment on several MRI markers of MS activity and disease burden, including absolute and normalized cerebrospinal fluid (CSF) volumes, which can be viewed as "inverse" measures of the extent of brain atrophy. Data from 54% of the original cohort of patients entered this analysis. At the time of MRI follow-up, the mean duration of active drug exposure was 2433 days for patients originally randomized to GA and 1476 days for those randomized to placebo. Absolute and normalized CSF volumes were found to be significantly lower for patients who had longer exposure to GA treatment and the group difference remained statistically significant after correcting for patients' age, disability and disease duration. Despite the methodological limitations related to an open-label study, this analysis seems to indicate that long-term treatment with GA might prevent the loss of brain parenchyma in RRMS patients.

The European/Canadian MRI trial was designed to assess the efficacy of GA on MRI-derived measures of RRMS activity and consisted of a nine month, double-blind, placebo-controlled phase followed by a nine month open-label phase (Comi et al., 2001b; Wolinsky et al., 2002). In an ancillary study (Rovaris et al., 2001), brain volume was measured from the scans obtained at baseline, at the end of the double-blind phase and at the end of the study. A seed growing technique for brain tissue segmentation was used (Rovaris et al., 2000). The absolute brain parenchymal volume was calculated for a slab of tissue including the seven contiguous slices rostral to the velum interpositum. Comparison with subsequent scans from each individual patient allowed consistent slice choice and reduced the effects of volume variation due to patient positioning on serial scans. PBVC between two subsequent scans was computed from the corresponding absolute values. From the original trial cohort, image sets from 113/119 patients randomized to GA and 114/120 randomized to placebo treatment were evaluated for brain atrophy analysis. The average brain volume at study entry was not significantly different between patients in the two study arms. During the double-blind phase, an average brain volume reduction of 0.7% and 0.8% was seen in placebo- and GA-treated patients. The rate of brain volume decrease was lower during the open-label phase for the subjects that had been on continuous GA treatment from randomization (0.6% loss for those originally on placebo, 0.4% for those always on GA), but these differences were not significant. After 18 months, brain volume was decreased by 1.4% and 1.2% in patients originally randomized to placebo and GA treatment, respectively. Neither the absolute nor the percentage changes of brain volume were significantly different between the two study arms. Covariate analysis was performed that included age, gender, center, disease duration and brain volume at baseline. No significant treatment effect was found on PBVC during the double-blind phase of the study, even when the analysis was repeated after adding the number of Gd-enhancing lesions at baseline to the covariates.

More recently, a post hoc analysis (Sormani et al., 2004) was run in which the atrophy dataset of the European/Canadian GA trial was reassessed using the normalized, fully-automated SIENA technique (Smith et al., 2001). These results were compared with those of the semi-automated, non-normalized technique with partial brain coverage (OLD) used for the original study (Rovaris et al., 2001). PBVC between month 18 and months 9 and baseline was measurable with both the techniques for 97 placebo and 97 GA patients. In this subcohort of patients, the average PBVC values calculated using the OLD technique did not differ from those of the larger cohort of the original study (Rovaris et al., 2001). No significant differences in PBVC values were found between the OLD and the SIENA methods during the double-blind and the open-label phase of the study, as well as over the whole study period. Using the SIENA technique, PBVC during the double-blind phase was slightly, but not significantly, lower in GA-treated than in placebo patients. During the open-label phase, the mean SIENA-calculated PBVC was significantly lower for patients who had been treated with GA since randomization (-0.6%) than for those originally on placebo (-1.0%, $P = 0.015$). The between-group difference that favored patients who had always been treated with GA was also found to be significant over the entire study period ($P = 0.037$). Using a simulation algorithm, the between-subject variability of PBVC from month 0 to month 9 of the study was estimated to be 0.84%. The variability due to measurement error of the OLD technique was estimated to be 2.05%, while that of the SIENA technique was estimated to be 0.80%.

This means that the between-subjects PBVC variability had the same magnitude as the measurement error of the SIENA technique, whereas the measurement error of the OLD technique was much higher and possibly responsible for a type II error in the previous study (Rovaris et al., 2001).

Corticosteroids

A recent, retrospective study (Rao et al., 2002) has shown that brain volume is significantly decreased at one month and, to a lesser extent, at two months after the administration of intravenous methylprednisolone (IVMP) given for MS clinical relapses, whereas no significant differences versus pre-treatment values were found after three months. These results conflict, at least partially, with those obtained by (Hoogervorst et al., 2002), who did not find any significant effect of IVMP pulse therapy on brain volume measures obtained on MRI scans in the subsequent months. However, in the latter study (Hoogervorst et al., 2002), a subcohort of patients receiving oral tapering after the IVMP pulse showed brain volume reductions that were significant immediately after treatment and persisted after a mean interval of one month. These studies suggest a transient but possibly confounding effect of short courses of steroid therapy on MRI measures of brain atrophy obtained in MS trials. Only one randomized, controlled, single-blind study (Zivadinov et al., 2001) has investigated the effect of chronic therapy with pulsed IVMP on clinical and MRI outcomes in 81 RRMS patients, who were followed up for five years. Patients who were randomized to active treatment received IVMP pulses every four months during the first three years and every six months during the subsequent two years. Brain parenchymal volumes were measured at baseline and at the end of the study period, using a home-developed semi-automated program for tissue segmentation, without normalization. Patients in the pulsed IVMP arm did not show significant changes in brain parenchymal volume after five years, whereas untreated patients had, on average, a 5.9% decrease in brain volume ($p=0.003$). Significant correlations were found between the decrease of brain parenchymal volume and an increase in MRI-visible lesion load.

Treatment Effect on Brain Atrophy in Progressive MS

Secondary Progressive MS

Several immunomodulating and immunosuppressive agents have been tested for the treatment of patients with secondary-progressive (SP) MS (Coles et al., 1999; ESG, 1998; Hommes et al., 2002; Rice et al., 2000; Wolinsky et al., 2000). However, to the best of our knowledge, data on brain volume changes have been published only for studies with INFβ-1b (Molyneux et al., 2000), cladribine (Filippi et al., 2000) and Campath 1H (Coles et al., 1999; Paolillo et al., 1999).

The European multicenter, double-blind, placebo-controlled, randomized trial of IFNβ-1b (Betaferon®), in which 718 patients with SPMS were enrolled, showed a significant delay in time to sustained clinical progression for treated vs. placebo patients, together with a beneficial effect on relapse rate and MRI lesion load (ESG, 1998; Miller et al., 1999). However, three other IFNβ trials in SPMS (Cohen et al., 2001; Goodkin and MS, 2000; Li et al., 2001; SPECTRIMS, 2001), one with the same treatment regimen and two with different dosages of IFNβ-1a (Avonex® and Rebif®), failed to demonstrate any treatment efficacy on disability progression, despite significant effects on relapses and MRI measures of disease activity (Li et al., 2001; SPECTRIMS, 2001). In a subcohort of 95 patients participating in the European IFNβ-1b trial who underwent a more extensive MRI evaluation in selected centers, the impact of IFNβ treatment on brain atrophy was assessed (Molyneux et al., 2000). The absolute volume of a slab of central brain slices was measured on T1-weighted MRI scans obtained at baseline and every six months for the three-year study period, using a semi-automated technique for tissue segmentation characterized by a limited amount of human intervention (Losseff et al., 1996a). As a consequence, such a technique has a high level of reproducibility and is sensitive to brain volume changes in MS patients (Losseff et al., 1996a). A significant and progressive reduction of cerebral volume was observed in both placebo and IFNβ-treated SPMS patients, with an average reduction of about 4% and 3% at three years, respectively, without any significant treatment effect. This fits with the more recent observation that IFNβ-1b was unable to affect brain magnetization transfer ratio (MTR) deterioration in a subgroup of patients of the same trial (Inglese et al., 2003). Two lines of evidence suggest that some of the atrophy in the IFNβ-1b group may have been due to the anti-inflammatory effect of the drug, causing a decrease in brain water content: a) brain volume reduction in the first six months was greater in the IFNβ-1b than in the placebo group, even though the difference was not significant; b) patients without MRI evidence of ongoing inflammatory activity (i.e., without contrast-enhancing lesions) at baseline had a greater reduction of cerebral volume in the placebo than in the IFNβ-1b arm, whereas the reverse was true for patients with enhancing lesions. Such an anti-edema effect might also contribute to the lack of any relationship between cerebral volume and neuropsychological function change observed in the IFNβ-1b arm.

Cladribine (2-chlorodeoxyadenosine) is a lymphocytotoxic drug with a long-lasting action (Sipe et al., 1994). A multicenter, randomized, double-blind, placebo-controlled trial of patients with progressive MS (Rice et al., 2000) has shown that cladribine has a dramatic effect on the volume and number of active MRI lesions, a modest effect on the accumulation of T2-hyperintense lesion volume and no effect on the accumulation of disability. A post hoc analysis of cladribine efficacy on brain volume changes was also performed in the same cohort of 159 progressive MS patients, 70% of whom had a SP disease course (Filippi et al., 2000). Using a semi-automated segmentation technique based on local thresholding, absolute whole brain parenchymal volume was calculated on scans obtained at study entry, after six and after 12 months. A significant decrease of brain volume over the study period was observed independent of treatment assignment (placebo vs. 0.7 or 1.2 mg/Kg cladribine). The average brain volume percentage change was –0.7% per year in the whole patient sample and no significant correlation was found between brain volume decrease and other MRI measures of MS lesion load accumulation.

Campath-1H is a humanized monoclonal antibody which targets the CD52 antigen and leads to sustained lymphocyte depletion (Coles et al., 1999). The effects of Campath-1H on clinical and MRI outcomes of disease progression have been tested in a cross-over trial of 25 SPMS patients (Paolillo et al., 1999). In this trial, patients were followed up with monthly

MRI scans of the brain for a three-month run-in period, and then for six months following a single-pulse course of Campath 1H, and again for another semester beginning one year after treatment administration. A measure of cerebral volume was obtained from the four central slices of the T1-weighted image sets, following the same methodology used in the European IFNβ-1b SPMS trial (Losseff et al., 1996a). Substantial decrease in brain volume was regarded as having occurred if the measured change exceeded the 95% confidence intervals of measurement variation for this technique (Losseff et al., 1996a). Campath 1H treatment was associated with a reduction in the number and volume of enhancing lesions, but a significant decrease in cerebral volume was observed in 52% of patients one-and-a-half years after administration of treatment. There was a strong correlation (r = -0.77) between pre-treatment MRI-measured inflammatory activity and subsequent brain volume decrease. Interestingly, more than 70% of patients with a significant brain volume reduction also experienced a progression of clinical disability, whereas this was the case only for 25% of patients with stable cerebral volume (Paolillo et al., 1999). In a subcohort of 12 patients who also underwent brain MR spectroscopy, a significant correlation was detected between brain volume at 18 months and N-acetyl-aspartate (NAA) levels (r = 0.73), suggesting that axonal loss is an important cause of cerebral atrophy (Coles et al., 1999).

Preliminary data from a subcohort of 43 patients participating in the European-Canadian, randomized, placebo-controlled trial of intravenous immunoglobulin (IVIG) treatment in SPMS (Lin et al., 2002) report that, over the two-year study period, brain volume reduction was smaller in IVIG- than in placebo-treated patients, with a statistically significant difference regarding changes in infratentorial brain volume.

Primary Progressive MS

To the best of our knowledge, only one exploratory, randomized, placebo-controlled trial (Leary et al., 2003) has been published investigating the effect of IFNβ-1a (30 or 60 mcg weekly) on brain atrophy in 50 patients with PPMS. No significant treatment effect was seen on the primary clinical outcome of disability progression over the two years of study, nor was the rate of brain atrophy progression, as measured on yearly scans, found to be different between placebo and treated patients. Surprisingly, patients on IFNβ-1a 60 mcg showed a greater rate of ventricular enlargement than those in the placebo arm. Preliminary data from a single-center, randomized, placebo-controlled trial of IFNβ-1b (Betaferon®) in 49 primary and 24 transitional progressive MS (Montalban et al., 2003) did not report any treatment effect on brain volume decrease over the two-year study period, even though statistically significant differences were found for MRI lesion load increase and the number of active lesions in favor of the IFN-treated group. Atrophy results from the randomized, placebo-controlled trial of GA in PPMS are pending (Wolinsky et al., 2003).

As already mentioned, about 30% of patients participating in the cladribine US trial (Rice et al., 2000) were affected by PPMS. A subgroup analysis of this cohort confirmed the lack of any treatment effect on brain volume decrease (Filippi et al., 2000).

Treatment Effect on Cord Atrophy in MS

In the last few years, there has been increasing interest in measuring cervical cord atrophy as an MRI marker of irreversible MS pathology in a CNS site whose damage may significantly contribute to locomotor disability. Current measurement techniques are mostly based upon the segmentation of cord tissue from axially reconstructed 3D MR images and the subsequent computation of cross-sectional cord areas at the upper cervical cord level as a measure reflecting cord atrophy (Losseff et al., 1996b). This method seems to be reproducibile and sensitive to longitudinal changes in patients with chronic progressive MS (Stevenson et al., 1998; Stevenson et al., 2000).

In the IFNβ-1a PPMS trial (Leary et al., 2003), cervical cord area reduction over the two-year study period was similar in placebo and treated patients. In another study of a subcohort of 20 RR and 18 SPMS patients participating in two treatment trials of high dose IFNβ-1a (Rebif®) (Lin et al., 2003), the average upper cervical cord area reduction after four years was 5.7% for patients initially on placebo, who received treatment at 24 (RRMS) or 36 months (SPMS), while it was 4.5% for those on IFNβ-1a throughout the study ($p=0.35$). A pilot study (Kalkers et al., 2002b) of the efficacy of the neuroprotective agent riluzole (which is an approved treatment for amyotrophic lateral sclerosis) has been performed in 16 PPMS patients using a baseline-versus-treatment design and including cervical cord atrophy as an MRI outcome. Interestingly, an average decrease of 2.0% was observed in the cord area after the first year without treatment, while the change was reduced to –0.2% during the second year with treatment, suggesting a favorable effect by riluzole on MS-related irreversible cord damage.

Treatment Effects on Brain Atrophy in MS: Explanations for a (Partial) Failure

The vast majority of currently available placebo-controlled trials (Filippi et al., 2000; Molyneux et al., 2000; Rovaris et al., 2001) consistently showed that the effect of treatment in reducing the rate at which brain atrophy develops in RRMS and SPMS patients was absent or only modest at best, even though the same treatments were highly effective in favorably modifying other MRI measures of MS activity (Comi et al., 2001b; Miller et al., 1999; Paolillo et al., 1999; Simon et al., 1998). These findings prompt speculation on the correlation between various aspects of MS pathology and on the impact that available treatments may have on the most severe and disabling pathological substrates of the disease.

There are several potential reasons why treatments able to significantly reduce clinical and MRI-measured MS activity did not show a substantial efficacy on the development of brain atrophy. These include the inadequacy of trial design, the limitations of brain volume measurement strategies and the "real" lack of a treatment effect.

Inadequacy of Trial Design

All published trials (Jones et al., 2001; Rudick et al., 1999; Filippi et al., 2000; Gasperini et al., 2002; Molyneux et al., 2000; Paolillo et al., 1999; Rovaris et al., 2001; Rudick et al., 1999; Zivadinov et al., 2001) were not originally designed and powered to test the treatment efficacy on brain atrophy. Brain tissue loss is an end-stage phenomenon of MS pathology, which is known to occur at an average 1% yearly rate in patients with established MS. The relatively small magnitude of this variation might render it difficult to reliably detect any difference between treatment arms. Moreover, sample size estimations for MS trials are based on clinical and MRI measures that are more sensitive to disease-related changes than brain volume assessment is (Rovaris and Filippi, 1999). This might be an additional factor contributing to a failure of treatment efficacy detection. The short duration of the follow-up periods, ranging from nine months to two years for most of the published trials, may also limit the sensitivity for detecting any effect of treatment on brain volume changes.

Limitations of Brain Volume Measurement Strategies

Published MS trials have used a wide range of techniques to measure brain volume, and this renders a comparison between different studies challenging. A correct interpretation of brain atrophy results is also limited by the potential role played by "technical" issues. Ideally, high resolution volumetric acquisitions would be more attractive than 2D sequences used so far in MS trials, since a 3D acquisition allows more accurate re-slicing of datasets when registering volumes between serial scans, thus reducing partial volume errors due to poor repositioning. Moreover, each of the various postprocessing techniques used for brain volume assessment has its own different pros and cons in terms of feasibility, speed and reproducibility of measurements. The results of the recent post hoc analysis of the European/Canadian GA trial (Sormani et al., 2004) highlight the fact that interpretation of atrophy measurement results in MS trials must account for non-biological technical factors. Fully-automated, normalized techniques with whole brain coverage, such as SIENA, seem to reduce the measurement error so that it falls below the between-patient variability of brain volume changes observed in RRMS patients over a short period of time, thus increasing the statistical power of a given study. All these "technical" considerations (Miller et al., 2002; Zivadinov and Bakshi, 2004) (see also related chapters in this book presented by the University of Rome and the University of San Francisco group) (Gasperini, 2004; Garrison et al., 2004) indicate that, prior to drawing ultimate conclusions on the effect of MS treatments on brain atrophy progression, further studies would be desirable. These studies should be designed with the appropriate image acquisition and postprocessing protocols.

Real Lack of a Treatment Effect

An additional explanation for the substantial inefficacy of available treatments on brain atrophy development might be the limited ability of these therapies to modify the pathological mechanisms leading to tissue loss in MS. Both immunomodulating and immunosuppressive treatments primarily exert an anti-inflammatory action (Li and Paty, 1999; Yong et al., 1998), as also indicated by their dramatic impact on MRI measures of disease activity (i.e., enhancing lesions and T2-hyperintense lesion load) (Coles et al., 1999; Comi et al., 2001b; IFNßMSSG, 1995; Li and Paty, 1999; Miller et al., 1999; Rice et al., 2000; Simon et al., 1998; Wolinsky et al., 2000). The modest magnitude of the correlation between contrast enhancement and brain tissue loss (Leist et al., 2001; Lin and Blumhardt, 2001) supports the hypothesis that the latter action may not necessarily be rapidly or fully translated into a beneficial effect on other MRI measures which reflect tissue loss. The temporal dissociation between a significant reduction of the inflammatory components of MS-related damage and the prevention of subsequent neurodegeneration might also contribute to the apparent failure of treatment efficacy on brain atrophy progression. The latter phenomenon merely reflects the "end-stage" loss of brain parenchyma, which may take place years after the beginning of more subtle neurodegenerative processes, such as irreversible demyelination and axonal loss. On the other hand, pathological data (Trapp et al., 1998) have shown that axonal damage occurs in inflammatory MS lesions, thus suggesting that preventing brain inflammation should have at least a partial effect on the progressive loss of tissue seen in MS patients. The magnitude of this effect might be, however, too small to be detected by measurements of brain tissue volume over relatively short intervals. Some reparative mechanisms following MS injury, such as remyelination and axonal sprouting, can also occur over relatively long periods. Therefore, the effects of repair in preventing cerebral atrophy might only be apparent late, after a prolonged reduction in inflammatory activity is well established. This hypothesis is also supported by a recent follow-up study of MS patients (Chard et al., 2003), where it was found that change in MRI lesion load in the first five years was more closely correlated to brain atrophy at 14 years than later changes in lesion load, although the correlation was only moderate ($r = -0.53$). An alternative explanation for treatment inefficacy on brain atrophy progression is that the relationship between brain inflammation and neurodegeneration might be stronger soon after the onset of MS but become tenuous with increasing disease duration. Thus, the effect of any immunomodulating agent on the prevention of brain atrophy might be stronger if treatment was instituted early. Evidence supporting this hypothesis comes from the results of the ETOMS trial (Comi et al., 2002). Moreover, a recent post mortem study (Kuhlmann et al., 2002) showed that acute axonal damage in MS lesions and normal-appearing white matter is more pronounced during the initial stages of the disease than later, thus suggesting that treatment aimed at protecting axons should be initiated as soon as possible.

Conclusions

The results of MS trials testing the efficacy of disease-modifying treatments in the prevention of brain atrophy confirm that the assessment of brain volume on serial MRI provides a reliable measure of an important component of MS pathology. Among MS patients selected for high clinical and MRI disease activity, the loss of cerebral volume can be significant even over relatively short periods of time (Hardmeier et al., 2003) and during the "non-disabling" phases of the disease. Data from patients enrolled in the placebo arms indicate that MS inflammatory activity is only in part responsible for the development of brain atrophy. Consistent with this, several immunomodulating and immunosuppressive treatments that are known to reduce MRI-measurable MS inflammatory activity and lesion accumulation did not exert a similar effect on progressive tissue loss, either in RR or in SP

MS patients. The failure to find a significant treatment benefit in preventing brain atrophy in MS might be the result of inadequate trial power and duration, which may not allow for the detection of beneficial effects in such a long-lasting disease. Conversely, this failure might indicate that treatments able to reduce MS-related inflammation are unable to act with the same efficacy on the most severe pathological substrates of the disease. The modest correlation between enhancement and brain atrophy observed in the placebo groups of several trials also fits with the concept that the suppression of inflammatory activity in MS patients is not fully and rapidly associated with a similar effect on the global neurodegenerative process of the disease.

All of this suggests that brain volume measurements should always be considered as an adjunctive outcome of MS trials and that they might be best suited to test the efficacy of new MS treatments targeted to counteract the non-inflammatory components of the disease.

References

Chard DT, Brex PA, Ciccarelli O, Griffin CM, Parker GJ, Dalton C, et al. The longitudinal relation between brain lesion load and atrophy in multiple sclerosis: a 14 year follow up study. *J Neurol Neurosurg Psychiatry* 2003; 74: 1551-4.

Cohen JA, Goodman DA, Heidenreich FR. Results of IMPACT, a phase 3 trial of interferon beta-1a in secondary progressive multiple sclerosis. *Neurology* 2001; 56: A148.

Coles AJ, Wing MG, Molyneux P, Paolillo A, Davie CM, Hale G, et al. Monoclonal antibody treatment exposes three mechanisms underlying the clinical course of multiple sclerosis. *Ann Neurol* 1999; 46: 296-304.

Comi G, Filippi M, Barkhof F, Durelli L, Edan G, Fernandez O, et al. Effect of early interferon treatment on conversion to definite multiple sclerosis: a randomised study. *Lancet* 2001a; 357: 1576-82.

Comi G, Filippi M, Wolinsky JS. European/Canadian multicenter, double-blind, randomized, placebo-controlled study of the effects of glatiramer acetate on magnetic resonance imaging--measured disease activity and burden in patients with relapsing multiple sclerosis. European/Canadian Glatiramer Acetate Study Group. *Ann Neurol* 2001b; 49: 290-7.

Comi G, Inglese M, De Stefano N, Smith S, Barkhof F, Durelli L, et al. Brain volume changes in patients at presentation with suspected multiple sclerosis: results from the ETOMS study. *Multiple Sclerosis* 2002; 8: S10.

ESG. Placebo-controlled multicentre randomised trial of interferon beta-1b in treatment of secondary progressive multiple sclerosis. European Study Group on interferon beta-1b in secondary progressive MS. *Lancet* 1998; 352: 1491-7.

Filippi M, Grossman RI. MRI techniques to monitor MS evolution: the present and the future. *Neurology* 2002; 58: 1147-53.

Filippi M, Rovaris M, Iannucci G, Mennea S, Sormani MP, Comi G. Whole brain volume changes in patients with progressive MS treated with cladribine. *Neurology* 2000; 55: 1714-8.

Fisher E, Rudick RA, Cutter G, Baier M, Miller D, Weinstock-Guttman B, et al. Relationship between brain atrophy and disability: an 8-year follow-up study of multiple sclerosis patients. *Mult Scler* 2000; 6: 373-7.

Garrison K, Henry R, Pelletier D. In: Zivadinov R, Bakshi R, eds. *Brain and Spinal Cord Atrophy in Multiple Sclerosis. Technical Aspects of Brain Atrophy Measurement.* New York: Nova Science Publisher 2004; (p39-61).

Gasperini C, Paolillo A, Giugni E, Galgani S, Bagnato F, Mainero C, et al. MRI brain volume changes in relapsing-remitting multiple sclerosis patients treated with interferon beta-1a. *Mult Scler* 2002; 8: 119-23.

Gasperini C. In: Zivadinov R, Bakshi R, eds. *Brain and Spinal Cord Atrophy in Multiple Sclerosis. Whole Brain Atrophy Measurement and Short-term Brain Volume Changes.* New York: Nova Science Publisher 2004; (p29-38).

Ge Y, Grossman RI, Udupa JK, Wei L, Mannon LJ, Polansky M, et al. Brain atrophy in relapsing-remitting multiple sclerosis and secondary progressive multiple sclerosis: longitudinal quantitative analysis. *Radiology* 2000; 214: 665-70.

Goodkin DE, MS NASGolb-biSP. Interferon Beta-1b in Secondary Progressive MS: Clinical and MRI Results of a 3-Year Randomized Controlled Trial. *Neurology* 2000; 54: 2350.

Hardmeier M, Wagenpfeil S, Freitag P, Fisher E, Rudick RA, Kooijmans-Coutinho M, et al. Atrophy is detectable within a 3-month period in untreated patients with active relapsing remitting multiple sclerosis. *Arch Neurol* 2003; 60: 1736-9.

Hommes O, Filippi M, Lin X, Petereit H. Results of the European-Canadian clinical trial of IVIG-treatment in secondary progressive multiple sclerosis. *Journal of Neurology* 2002; 249: I/60.

Hoogervorst EL, Polman CH, Barkhof F. Cerebral volume changes in multiple sclerosis patients treated with high-dose intravenous methylprednisolone. *Mult Scler* 2002; 8: 415-9.

IFNßMSSG. Interferon beta-1b in the treatment of multiple sclerosis: final outcome of the randomized controlled trial. The IFNB Multiple Sclerosis Study Group and The University of British Columbia MS/MRI Analysis Group. *Neurology* 1995; 45: 1277-85.

Inglese M, Rovaris M, Giacomotti L, Mastronardo G, Comi G, Filippi M. Quantitative brain volumetric analysis from patients with multiple sclerosis: a follow-up study. *J Neurol Sci* 1999; 171: 8-10.

Inglese M, van Waesberghe JH, Rovaris M, Beckmann K, Barkhof F, Hahn D, et al. The effect of interferon beta-1b on quantities derived from MT MRI in secondary progressive MS. *Neurology* 2003; 60: 853-60.

Jacobs LD, Beck RW, Simon JH, Kinkel RP, Brownscheidle CM, Murray TJ, et al. Intramuscular interferon beta-1a therapy initiated during a first demyelinating event in multiple sclerosis. CHAMPS Study Group. *N Engl J Med* 2000; 343: 898-904.

Jacobs LD, Cookfair DL, Rudick RA, Herndon RM, Richert JR, Salazar AM, et al. Intramuscular interferon beta-1a for disease progression in relapsing multiple sclerosis. The Multiple Sclerosis Collaborative Research Group (MSCRG). *Ann Neurol* 1996; 39: 285-94.

Johnson KP, Brooks BR, Cohen JA, Ford CC, Goldstein J, Lisak RP, et al. Copolymer 1 reduces relapse rate and improves disability in relapsing-remitting multiple sclerosis: results of a phase III multicenter, double-blind placebo-controlled trial. The Copolymer 1 Multiple Sclerosis Study Group. *Neurology* 1995; 45: 1268-76.

Johnson KP, Brooks BR, Cohen JA, Ford CC, Goldstein J, Lisak RP, et al. Extended use of glatiramer acetate (Copaxone) is well tolerated and maintains its clinical effect on multiple sclerosis relapse rate and degree of disability. Copolymer 1 Multiple Sclerosis Study Group. *Neurology* 1998; 50: 701-8.

Jones CK, Riddehough A, Li DKB, Zhao G, Paty DW, Group PSGUMMR. MRI cerebral atrophy in relapsing-remitting MS: results from the PRISMS trial (abstract). *Neurology* 2001; 56: A379.

Kalkers NF, Ameziane N, Bot JC, Minneboo A, Polman CH, Barkhof F. Longitudinal brain volume measurement in multiple sclerosis: rate of brain atrophy is independent of the disease subtype. *Arch Neurol* 2002a; 59: 1572-6.

Kalkers NF, Barkhof F, Bergers E, van Schijndel R, Polman CH. The effect of the neuroprotective agent riluzole on MRI parameters in primary progressive multiple sclerosis: a pilot study. *Mult Scler* 2002b; 8: 532-3.

Kuhlmann T, Lingfeld G, Bitsch A, Schuchardt J, Bruck W. Acute axonal damage in multiple sclerosis is most extensive in early disease stages and decreases over time. *Brain* 2002; 125: 2202-12.

Leary SM, Miller DH, Stevenson VL, Brex PA, Chard DT, Thompson AJ. Interferon beta-1a in primary progressive MS: an exploratory, randomized, controlled trial. *Neurology* 2003; 60: 44-51.

Leist TP, Gobbini MI, Frank JA, McFarland HF. Enhancing magnetic resonance imaging lesions and cerebral atrophy in patients with relapsing multiple sclerosis. *Arch Neurol* 2001; 58: 57-60.

Li DK, Paty DW. Magnetic resonance imaging results of the PRISMS trial: a randomized, double-blind, placebo-controlled study of interferon-beta1a in relapsing-remitting multiple sclerosis. Prevention of Relapses and Disability by Interferon-beta1a Subcutaneously in Multiple Sclerosis. *Ann Neurol* 1999; 46: 197-206.

Li DK, Zhao GJ, Paty DW. Randomized controlled trial of interferon-beta-1a in secondary progressive MS: MRI results. *Neurology* 2001; 56: 1505-13.

Lin X, Blumhardt LD. Inflammation and atrophy in multiple sclerosis: MRI associations with disease course. *J Neurol Sci* 2001; 189: 99-104.

Lin X, Tench CR, Turner B, Blumhardt LD, Constantinescu CS. Spinal cord atrophy and disability in multiple sclerosis over four years: application of a reproducible automated technique in monitoring disease progression in a cohort of the interferon beta-1a (Rebif) treatment trial. *J Neurol Neurosurg Psychiatry* 2003; 74: 1090-4.

Lin X, Turner B, Constantinescu CS. Cerebral volume change in secondary progressive multiple sclerosis: effects of intravenous immunoglobulins. *Journal of Neurology* 2002; 249: I/169.

Losseff NA, Wang L, Lai HM, Yoo DS, Gawne-Cain ML, McDonald WI, et al. Progressive cerebral atrophy in multiple sclerosis. A serial MRI study. *Brain* 1996a; 119: 2009-19.

Losseff NA, Webb SL, O'Riordan JI, Page R, Wang L, Barker GJ, et al. Spinal cord atrophy and disability in multiple sclerosis. A new reproducible and sensitive MRI method with potential to monitor disease progression. *Brain* 1996b; 119: 701-8.

Miller DH, Barkhof F, Frank JA, Parker GJ, Thompson AJ. Measurement of atrophy in multiple sclerosis: pathological basis, methodological aspects and clinical relevance. *Brain* 2002; 125: 1676-95.

Miller DH, Molyneux PD, Barker GJ, MacManus DG, Moseley IF, Wagner K. Effect of interferon-beta1b on magnetic resonance imaging outcomes in secondary progressive multiple sclerosis: results of a European multicenter, randomized, double-blind, placebo-controlled trial. European Study Group on Interferon-beta1b in secondary progressive multiple sclerosis. *Ann Neurol* 1999; 46: 850-9.

Molyneux PD, Kappos L, Polman C, Pozzilli C, Barkhof F, Filippi M, et al. The effect of interferon beta-1b treatment on MRI measures of cerebral atrophy in secondary progressive multiple sclerosis. European Study Group on Interferon beta-1b in secondary progressive multiple sclerosis. *Brain* 2000; 123: 2256-63.

Montalban X, Brieva L, Tintore M. Single centre, DBPC, randomised trial of interferon beta-1b in primary progressive and transitional progressive multiple sclerosis: an exploratory phase II study. *Neurology* 2003; 60: A483.

Neuhaus O, Farina C, Wekerle H, Hohlfeld R. Mechanisms of action of glatiramer acetate in multiple sclerosis. *Neurology* 2001; 56: 702-8.

Paolillo A, Coles AJ, Molyneux PD, Gawne-Cain M, MacManus D, Barker GJ, et al. Quantitative MRI in patients with secondary progressive MS treated with monoclonal antibody Campath 1H. *Neurology* 1999; 53: 751-7.

Paolillo A, Pozzilli C, Giugni E, Tomassini V, Gasperini C, Fiorelli M, et al. A 6-year clinical and MRI follow-up study of patients with relapsing-remitting multiple sclerosis treated with Interferon-beta. *Eur J Neurol* 2002; 9: 645-55.

Paty DW, Li DK. Interferon beta-1b is effective in relapsing-remitting multiple sclerosis. II. MRI analysis results of a multicenter, randomized, double-blind, placebo-controlled trial. UBC MS/MRI Study Group and the IFNB Multiple Sclerosis Study Group. *Neurology* 1993; 43: 662-7.

PRISMS. Randomised double-blind placebo-controlled study of interferon beta-1a in relapsing/remitting multiple sclerosis. PRISMS (Prevention of Relapses and Disability by Interferon beta-1a Subcutaneously in Multiple Sclerosis) Study Group. *Lancet* 1998; 352: 1498-504.

Rao AB, Richert N, Howard T, Lewis BK, Bash CN, McFarland HF, et al. Methylprednisolone effect on brain volume and enhancing lesions in MS before and during IFNbeta-1b. *Neurology* 2002; 59: 688-94.

Rice GP, Filippi M, Comi G. Cladribine and progressive MS: clinical and MRI outcomes of a multicenter controlled trial. Cladribine MRI Study Group. Neurology 2000; 54: 1145-55.

Rovaris M, Comi G, Rocca MA, Wolinsky JS, Filippi M. Short-term brain volume change in relapsing-remitting multiple sclerosis: effect of glatiramer acetate and implications. *Brain* 2001; 124: 1803-12.

Rovaris M, Filippi M. Magnetic resonance techniques to monitor disease evolution and treatment trial outcomes in multiple sclerosis. *Curr Opin Neurol* 1999; 12: 337-44.

Rovaris M, Inglese M, van Schijndel RA, Sormani MP, Rodegher M, Comi G, et al. Sensitivity and reproducibility of volume change measurements of different brain portions on magnetic resonance imaging in patients with multiple sclerosis. *J Neurol* 2000; 247: 960-5.

Rudick RA, Fisher E, Lee JC, Duda JT, Simon J. Brain atrophy in relapsing multiple sclerosis: relationship to relapses, EDSS, and treatment with interferon beta-1a. *Mult Scler* 2000; 6: 365-72.

Rudick RA, Fisher E, Lee JC, Simon J, Jacobs L. Use of the brain parenchymal fraction to measure whole brain atrophy in relapsing-remitting MS. Multiple Sclerosis Collaborative Research Group. *Neurology* 1999; 53: 1698-704.

Simon JH, Jacobs LD, Campion M, Wende K, Simonian N, Cookfair DL, et al. Magnetic resonance studies of intramuscular interferon beta-1a for relapsing multiple sclerosis. The Multiple Sclerosis Collaborative Research Group. *Ann Neurol* 1998; 43: 79-87.

Simon JH, Jacobs LD, Campion MK, Rudick RA, Cookfair DL, Herndon RM, et al. A longitudinal study of brain atrophy in relapsing multiple sclerosis. The Multiple Sclerosis Collaborative Research Group (MSCRG). *Neurology* 1999; 53: 139-48.

Sipe JC, Romine JS, Koziol JA, McMillan R, Zyroff J, Beutler E. Cladribine in treatment of chronic progressive multiple sclerosis. *Lancet* 1994; 344: 9-13.

Smith SM, De Stefano N, Jenkinson M, Matthews PM. Normalized accurate measurement of longitudinal brain change. *J Comput Assist Tomogr* 2001; 25: 466-75.

Sormani MP, Rovaris M, Valsasina P, Wolinsky JS, Comi G, Filippi M. Measurement error of two different techniques for brain atrophy assessment in multiple sclerosis. *Neurology* 2004; 62:1432-34.

SPECTRIMS. Randomized controlled trial of interferon- beta-1a in secondary progressive MS: Clinical results. *Neurology* 2001; 56: 1496-504.

Stevenson VL, Leary SM, Losseff NA, Parker GJ, Barker GJ, Husmani Y, et al. Spinal cord atrophy and disability in MS: a longitudinal study. *Neurology* 1998; 51: 234-8.

Stevenson VL, Miller DH, Leary SM, Rovaris M, Barkhof F, Brochet B, et al. One year follow up study of primary and transitional progressive multiple sclerosis. *J Neurol Neurosurg Psychiatry* 2000; 68: 713-8.

Trapp BD, Peterson J, Ransohoff RM, Rudick R, Mork S, Bo L. Axonal transection in the lesions of multiple sclerosis. *N Engl J Med* 1998; 338: 278-85.

Wolinsky JS, Comi G, Filippi M, Ladkani D, Kadosh S, Shifroni G. Copaxone's effect on MRI-monitored disease in relapsing MS is reproducible and sustained. *Neurology* 2002; 59: 1284-6.

Wolinsky JS, Narayana PA, Johnson KP. United States open-label glatiramer acetate extension trial for relapsing multiple sclerosis: MRI and clinical correlates. Multiple Sclerosis Study Group and the MRI Analysis Center. *Mult Scler* 2001; 7: 33-41.

Wolinsky JS, Narayana PA, Noseworthy JH, Lublin FD, Whitaker JN, Linde A, et al. Linomide in relapsing and secondary progressive MS: part II: MRI results. MRI Analysis Center of the University of Texas-Houston, Health Science Center, and the North American Linomide Investigators. *Neurology* 2000; 54: 1734-41.

Wolinsky JS, Pardo L, Stark Y, Zak B, Kadosh S, Ladkani D. Primary progressive MS: what can we learn from the PROMiSe trial? *Multiple Sclerosis* 2003; 9: S5.

Yong VW, Chabot S, Stuve O, Williams G. Interferon beta in the treatment of multiple sclerosis: mechanisms of action. *Neurology* 1998; 51: 682-9.

Zivadinov R, Bakshi R. Role of MRI in multiple sclerosis II: brain and spinal cord atrophy. *Front Biosci* 2004; 9: 647-64.

Zivadinov R, Rudick RA, De Masi R, Nasuelli D, Ukmar M, Pozzi-Mucelli RS, et al. Effects of IV methylprednisolone on brain atrophy in relapsing-remitting MS. *Neurology* 2001; 57: 1239-47.

Index

#

3DVIEWNIX, 45-46, 50

A

activated microglia, 76
adhesion molecules, 13, 170-171
alcohol, 3, 30, 34, 52
alcohol use, 34
Alfano method, 42, 46, 50, 55-56
algorithms, 30, 40, 45, 48, 54, 60, 66, 92
altered electrical conduction, 3, 126
amyloid precursor protein (APP), xv, 6, 9
angulation of the brain, 54
anorexia nervosa, 3, 35, 38, 52, 58
antiganglioside antibodies, 171, 174
Apo E genotype, 168-169
apoptosis, 3, 23, 35, 100
apparent diffusion coefficient (ADC), xv, 87
atrophy, xix-xx, 1-6, 10-11, 15, 17-18, 20-26, 29-37, 39-49, 51-59, 61, 63-65, 68-71, 73-81, 83-86, 88, 90-94, 96, 98-100, 103-104, 106-111, 113-115, 118-135, 145, 147-152, 154-160, 163-164, 168-170, 173, 175-179, 181-190
atrophy-related tissue changes, 74
automated techniques, 16, 30, 41
axial slice, 67-68, 150
axonal and neuronal degeneration, 2, 8
axonal damage, 8-10, 12-13, 59, 84, 93, 105-106, 109, 124, 133, 135, 144, 168, 171-173, 185, 188
axonal density, 9, 19, 21, 79, 90-92
axonal dysfunction, 1, 8, 90
axonal injury, 3, 8, 10-11, 45, 107, 169
axonal loss, xix, 2, 6-10, 12, 18, 20, 23, 25, 29, 55, 68-69, 74-77, 81, 86, 88, 91-92, 95, 98-101, 104-106, 121, 126, 144, 148, 167-168, 170-173, 182, 185
axonal spheroids, 6
axonal transection, 2-3, 76, 91
axonal transport, 9
axons, xix, 3, 6, 8-9, 10, 12-13, 34-35, 55, 91-93, 98, 126, 185

B

bacterial lipopolysaccharides, 5
Bayesan, 32, 50
Beta-2 Microglobulin, 173
bicaudate ratio (BCR), xv, 21-22, 24, 33, 129, 147, 149, 152, 154, 159
black holes, 59, 83-84, 86-88, 100, 108, 111, 133, 143, 165, 168-169, 174
bladder, 119
blood-brain barrier (BBB), xv, 6-7, 34, 59, 83, 86, 100, 170
BPF algorithm, 42-43
brain atrophy, 1-3, 6, 10, 20, 23-24, 26-27, 30, 34-47, 50-61, 71, 73, 78-80, 84, 103, 105-107, 109-110, 112-115, 118-136, 145, 148-149, 151-152, 155, 159, 164-165, 168-171, 174, 176-186, 188-190
brain boundary shift integral (BBSI), xv, 47, 50, 116-117
brain bulk, 73
brain parenchyma, xv, 16, 24, 26, 31, 36-37, 39-43, 45-46, 50-52, 58, 60, 98, 109, 115, 117, 122-123, 134, 148-149, 164, 168, 172, 177-181, 185, 189
brain parenchyma image, 46
brain parenchymal fraction (BPF), xv, 16, 24, 26, 33, 36-37, 41-45, 48, 50, 55, 58, 60, 78, 81, 98, 109, 115-118, 120, 122-123, 126-127, 134, 147-150, 152, 154-155, 157, 164, 168, 170, 177, 189
brain parenchymal tissue, 39, 42-43, 177
brain size, 40, 50, 94
brain tissue, xix, 31-32, 35, 40, 45, 47-48, 55, 57, 89, 121, 169, 174, 177, 179, 185

brain to intracranial capacity ratio (BICCR), xv, 33, 42, 44-45, 50, 57
brain volume, 6, 24, 29-37, 39, 41-42, 45-48, 51-54, 57-58, 60, 75, 81, 84, 97-98, 101-102, 107, 109, 117, 119, 122-124, 126-127, 130-135, 148-149, 151, 169, 171, 175-189
brain volumetry, 75, 98
brain width, 33
brainstem, 6, 16, 23, 119, 168
Brief Visuospatial Memory Test – Revised (BVMT-R), xv, 139, 147-149

C

California Verbal Learning Test (CVLT II), xv, 139, 141, 148, 160
caudal slice, 21, 65
caudate nucleus, 21-22, 153-154
central nervous system (CNS), xv, 1-13, 16, 21, 26, 30, 32, 35, 46, 52, 61, 64, 68, 76, 94, 103-104, 113-114, 118-122, 124-128, 133-135, 137, 168, 173, 176, 183
cerebellar dysfunction, 1
cerebellum, 16, 23-24, 30, 49, 168
cerebral atrophy, 26, 29, 33-37, 41-42, 47, 56-59, 105, 107, 110-111, 130-135, 137, 157, 174, 182, 185, 188-189
cerebral dehydration, 52
cerebral volume loss, 167
cerebrospinal fluid (CSF), xv, 2, 23, 31-34, 39-48, 50-52, 65-67, 74, 79-80, 92, 94, 101, 107, 114, 118, 143, 148-149, 151, 170, 172-174, 178
cerebrospinal fluid spaces, 107
cervical spinal cord, 12, 63-64, 66-71, 130
clinical deterioration, 2, 41
clinical disability, xix, 9, 59, 77, 102, 108, 129, 133, 182
clinically isolated syndrome (CIS), xv, xix, 17, 25-26, 77, 79, 86, 91, 97, 101, 104, 106, 116-117, 121-123, 128-130, 133-134, 178
CNS atrophy, 1-4, 6-10, 113-114, 118, 120-122, 124-128, 173
coefficient of variation (COV), xv, 42, 44-45, 53-54, 65
cognition, 140, 142, 150-151, 164
cognitive decline, 10, 162
cognitive impairments, 140
computerized tomography (CT), xv, 1, 15, 17, 56, 137, 145-147
confocal microscopy, 6
contrast agents, 83
contrast weighting methods, 32
Controlled High-Risk Subjects Avonex Multiple Sclerosis Prevention Study (CHAMPS), xv, 17, 187
Controlled Oral Word Association Test (COWAT), xv, 140-141, 146, 148-149
corpus callosum, 3, 12, 16-21, 24-26, 69, 78, 89, 117, 127, 145, 148, 151, 164, 169
corpus callosum width, 33
cortex, 21, 24, 26, 29, 45, 57, 59, 80, 93, 103, 105, 110, 119, 134, 144, 150, 159, 161
cortical atrophy, 23, 25, 57, 105, 130, 145, 150, 155-156, 172
cortical thinning, 80-81, 98
corticospinal tract, 49, 59, 111
corticosteroids, 30, 34, 84
cross-sectional area (CSA), 63-66, 68-69
CSF compartments, 2, 31, 118
CSF fluid, 45
CSF volumes, 33, 42, 151, 178
CT literature, 17
cytokines, 7, 13, 91, 170
cytosine-adenosine (CA), xii-xiii, xv, 4, 24-25, 39, 57, 104-106, 111, 117, 122, 147, 161, 165, 170
cytotoxic T lymphocyte (CTL), xv, 6

D

degeneration, 3, 8-13, 16, 18-19, 21, 26, 73, 75-78, 80-81, 88, 92-94, 96, 99, 101, 111, 168, 173
dehydration, 3, 52, 59
Delis-Kaplan Executive Function System (D-KEFS), xv, 140-141, 160
dementia, 1, 4, 21, 25, 104, 138, 143-144, 154, 160, 162-163, 165
demyelinated neurites, 8
demyelinating disease, 11-12, 143
demyelinating lesions, 64, 106, 163
demyelination, 1, 3, 6, 10-13, 23-24, 29, 34-35, 39, 57, 74-77, 81, 86, 88, 92, 95-96, 99-101, 103-104, 126, 134, 137, 170, 185
diffuse low-grade inflammation, 29
diffusion imaging (DI), xv, 87-88, 102
diffusion tensor imaging (DTI), xv, 24, 55, 78, 88, 101, 103
diffusion weighted imaging, 137, 144
direct microscopic injury, 3
disease activity, xix, 3, 75, 77, 79, 84-85, 94, 96-98, 107, 110, 121, 148, 168-170, 172-176, 178, 181, 184-186

E

edema, 3, 52, 75-76, 78, 81, 84, 86, 88, 95-96, 98, 100, 106, 108, 126, 144, 175
EDSS scores, 43, 68
endothelial cell adhesion molecule (ECAM), xv, 7
environmental factors, 5
Epstein-Barr virus, 7
estimated premorbid intelligence, 141
executive function, 141
Expanded Disability Status Scale (EDSS), xv, 21, 34, 43-45, 48-49, 63, 66, 68, 70, 77, 99, 109, 115, 118-119, 122-123, 126, 129, 134, 143, 149, 152, 154, 168-169, 171, 189
extension of SIENA (SIENAX), xvii, 33, 42, 46, 50

F

fiber anatomy, 88
fiber loss, 17, 88
field of view (FOV), xv, 92
F-labeled fluorodeoxyglucose positron emission tomography (FDG PET), xv
FLAIR images, 43, 79, 152-154
FLAIR lesion volume (FLV), xv, 149, 151
fluid attenuated inversion recovery (FLAIR), xv, 32, 43, 51, 79-80, 143, 145, 149-154
frontal, 23, 93, 104, 119, 142-145, 148, 151, 158, 161, 165
fuzzy connectedness, 33, 42, 46, 60

G

genetically susceptible individuals, 5
genetic-immunologic components, 2
glatiramer acetate, 6, 84, 109, 123, 134-135, 176, 186-187, 189-190
glial cell proliferation, 92, 98
glial cells, 6, 10, 55, 90, 92-93, 133
glial scars, 34, 84
global atrophy, 16, 42, 75, 78, 93-94, 97
global brain volume, 81, 169
global volume loss, 16
gray matter (GM), xv, 2-3, 6, 11, 21, 23-24, 32, 34-35, 40, 43, 45, 47-50, 53-56, 58, 63, 73, 76, 78, 80, 90-92, 94, 98, 100, 103, 106-107, 118, 129, 131, 143, 145, 148, 151, 161-162, 165

H

HLA-DR2, 7
hydration, 34, 85, 126
hypointense lesions, 81, 103, 111, 165, 167

I

image analysis procedures, 64, 68
image contrast, 32, 51, 65
immune-mediated disease, 5
index of brain atrophy (IBA), xv, 42, 44, 50
inducible nitric oxide synthase (iNOS), xvi, 8
inflammation, 3, 5-6, 9-11, 18, 23, 34, 36, 52, 55, 73, 75-77, 83-86, 90-91, 95-96, 98, 100, 109, 124, 126, 128, 144, 170, 173, 185-186
inflammatory mediators, 8
inflammatory tissue injury, 2
infratentorial atrophy, 23, 98
insulin-like growth factor, 35, 59
intensity gradient magnitude, 66
intercaudate distance, 21-22, 149
intercaudate ratio, 22
intercellular adhesion molecule 1 (ICAM-1), xv, 7, 170-171
interferon (IFN), xv, 6, 9, 13, 17-18, 37, 59, 66, 69-70, 103, 109-110, 121, 129-134, 161, 163, 173, 176-178, 180, 182-183, 186-190
interleukin (IL), xv
intracranial hypertension, 3, 52, 59
intravenous immunoglobulin (IVIG), xvi, 182, 188
intravenous methylprednisolone (IVMP), xvi, 34-36, 52, 58, 124, 131, 180, 187
inversion recovery (IR), xvi, 9, 11, 32, 51, 56, 58, 79, 103, 115, 128, 143, 158, 165, 177
iron deposition, 3, 8, 11, 80, 100, 126
iron-containing material, 21
irreversible tissue destruction, 2, 75, 83
ischemic episodes, 8
isomorphic gliosis, 98
IVMP limits, 35, 52

J

Judgment of Line Orientation (JLO), xvi, 140-141, 146, 148-149

L

language, 140
lateral ventricle, 17-19, 21, 44, 115, 117, 119, 145, 153-154
learning and recent memory, 141
lesion burden, 56, 59, 75-79, 81, 83-84, 93, 96, 102, 110, 143-145, 148-149, 151, 155, 157, 159

lesion load (LL), xvi, 9, 12, 31, 46, 60, 76-77, 79, 84-85, 98, 104, 109-110, 118-121, 129-130, 133-135, 143-144, 167-168, 170, 173, 180-182, 185-186
lymphocyte function associated antigen (LFA-1), xvi, 170
linear measures, 15-16, 19, 24, 145, 149

M

MACFIMS battery, 153-155
macrophages, 6-8
macrophages/microglia release, 8
magnetic field inhomogeneity, 46, 53
magnetic resonance (MR), xvi, xix, 1, 6, 9, 11, 13, 16, 20, 22, 24-26, 29, 34, 36-39, 47-48, 50-51, 53-61, 63, 69-71, 73, 75, 78, 81, 87-88, 103-111, 113, 128-132, 134-137, 144, 149, 158-165, 169, 174, 182-183, 186, 188-189
magnetic resonance imaging (MRI), viii, xvi, xix, 1-4, 6, 11, 15-17, 21, 23-26, 29, 31, 34-45, 47-49, 51-53, 55-61, 63-64, 66-71, 73-81, 83-85, 89, 91-96, 98-115, 118-122, 124-137, 143-152, 154-190
magnetic resonance spectroscopy (MRS), xvi, 1, 13, 26, 78, 80, 89-92, 101-102, 107-108, 111, 144, 149-150, 158, 161, 169
magnetization transfer (MT), xvi, 52, 59, 61, 75, 78, 85-88, 102, 104-110, 111, 133, 137, 144, 165, 181, 187
magnetization transfer imaging (MTI), 16, 61, 85, 86, 99, 101-102, 104-107, 110, 137, 144, 165
magnetization transfer ratio (MTR), xvi, 20, 59, 78, 86-87, 96, 107, 109, 144, 155, 181
major histocompatibility complex (MHC), xvi, 6-7
Markov random field (MRF), xvi, 47, 61
matalloproteinases (MMPs), 7
matrix metalloproteinase-9 (MMP-9), 169-170, 173-174
mechanical trauma, 8
medial dorsal nucleus, 21
Medical Image Display Analysis Software (MIDAS), xvi, 33, 47
messenger RNA (mRNA), xvi, 10
metabolic investigation, 89
metabolic stress, 5
methylprednisolone, 38, 61, 112, 136, 174, 190
microglia, 7-8
Minimal Assessment of Cognitive Function in Multiple Sclerosis (MACFIMS), xvi, 140, 142, 149, 152-155
mitochondrial respiration, 8
mitoxantrone, 6
Montreal Neurological Institute, 45, 49, 55
morphological changes, 39
morphometry, 33, 45, 73-75, 79, 94, 98, 108
MR spectroscopy, xix, 16, 20, 55, 75, 88, 103-106, 108, 182
MRI metrics, 2-3, 73-75, 85, 99-100
MRI morphometric variables, 74
MRI sequences, xix, 36, 39, 48, 51, 58, 106, 120
MRS spectrum, 89
MR-spectroscopic studies, 9
MS lesions, 6, 8-10, 16, 18, 21, 31, 46, 50, 60, 76, 85, 91-92, 105, 110, 137, 144, 169, 185
MS pathogenesis, 7, 10
mucosal addressin cell adhesion molecule 1 (MACAM-1), xvi, 7
multiple sclerosis (MS), xvi, xix, 1-13, 15-19, 21-27, 29, 31-39, 41-61, 63-66, 68-71, 73-80, 83-92, 94, 96-98, 102-115, 118-122, 124-146, 148-152, 154-178, 180-190
Multiple Sclerosis Functional Composite (MSFC), xvi, 118, 122, 134, 139, 157, 161
myelin, xvi, xix, 1, 3, 6-8, 10, 12, 18, 20, 35, 55, 76, 85-86, 90, 92-93, 103, 144, 172, 175-176
myelin basic protein (MBP), xvi, 7, 176
myelin debris, 8
myelin oligodendrocyte glycoprotein (MOG), xvi, 7
myelin-specific CD4+ T lymphocytes, 7

N

N-acetyl aspartate (NAA), xvi, xix, 1, 9, 20-21, 44-45, 47, 55, 89-92, 99, 101-102, 104, 144, 149, 169, 182
NEO Personality Inventory (NEO-PI), xvi, 141-142
neurobehavioral, 2-3, 156, 161
neurodegeneration, 6, 10, 24, 29, 57, 100, 109, 129, 185
neurodegenerative, xix, 3, 10, 58, 74, 78-80, 84, 185-186
neurodegenerative process, xix, 3, 10, 74, 79, 185-186
neurofilament heavy (NfH), xvi, 172
neurofilament light (NfL), xvi, 172, 174
neurofilaments, 172
neurological deficits, 5, 8
neuronal fibers, 3, 24
neuronal loss, xix, 2, 10, 18
neuronal synapses, 8
neuronal tracts, 15
neuronal transection, 23
Neuropsychiatric Inventory (NPI), xvi, 141-142, 152, 154, 156, 160
neuropsychological impairment, 25, 56, 109, 114, 145, 156, 159, 162, 164

neuropsychological measures, 146-148, 157
neuropsychology (NP), xvi, 137-138, 140, 143, 145, 149-150
non-frontal, 143
normal appearing brain tissue (NABT), xvi, 161
normal appearing white matter (NAWM), xvi, xix, 9-10, 16, 19, 25, 29, 55, 63, 78-79, 86-89, 91, 96, 101, 105-107, 110-111, 144, 155
normalization, 24, 34, 38, 40, 42, 44-46, 48, 90, 92-94, 180
normalized brain parenchymal volume or normalized brain volume (NBV), xvi, 169, 178
NP syndromes, 137
nuclear magnetic resonance (NMR), xvi, 51, 111
nutrition, 34, 52
nutritional status, 3, 52

O

oligodendrocytes, 6, 8-13, 34-35, 132, 172
oxidative stress, 8

P

Paced Auditory Serial Addition Test (PASAT), xvi, 138, 141, 146-149, 157
parallel fibers, 88
parenchymal tissue, 42, 73, 84
parenchymal volume, 45, 73, 78, 84, 94, 99, 117, 148, 177, 180
pathological laughter-crying (PLO), xvi, 142
patients, xix, 1-2, 4-6, 8-13, 16-18, 22-26, 32-33, 35-38, 41, 44-49, 51, 54-60, 63, 65-66, 68-71, 77, 79, 84, 89, 91-93, 96-97, 103-111, 113-114, 117-134, 137-140, 142-145, 148-149, 151-152, 156-160, 162-165, 167-174, 176-189
percentage brain volume change (PBVC), xvi, 48, 116-117, 178-179
permanent disability, 8, 10
personality, 140-141, 159
personality/behavior disorder, 154
phagocytosis, 8
platelet endothelial cell adhesion molecule-1 (PECAM-1), xvi, 7, 12
PP MS, 44, 54, 69, 93, 124
primary progressive (PP), xvi, 44, 47, 54-55, 59-60, 65, 68-70, 79, 93, 98, 107, 109-110, 117-118, 124, 132-135, 160, 169-172, 174, 188-189
probabilistic segmentation, 33
Processing Speed/Working Memory, 141
proteolipid protein (PLP), xvi, 7
proteolytic enzymes, 7
proton density (PD), xvi, 19, 32, 34, 37, 43-46, 51, 59, 70, 104, 108, 133, 137, 188-189
pulse sequences, 32, 37, 51, 59

R

radio frequency (RF), xvi, 52
reactive metabolites, 5
recombination activating gene 1 (Rag-1), xvi
regional atrophy, 16-17, 20, 78, 84, 88, 94, 98
regional measures, 3, 15-16, 24, 33-34, 40, 73, 110, 148
relapsing remitting (RR), xvi, 5-6, 23, 35, 42, 44-45, 47-49, 51-52, 54-55, 65, 68-69, 76, 84, 86, 91, 93, 96-98, 106, 116-117, 121, 128, 131, 144-145, 149, 151-152, 157-158, 160, 169-172, 176, 183, 185, 187
remyelination, 3, 9-13, 34, 81, 86, 176, 185
repair, 9-10, 12, 73, 76, 83, 91-92, 169, 185

S

secondary progressive (SP), xvii, 5-6, 18, 23, 37, 45, 48, 54-55, 58-60, 65, 68-70, 76, 83-84, 86, 98, 103, 106, 108, 111, 117-118, 122, 128, 130-131, 133, 135, 142, 145, 149, 156, 169-172, 174, 180-181, 185-190
semi-automated, non-normalized technique with partial brain coverage (OLD), xvi, 179
sexual function, 119
signal to noise ratio (SNR), xvii, 66, 68, 90, 92, 101
skull, 21-23, 42, 46-47, 50, 64
Sobel image, 66
spatial, 31, 45-46, 75, 77, 92, 128, 139, 145
spatial processing, 141
spatiotemporal propagation, 82
spatio-temporal variability, 77
spinal cord, xix, 2-4, 6, 10, 15-16, 26, 30-31, 37-38, 59, 61, 63-66, 68-70, 79, 98, 104, 107-108, 112, 114, 118-120, 122, 125, 128-129, 132, 134-135, 145, 168, 172-173, 190
spinal cord atrophy, xix, 2-4, 26, 37-38, 59, 61, 64, 66, 68-70, 107, 112, 114, 118-120, 122, 125, 128, 132, 134-135, 168, 173, 190
spinal parenchyma, 2
SP MS, 49, 83, 91, 118-119, 124-125, 128, 170-172, 180-183
statistical parametric mapping (SPM), xvii, 31, 47-50, 55
stereology, 33
steroid therapy, 3, 52, 180

Structural Image Evaluation, using Normalization, of Atrophy (SIENA), xvi, 33, 46-47, 50, 178-179, 184
subcortical structures, 21
subject head placement, 54
subject head size, 54
sublethal axonal injury, 3, 176
superantigens, 5
supratentorial brain parenchyma, 44
supratentorial parenchyma + ventricles, 44
swelling, 9, 84, 100
Symbol Digit Modalities Test (SDMT), xvi, 138, 141, 146-150, 155, 157
systemic illnesses, 34

T

T1 hypointense lesions, 81, 83-84, 110
T1 lesion volume (T1LV), xvii, 149-150
T1-weighted images, 30, 48, 106, 177
T1-weighted magnetic resonance, 167
T2 lesion, 22, 44, 59, 63, 68, 76-79, 81, 83-84, 96-97, 100, 118-119, 143, 149-150
T2 lesion appearance, 77
T2 lesion morphometry, 77, 79
T2 shortening, 21, 80, 103, 110
T2-weighted images, 30, 44-46, 51, 79, 177
targeted neurological deficit (TND), xvii, 98
template-driven segmentation (TDS), xvii, 33, 47-48, 50
thalamus, 15, 17, 19, 21, 24, 55, 80, 105, 145
third ventricle width (TVW), xvii, 16-17, 19, 21, 33, 117, 149-152, 154-155
tissue atrophy, 2
tissue destruction, 2, 10, 77, 81, 83-84, 86, 88, 96, 99-100, 169
tissue loss, 3, 6, 10, 23, 35, 55-56, 73-74, 80, 86, 100, 126, 184-185
total lesion area (TLA), xvii, 143, 145, 147-148
transcallosal bands, 16-17, 19
transendothelial migration, 5, 7
trans-neuronal degeneration, 8
transverse width, 22
typical lesions, 16

U

urodynamic abnormalities, 119

V

vascular cell adhesion molecule (VCAM), xvii, 7, 170
vascular cell adhesion molecule 1 (VCAM-1), xvii, 170-171
VE-cadherin, 7, 13
ventricle, 15-17, 19, 21, 24, 30, 33, 44, 80, 100, 145, 149-150, 152-156
ventricular fraction (VF), xvii, 30, 116-117, 123, 172
very late activation antigen 4 (VLA-4), xvii, 170
viral infection, 5
visual criteria, 17
volume measurements, 32, 40, 46, 52-53, 56-57, 178
volume on central brain slices, 33
voxel drift, 53
voxel-based, 33, 36, 56
voxel-based map, 42
voxel-based morphometry (VBM), xvii, 47-50
voxels, 42, 46, 48, 50-51, 65-66, 68, 78

W

Wallerian degeneration, 2, 6, 8, 11, 29, 35, 85, 91, 109
white and gray matter, 31, 40, 42, 48, 55, 60, 73, 134, 155
white matter (WM), xvii, xix, 2, 6-7, 9, 12, 23-25, 30-32, 34-36, 38-40, 45, 47-51, 54-59, 63, 69, 78-81, 86, 88-89, 92-94, 96, 98, 101, 103-109, 118-119, 130-131, 144, 148, 151, 163, 167, 185
white matter composition, 93
white matter signal abnormalities (WMSA), xvii, 76-77, 96
white-matter cerebral lesions, 143
whole brain ratio (WBR), xvii, 33, 42, 44-45, 50, 116-117
whole-brain, 2, 30, 32-33, 36, 57, 94, 119, 123-124, 129, 148, 159, 176
whole-brain atrophy, 32, 36, 57, 119, 123-124, 129, 148, 159
whole-brain parenchyma, 30, 94
width of the brain, 17, 22, 145
Wisconsin Card Sorting Test (WSCT), xvii, 139, 143, 149, 158
women, 5

Y

young adults, 5